T0264543

RELIGION, MEDICINE AND THE HUMAN EMBRYO IN TIBET

This book explores the fascinating history of embryology in Tibet, in culture, religion, art and literature. It reveals the prevalence of descriptions of the development of the human body – from conception to birth – found in all forms of Tibetan religious literature, as well as in medical texts and in art. By analyzing stories of embryology, Frances Garrett explores questions of cultural transmission and adaptation: how did Tibetan writers adapt ideas inherited from India and China for their own purposes? What original views did they develop on the body, on gender, on creation, and on life itself?

The transformations of embryological narratives over several centuries illuminate key turning points in Tibetan medical history, and its relationship with religious doctrine and practice. Embryology was a site for both religious and medical theorists to contemplate profound questions of being and becoming, where topics such as pharmacology and nosology were left to shape secular medicine. The author argues that stories of human development comment on embodiment, gender, socio-political hierarchy, religious ontology, and spiritual progress. Through the lens of embryology, this book examines how these concerns shift as Tibetan history moves through the formative period of the twelfth to seventeenth centuries.

Frances Garrett is Assistant Professor of Buddhist Studies at the University of Toronto. She is a historian whose research addresses doctrinal, ritual and textual practice in Tibetan Cultures.

ROUTLEDGE CRITICAL STUDIES IN BUDDHISM

Founding Editors:
Charles S. Prebish and Damien Keown

Routledge Critical Studies in Buddhism is a comprehensive study of the Buddhist tradition. The Series explores this complex and extensive tradition from a variety of perspectives, using a range of different methodologies.

The Series is diverse in its focus, including historical studies, textual translations and commentaries, sociological investigations, bibliographic studies, and considerations of religious practice as an expression of Buddhism's integral religiosity. It also presents materials on modern intellectual historical studies, including the role of Buddhist thought and scholarship in a contemporary, critical context and in the light of current social issues. The Series is expansive and imaginative in scope, spanning more than two and a half millennia of Buddhist history. It is receptive to all research works that inform and advance our knowledge and understanding of the Buddhist tradition.

A SURVEY OF VINAYA LITERATURE
Charles S. Prebish

THE REFLEXIVE NATURE OF AWARENESS
Paul Williams

ALTRUISM AND REALITY
Paul Williams

BUDDHISM AND HUMAN RIGHTS
Edited by Damien Keown, Charles Prebish and Wayne Husted

WOMEN IN THE FOOTSTEPS OF THE BUDDHA
Kathryn R. Blackstone

THE RESONANCE OF EMPTINESS
Gay Watson

AMERICAN BUDDHISM
Edited by Duncan Ryuken Williams and Christopher Queen

IMAGING WISDOM
Jacob N. Kinnard

PAIN AND ITS ENDING
Carol S. Anderson

EMPTINESS APPRAISED
David F. Burton

THE SOUND OF LIBERATING TRUTH
Edited by Sallie B. King and Paul O. Ingram

BUDDHIST THEOLOGY
Edited by Roger R. Jackson and John J. Makransky

THE GLORIOUS DEEDS OF PURNA
Joel Tatelman

EARLY BUDDHISM – A NEW APPROACH
Sue Hamilton

CONTEMPORARY BUDDHIST ETHICS
Edited by Damien Keown

INNOVATIVE BUDDHIST WOMEN
Edited by Karma Lekshe Tsomo

TEACHING BUDDHISM IN THE WEST
Edited by V. S. Hori, R. P. Hayes and J. M. Shields

EMPTY VISION
David L. McMahan

SELF, REALITY AND REASON IN TIBETAN PHILOSOPHY
Thupten Jinpa

IN DEFENSE OF DHARMA
Tessa J. Bartholomeusz

BUDDHIST PHENOMENOLOGY
Dan Lusthaus

RELIGIOUS MOTIVATION AND THE ORIGINS OF BUDDHISM
Torkel Brekke

DEVELOPMENTS IN AUSTRALIAN BUDDHISM
Michelle Spuler

ZEN WAR STORIES
Brian Victoria

THE BUDDHIST UNCONSCIOUS
William S. Waldron

INDIAN BUDDHIST THEORIES OF PERSONS
James Duerlinger

ACTION DHARMA
Edited by Christopher Queen, Charles Prebish and Damien Keown

TIBETAN AND ZEN BUDDHISM IN BRITAIN
David N. Kay

THE CONCEPT OF THE BUDDHA
Guang Xing

THE PHILOSOPHY OF DESIRE IN THE BUDDHIST PALI CANON
David Webster

THE NOTION OF *DITTHI* IN THERAVADA BUDDHISM
Paul Fuller

THE BUDDHIST THEORY OF SELF-COGNITION
Zhihua Yao

MORAL THEORY IN SANTIDEVA'S SIKSAMUCCAYA
Barbra R. Clayton

BUDDHIST STUDIES FROM INDIA TO AMERICA
Edited by Damien Keown

DISCOURSE AND IDEOLOGY IN MEDIEVAL JAPANESE BUDDHISM
Edited by Richard K. Payne and Taigen Dan Leighton

BUDDHIST THOUGHT AND APPLIED PSYCHOLOGICAL RESEARCH
Edited by D. K. Nauriyal, Michael S. Drummond and Y. B. Lal

BUDDHISM IN CANADA
Edited by Bruce Matthews

BUDDHISM, CONFLICT AND VIOLENCE IN MODERN SRI LANKA
Edited by Mahinda Deegalle

THERAVĀDA BUDDHISM AND THE BRITISH ENCOUNTER
Religious, missionary and colonial experience in nineteenth century Sri Lanka
Elizabeth Harris

BEYOND ENLIGHTENMENT
Buddhism, religion, modernity
Richard Cohen

BUDDHISM IN THE PUBLIC SPHERE
Reorienting global interdependence
Peter D. Hershock

BRITISH BUDDHISM
Teachings, practice and development
Robert Bluck

BUDDHIST NUNS IN TAIWAN AND SRI LANKA
A critique of the feminist perspective
Wei-Yi Cheng

NEW BUDDHIST MOVEMENTS IN THAILAND
Toward an understanding of Wat Phra Dhammakåya and Santi Asoke
Rory Mackenzie

BUDDHIST RITUALS OF DEATH AND REBIRTH
Contemporary Sri Lankan practice and its origins
Rita Langer

BUDDHISM, POWER AND POLITICAL ORDER
Edited by Ian Harris

ENVIRONMENTAL ETHICS IN BUDDHISM
A virtues approach
Pragati Sahni

THE CULTURAL PRACTICES OF MODERN CHINESE BUDDHISM
Attuning the Dharma
Francesca Tarocco

MINDFULNESS IN EARLY BUDDHISM
New approaches through psychology and textual analysis of Pali, Chinese and Sanskrit sources
Tse-fu Kuan

RELIGION, MEDICINE AND THE HUMAN EMBRYO IN TIBET
Frances Garrett

The following titles are published in association with the *Oxford Centre for Buddhist Studies*

The *Oxford Centre for Buddhist Studies* conducts and promotes rigorous teaching and research into all forms of the Buddhist tradition.

EARLY BUDDHIST METAPHYSICS
Noa Ronkin

MIPHAM'S DIALECTICS AND THE DEBATES ON EMPTINESS
Karma Phuntsho

HOW BUDDHISM BEGAN
The conditioned genesis of the early teachings
Richard F. Gombrich

BUDDHIST MEDITATION
An anthology of texts from the Pāli Canon
Sarah Shaw

REMAKING BUDDHISM FOR MEDIEVAL NEPAL
The fifteenth-century reformation of Newar Buddhism
Will Tuladhar-Douglas

METAPHOR AND LITERALISM IN BUDDHISM
The doctrinal history of Nirvana
Soonil Hwang

THE BIOGRAPHIES OF RECHUNGPA
The evolution of a Tibetan hagiography
Peter Alan Roberts

THE ORIGIN OF BUDDHIST MEDITATION
Alexander Wynne

RELIGION, MEDICINE AND THE HUMAN EMBRYO IN TIBET

Frances Garrett

Routledge
Taylor & Francis Group
LONDON AND NEW YORK

First published 2008
by Routledge
2 Park Square, Milton Park, Abingdon, Oxfordshire OX14 4RN

Simultaneously published in the USA and Canada
by Routledge
711 Third Avenue, New York, NY 10017

First issued in paperback 2014

Routledge is an imprint of the Taylor & Francis Group, an informa business

© 2008 Frances Garrett

Typeset in Times by Wearset Ltd, Boldon, Tyne and Wear

All rights reserved. No part of this book may be reprinted or reproduced or utilized in any form or by any electronic, mechanical, or other means, now known or hereafter invented, including photocopying and recording, or in any information storage or retrieval system, without permission in writing from the publishers.

British Library Cataloguing in Publication Data
A catalogue record for this book is available from the British Library

Library of Congress Cataloging in Publication Data
Garrett, Frances Mary.
Religion, Medicine and the Human Embryo in Tibet/Frances Garrett.
p. cm. – (Routledge critical studies in Buddhism)
Includes bibliographical references and index.
1. Medicine–Religious aspects–Buddhism. 2. Embryology, Human–Religious aspects–Buddhism. 3. Embryology, Human–China–Tibet. 4. Buddhism–China–Tibet. I. Title.
BQ4570.M7G37 2008
294.3′661–dc22
2007046155

ISBN13: 978-1-138-86225-8 (pbk)
ISBN13: 978-0-415-44115-5 (hbk)

FOR MY PARENTS

CONTENTS

FIGURES

TABLES

ACKNOWLEDGMENTS

For generously sharing their scholarly expertise in the course of writing this book, I am grateful to Ngawang Jinpa and Jampa in Darjeeling, Dorjé Dramdül in Sarnath, and Yangga Trarong, Dawa, and Jampa Trinlé in Lhasa. In the U.S., I deeply appreciate the substantial advice of Paul Groner, Jeffrey Hopkins, Anne Kinney, Karen Lang, Anne Monius and Ann Gill Taylor. I am especially grateful to David Germano for many years of support and kindness. This book has benefitted also from suggestions by Janet Gyatso, Dan Martin, Robert Kritzer, Dominik Wujastyk, Charles Burnett, Jonathan Silk, John Kloppenborg, Amy Langenberg and several anonymous reviewers. The largest debts of gratitude are owed to my parents, for their unfailing generosity, to Travis, for his affection, and to Sivert, for getting me interested in embryos in the first place

I would also like to acknowledge Fulbright-Hays, the U.S. National Institutes for Health, the U.S. Department of Education, and the Weedon Foundation for supporting me in my research and writing, as well as the University of Virginia's Center for South Asian Studies, its Center for the Study of Complementary and Alternative Therapies, and its Tibetan and Himalayan Digital Library. The assistance of the Tibetan Academy of Social Sciences faciliated productive research time in Tibet.

The following editors and publishers have allowed me to use extracts of my writing from their publications in this book:

"Embodiment and Embryology in Tibetan Literature," in *Soundings in Tibetan Medicine: Historical and Anthropological Perspectives*, ed. Mona Schrempf, Leiden: Brill Publishers, 2007, 411–426.

"The Three Channels in Tibetan Medical and Religious Texts, including a translation of Tsultrim Gyaltsen's 'Treatise on the Three Channels in Tibetan Medicine'," with Vincanne Adams, in *Traditional South Asian Medicine*, forthcoming in 2008.

"Ordering human growth in Tibetan medical and religious embryologies," in *Textual Healing: Essays on Medieval and Early Modern Medicine*, ed. Elizabeth Furdell, Leiden: Brill Publishers, 2005, 31–52.

Illustrations of the Tibetan medical paintings on embryology are printed here from images held by the Tibetan and Himalayan Digital Library, made available under the THDL Public License. These photographs reproduce the collection of paintings held at the Museum of Medical History at the Traditional Medicine Factory on Nyangré Road in Lhasa. An entire set of medical paintings (slightly different in detail than those presented here) are beautifully reproduced in Gyurme Dorje and Fernand Meyer, eds. *Tibetan Medical Paintings: Illustrations to the "Blue Beryl" Treatise of Sangye Gyamtso (1653–1705)*, 2 vols, New York: Harry N. Abrams, Inc. Publishers, 1992.

Tibetan transcription and transliteration

This book uses the system of phonetic transcription of Tibetan words that is described at the Tibetan and Himalayan Digital Library's "THDL Simplifie Phonetic Transcription of Standard Tibetan," by David Germano and Nicolas Tournadre (2003), available at http://www.thdl.org/xml/showEssay.php?xml=/collections/langling/THDL_phonetics.xml. At the end of this book, a guide to transliteration of Tibetan provides the exact spelling for each phoneticized term. In the body of the book, when Tibetan and Sanskrit terms are provided in parentheses, the Tibetan term will always be provided first, followed by the Sanskrit term; Sanskrit terms are preceded by the abbreviation "Skt."

1

BECOMING HUMAN IN TIBETAN LITERATURE

In 1479, the Tibetan physician Kyempa Tsewang suggested that during the early stages of a woman's pregnancy, a doctor should recommend certain procedures to ensure that the fetus will be a boy. On the astrologically auspicious day when the Victory star and the moon are aligned, he explains, a blacksmith should create the form of a male child out of three, five or seven types of metal. The form should be heated in a coal fire until it glows red, and then soaked in the milk of an animal who has given birth to male offspring, measuring an amount of milk that corresponds to however many types of metal were used. Two handfuls of cooled milk should be given to the woman. Alternatively, he continues, to achieve the same effect a medicinal concoction, a mixture of Seaberry, grape and molasses, could be administered to the pregnant woman. Finally, if these procedures are ineffective or impractical, the woman could try wearing an amulet. "Make three strands of thread with wool from the right shoulder of a breeding male sheep," Kyempa Tsewang explains, "and tie it around her waist with the tip hanging down."[1]

Kyempa Tsewang's text is a commentary on the *Four Tantras*, a work that came to be known in Tibetan medical circles in the thirteenth century and which is still the most influential textual authority on Tibetan medicine. Kyempa Tsewang's treatise is widely respected and studied in the halls of medical learning today, and yet some contemporary readers, Tibetan and non-Tibetan alike, are inclined to disregard recommendations such as those above. For many, these prescriptions are artifices now considered unscientific, arcane remnants of a foreign past. In the fifteenth century, however, Kyempa Tsewang was a leader among physicians, part of a community who saw these techniques as critical to medical practice and scholarship. If these intellectuals agreed, during the heyday of Tibet's scholarly renaissance, that such therapies were important to medical practice and knowledge, should we not take them seriously? What was medicine in the history of Tibet, if its recommendations included magical acts and amulets?

Roughly a hundred years earlier, an influential religious thinker known as Longchen Rabjampa composed a long treatise on Buddhist tantric practice. Early in that work, he discusses pregnancy and gestation. He explains how the embryo begins to form in the first few days after conception. During the firs days immediately after conception, the embryonic constituents are gathered together, dispersed, and reintegrated repeatedly by the actions of the natural elements, water, earth, fire, and so forth. On the very first day after conception, he writes, "an extremely subtle water-element circulatory channel originates by stretching straight out toward the right side of the woman, roughly the size of one-hundredth of a horse tail's hair. During this time, the woman feels cold." On the second day, another circulatory channel develops, and the woman feels of dizzy and sluggish. On the third day after conception, yet another channel emerges and the newly pregnant woman perspires and feels hot.[2]

Longchen Rabjampa was a prominent Buddhist scholar not known to have any training in medicine. His work covers what we may easily agree to be religious topics, such as contemplative and yogic practices and enlightened experience, and yet we also find a sizable portion of this text devoted to a detailed discussion of human gestation. Is it surprising to find data on embryology in an esoteric religious treatise? What was religion in the history of Tibet, if its treatises addressed conception, pregnancy and fetal growth?

This book reflects on these questions, considering a period of history when Tibetans themselves were negotiating similar matters. With the wide-scale dominance of "Western biomedicine" today, most of us assume we know what medicine is, and what it is that one must know to practice medicine. Topics such as anatomy and physiology, for instance, are unquestioned as the foundations of medicine in our day. In this book, however, we will recognize the fact that the categories of religion, medicine and science are products of particular times and places. In the past, in the history of Tibet just as in the history of European thought and practice, the disciplinary boundaries of knowledge were fluid or fixed in different ways than they are now. All of these terms, and the bodies of knowledge and action that surround them, have histories, their meanings changing often quite radically over time.

Medicine, science and religion in European thought

The history of disciplinary boundaries in Europe is intricate, and this has been a matter of interest for thinkers in all times. By the fourth century B.C.E., the Hippocratic school was pondering the role of philosophy in medicine. The writings of Plato and Aristotle had a strong shaping influence on the formulation of Greek medicine, and it was an influence that lasted: the discipline of biology in Europe was largely based on Aristotle until the eighteenth century.[3] While the close relationship of medicine to philosophy has been tolerable for most, medicine's connections to "religion" have been more problematic. For most historians, ancient Greek medicine was prized as a rational tradition that went beyond "superstitious" beliefs, which were seen to be part of religion. Until the 1970s, historians saw in the rationality of Greek medicine a precursor to modern scientific medicine: calling it rational was to say that, like contemporary scientifi medicine, it rejected a superstitious view of demons and gods as agents of harm and healing, and it fought disease by natural means, such as diet, drugs or surgery.[4] In recent decades, however, with a recognition of the cultural specificity of the very notion of rationality, the history of Greek medicine has been slowly revised. A distinction between "natural" and "supernatural" is no longer considered appropriate for the early Greek world. While its influence was lasting, the elite scholarly tradition of Greek medical texts is seen as but one tradition of knowledge in the Roman Empire and beyond. Temple medicine, for instance, with its emphasis on prayers and magical healing, is recognized as a key part of ordinary life for the Greeks.[5] Historians now realize that in the context of healing illness, religion, philosophy, astrology, alchemy, botany, magic and medicine all intermixed in the thoughts, practices and writings of various peoples around Europe.

Articulating the connections between the disciplines of religion, philosophy, medicine and science has been contentious for centuries.[6] By the thirteenth century, these subjects were formally investigated in the universities of Western Europe. Bringing students from all over Europe to towns such as Paris, Oxford and Bologna, medieval universities focused learning on four faculties, an arts degree forming a preliminary stage for professional degrees in theology, medicine or law. All university students were therefore similarly trained in the disciplines of the arts, which included a natural philosophy largely based on Aristotle.[7] While university educated Europeans received a comparable core schooling, defining the differences and interactions between these subdisciplines remained problematic, particularly when it came to the relationship between theology and science.[8]

While much has been written about cross-disciplinary scholarly exchange in Europe, less is known of such interactions in Asia. As in medieval Europe, large monastic universities in Tibet united students from around Central, East and South Asia to master a complex corpus of scholarly learning on topics as wide-ranging as logic, grammar, religious practice and medicine. This book will consider how portions of that vast body of literature came to be defined and differentiated during this formative period in Tibetan history.

The study of Asian medical traditions and their connections to religion has been troubled by a heritage of learning that divided disciplines of knowledge in particular ways. In European scholarship, Asian religions were initially define under the cloak of an Enlightenment concept of religion that placed emphasis on the cognitive, intellectual and doctrinal elements of religious traditions. With the nineteenth-century emphasis on rationality, and with the increasing availability of information about non-European religions from missionaries, cognitive accounts of religious belief, akin to a scientific description, served to objectify religion. The idealization of rationality used to define philosophical and other forms of scholarly thinking affected early Indologists such as Frauwaller, who attempted to prove Indian thought to be unconcerned with soteriology, for example, or Matilal, who tried to show Indian thought to be purely "scientific.[9]

Today, many scholars have noted that the epistemological frameworks that shape our conception of Asia and Asian religions are themselves shaped by the polemics and ideological concerns of our scholarly forebears. This is a cloak we have yet to shed. To this day, texts classified as medical or scientific are rarely consulted in the study of Indian religion. The study of Indian medicine largely consists of non-analytical descriptions aimed at identifying effective medical healing techniques. Some presentations of Āyurveda are still colored by the desire to prove it a "secular" and "empirically objective" science, and many translations from Sanskrit of seminal Āyurvedic treatises are purged of "magical" or "superstitious" elements that might lend doubt to the scientifi authority of the system as a whole.

For historians studying the relationship between science and religion generally, such a reading of present concerns into the past is known as "presentism." Today, however, influenced by the work of feminist and other theorists, this strategy has been largely dismissed in favor of "contextualism," a model that attempts to look at ideas or events on their own terms or in their own contexts, to the extent possible. Within this framework, rather than define the boundaries of Tibetan medicine and Tibetan religion by our own standards, we should instead try to think about how these lines were drawn by particular Tibetan thinkers at particular points in history. How did fifteenth-century Tibetan scholars themselves characterize the categories of "religion" and "medicine"? What sorts of topics did these disciplines contain? How can we describe the interactions between religion and medicine in Tibet at that point in history?

Models of comparison: science and religion, science and Buddhism

Characterizing the nature of the relationship between religion and science or medicine has been important to the historians of Europe. These thinkers have focused on models of conflict, mutual support, complementarity or total separation.[10] Recent scholars have criticized the long held dominance of the "conflic thesis," which claims conflict to be the defining mode of interaction between science and religion.[11] Richard Olson notes that in the early modern period, science, religion, law and history all used common language, methods, and concepts; he also observes that publishing scientists and religious thinkers were often the same individual. Science and religion were linked institutionally as well as conceptually or biographically, sharing or competing for resources, personnel, authority and prestige. Olson suggests that in general, projects of science and theology are driven by such differing concerns that a model of conflict is a misguided stereotype.

Colin Russell traces the expansion of this stereotype over nearly a century of writings on the relationship of science and religion, suggesting that while certainly there have been conflicts in the history of science and religion, a thesis of conflict as the defining characteristic in the relationship is inadequate for the "sensitive and realistic" historiography of science and religion.[12] He explains that the conflict thesis (1) occludes an understanding of any other sort of relationship between science and religion, (2) discounts many instances of a close alliance between science and religion, (3) emphasizes a Whiggish view of history as aiming at "victory", (4) ignores the richness of diversity of ideas in science and religion, and (5) exaggerates what were historically minor debates to the status of major conflicts [13] James Moore, likewise, criticizes the conflic thesis' "military metaphor" for promoting false dichotomies between science and religion, scientists and theologians, or scientific and religious institutions [14]

While some historians and scientists still accept the conflict thesis, most historians of science have rejected it as misleadingly presentist, now focusing instead on a "complexity thesis" that became the dominant methodology in the 1980s and 1990s.[15] With the complexity thesis, new studies of science and religion acknowledge a changing and multifaceted relationship between the two, and also recognize that specific and pervasive definitions for science and religion are unattainable, given that the terms have so many meanings in so many contexts. In this book I will agree with this position, seeing that in Tibetan history as in European history, the definitions of science and religion and the relationships between them are in flux and inherently contextual

The study of science and religion in European history is well developed. More recently, scholars have been considering the relationship between science and Buddhism specifically. In *Buddhism and Science: Breaking New Ground*, B. Alan Wallace surveys attitudes on the relationship between religion and science that emphasize either conflict or connection. At the outset he questions the applicability of the term "religion" to Buddhism, pointing out that definitions of religion are based on Judeo-Christian models of religion. Pressing Buddhism into these molds results in a distorting neglect of many key features of practice and thought that could, with a broader definition in action, be reasonably considered part of a continuous tradition; classifying Buddhism as religion encourages one to overlook aspects of that tradition that many may consider philosophy, psychology or science, for example.

For Wallace, science is a method more than a geographically and historically situated discipline: it is an "organized, systematic enterprise that gathers knowledge about the world and condenses the knowledge into testable laws and principles."[16] With this definition, he reasons that elements of Buddhism are strongly scientific: "Buddhism, like science, presents itself as a body of systematic knowledge about the natural world, and it posits a wide array of testable hypotheses and theories concerning the nature of the mind and its relation to the physical environment."[17] Recognizing the strict disjuncture between religion and science in both popular and scholarly attitudes, Wallace aims to capture Buddhism from the scientist's ghettoization of religion and demonstrate that Buddhism as a whole spans the Euro-American boundaries of science and religion. By definin science very broadly as method, moreover, he argues that Buddhism *is* science.

Taking another tack, but arguing similarly for an expansion beyond the particular limits of science and religion as defined by most Euro-Americans today, José Cabezón's essay in *Buddhism and Science* aims to categorize the relationship between Buddhism and science in "structural and typological, rather than in historical, terms."[18] He points out that while in fact the nature of this relationship has been largely one-sided, such that Buddhism is an object of scientific inquiry not the reverse, we can nevertheless speak of three modes of interaction between Buddhism and science: conflict/ambivalence similarity/identity, and complementarity. Until the recent scientific interest in limited aspects of Buddhism, he reports, the relationship has been one of ambivalence, not conflict, largely because Buddhism was simply "absent as a serious intellectual option" for scientists.[19] More recently, a similarity/identity model has operated, some writers considering Buddhism to be *like* science, others seeing Buddhism to *be* science. In the last model, that of complementarity, Buddhism and science offer either complementary *objects* of analysis, on the one hand, or complementary *methods* of analysis, on the other. In other words, Buddhism's focus on the mind complements science's expertise with the material world; or, Buddhism offers an ethical or embodied corrective to an ethically insensitive or disembodied scientific approach. Cabezón is critical of taking these metaphors too far, however, pointing out importantly that,

> Where the metaphor of Buddhism as an inner science is reified, it precludes a dialogue between Buddhism and science on the nature of matter; it prevents a serious engagement between Tibetan and Western medicine on the on the physical causes of illness. In short, it acts to silence Buddhism when it attempts to address any issue related to the material world.[20]

Cabezón highlights here a real risk of much contemporary work on Buddhism and science. If Buddhism is successfully captured as a "science of the mind," are the many volumes of Buddhist writing on the material world simply to be ignored because they are not scientific? And if they are not scientific, does this mean that they are not "systematic," not "objective," and somehow not "true"? And what about traditions of knowledge and practice that are commonly referred to as "Buddhist medicine," such as Tibetan medicine? If Tibetan medicine is considered "Buddhist," as it often is labeled, is it religion or science? If it is to be valued by the globalized world of contemporary researchers, it must be considered science. But what happens, then, to those aspects of Tibetan medicine that do not fall within the contemporary boundaries of science?

Such questions are not merely academic, as these issues have real and powerful effects on human lives and societies. The answers to these questions are matters of ideology and politics, today as much as in the past. The polemics of the Buddhism-as-science position, for example, have succeeded in publicizing the contemporary relevance of Tibetan Buddhism in particular, an important aim of the current Dalai Lama and others who recognize that for many, "religion" points to a static and outdated mode of knowing or practice. One effect of this position, however, involves the dismissal of the "religious" from Tibetan medicine in the twentieth century. For Tibetan doctors to gain the sort of prestige accorded to the popular Buddhism–science discussions, they must ally themselves with the science side of the equation, since Buddhism, in the complexities of that scheme, can be prized only for its expertise with the mind. "Science" in this dialogue means Euro-American science, moreover, and therefore Tibetan medicine must be fashioned after that model.

The elimination of Buddhism from Tibetan medicine has, therefore, occurred not only for Euro-American scholars, as discussed above, but it is also happening for many Tibetans, as has been documented by medical anthropologists. Vincanne Adams' work has examined the contemporary preoccupation among Tibetan doctors with defining what "science" and "religion" are and whether, or how, Tibetan medicine is science. This discussion has taken on new meanings in the last fifty years in Tibet, "brought about by recent political and social conditions that have made *science* a politically safe term at the same time that they have made *religion* politically unsafe."[21] Tibet has seen the gradual excising of content deemed "religious" from the curriculum of large state-sponsored medical schools, with the "religious" largely defined by guidelines set forth during the Cultural Revolution; the religious, including superstition and magic, is politically dangerous, primitive and nonscientific[22] As elsewhere in China, medical doctors in mid-twentieth-century Tibet were asked to use Marxist-Leninist principles of health care that distinguished between "the religious/superstitious and the materialist/scientific bases of their knowledge,"[23] and a generation of doctors was thus trained in a highly simplified version of Tibetan medicine. In a sense, this worked to the benefit of Tibetan medical institutions, which suffered far fewer deprivations over the ensuing decades than religious institutions. Ironically, this move also brings Tibetan medicine onto the world stage as a recognized tradition of medicine that may one day, with adequate research-based publications documenting its efficacy, stand alongside biomedicine.

As is proposed by the science historians' "complexity thesis," the relationships between medical and religious traditions are changing and multifaceted, determined in part by how the boundaries of those disciplines are articulated at different times, in different places, in different contexts, or for difference purposes. This is not only a phenomenon of modernity, or of European scholarship; it is also characteristic of the history of Buddhism and medical traditions in Asia. It is sometimes said that the practice of medicine is fully integrated with religious concerns in Tibet historically. But it is clear the two have been, in some way, individual disciplines and genres of literature for centuries. Although we must certainly be aware that the boundaries of these disciplines are not what they may be in Europe or North America, still it is the case that these were, and are, considered distinct disciplines in some sense. Obtaining a clearer understanding of just how these disciplines were understood at different points in history in Tibet is one important aim of this book, and we will do this by looking at embryology, a topic that for many Asian cultures spans the boundaries of medicine and religion. Tibetans in medical and religious communities alike were intrigued by the topic of human development, and as we study their perspectives on how life is created, we will also learn something about how they shaped the disciplines of knowledge that contextualized those perspectives.

Narratives of embryology

In 1688, Sanggyé Gyatso, the politically powerful regent of the Fifth Dalai Lama and a prolific scholar in his own right, completed the *Blue Beryl.* Like the work by Kyempa Tsewang cited above, this lengthy treatise is also a commentary on the *Four Tantras*. To accompany his commentary, Sanggyé Gyatso commissioned a series of eighty paintings. Corresponding directly to the chapters of his text, these paintings illustrate aspects of Tibetan medicine, including detailed drawings of anatomy and physiology, disease states, medicinal substances, diagnostic techniques and so on. One of these paintings illustrates human conception and the growth of the embryo.

The story of the embryo depicted in that painting begins with the soon-to-be mother and father lying in bed, and the mind, or "consciousness," of a transmigrating being entering the union of their reproductive substances. This is the moment of conception, an event that requires the confluence of three factors: reproductive substances emitted by a man and woman and a transmigrating consciousness, which is impelled by its own karma to that particular copulating couple. The text explains that if the reproductive substances of either the father or mother are faulty – if they are deficient in one of nine ways – conception will not occur. It also tells us when a woman is fertile and, moreover, that conception on odd days after the end of menstruation will result in a male child and on even days, a female child. It explains which aspects of the embryo's body are formed by which contributing factor (the reproductive substances of the parents or the consciousness), and how the body is formed also by the five natural elements (earth, water, fire, air and space

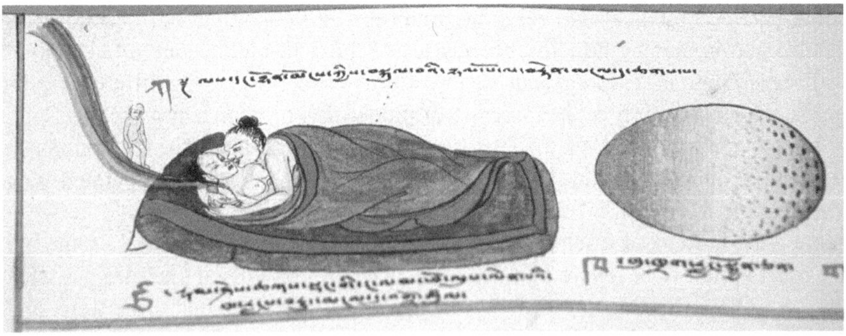

Figure 1.1 The seventeenth-century painting depicts the moment of conception.

During the first month after conception, the embryo is transformed from a substance that resembles curdled milk in week one, to a lengthened and thickened substance in week two, and by week three it resembles the semi-solid consistency of yogurt. After week three, rituals can be performed to transform the still undetermined sex of the embryo into that of a male. In the fourth week the embryo will take on a rounded, oval or elongated shape according to whether it will become male, female or indeterminate in sex. According to Sanggyé Gyatso's commentary and the associated images, these first nine weeks of development are known as the "fish stage.

The next period of gestation, weeks ten through seventeen, is the "tortoise stage": text and image describe precisely which aspects of the fetus' body develops during each of these weeks. In the fifth week of gestation the navel forms, and a week later the body's main circulatory channel extends from the navel. A preliminary form of the eyes develops in the seventh week around which the head grows the following week. In the ninth week the upper and lower torso form, followed by the shoulders and hips in the tenth week, the nine orifices of the body in the eleventh week, the five "solid organs" (heart, liver, kidney, spleen and lungs) in the twelfth week and the six "hollow organs" (stomach, small intestine, large intestine, urinary bladder, gall bladder and reproductive organs) in the thirteenth week. The third phase of development is the "pig stage," covering the eighteenth through thirty-fifth weeks. Following that period, the fetus begins to feel a sense of revulsion at being in the womb, additional signs of whether the fetus will be male or female are provided and, finally, the child is born.[24]

As clear and explicit as this text on early human development and its accompanying images may seem, in fact these details were controversial during the several hundred years of writing on human development preceding this text. Examining this controversy will tell us a great deal about intellectual history in Tibet, much as debates over embryology are a mirror into our own history. In Europe, embryological theories had a profound impact on the history of ideas, an influence that was felt in circles far beyond that of biologists and medical researchers. In the seventeenth and eighteenth centuries, for instance, the question of how the fetus developed was a contentious issue. Some embryologists favored a theory called epigenesis; others propounded a theory of preformation. In epigenesis, development of the human form within the womb was sequential, or cumulative. Conceptual difficulties in this view were centered around the problem of differentiation: what could be the stimulus that would convert nothing into something? This question caused many European embryologists of the late seventeenth and early eighteenth centuries to reject epigenesis in favor of preformation. In preformation, a tiny form of the human body was believed to exist from the very beginning of development; some preformationists even claimed they could see tiny human forms in ova or sperm. Conceptual troubles with this hypothesis, however, led to two schools of thought: the ovists, who placed the homunculus in ova, and the spermists who placed it in sperm.

Problems did not end there – if the homunculus was contained in the egg, then each homunculus must have another homunculus in an infinite regression, suggesting, in fact, that the entire human race was included in the ovaries of Eve.[25]

This debate cast its influence widely across European intellectual thought, art theory and literature. Eighteenth-century Europe saw a radically new orientation of thought, for instance, that brought about a change from a mimetic theory of art to an organic theory of art. Critics who searched widely for the origins of this transformation were led to focus on the importance of embryological research of a century earlier. Parallels had begun to be drawn between the production of a work of art and the conception and development of a living organism, such that organic imagery described the artist's creativity. Metaphors that drew on the processes of conception and fetal development were linked conceptually to that which is naturally conceived and developed. Rather than being manufactured from artificially conjoined substances and by means of strenuous effort in a figh against nature, the fruit borne by a means modeled after human conception and development bears quite different implications.[26]

In fact, the influence of embryology on intellectual life in Europe stretches back many centuries. In twelfth-century Europe, theologians used the anatomy and physiology of the body as proofs for divine perfection and intelligence. Theories of generation and embryology in particular were used in scholastic debates on a range of theological topics.[27] Earlier still, embryology proved an influential though controversial, topic for the philosophers of ancient Greece. Plato considered the embryo to be an animal, Hippocrates called it a plant, and Aristotle explained that in the process of gestation it began as a plant and later grew into an animal. Emerging Christian thinkers subsequently rejected the thought that the embryo could be a plant since, of course, plants have no souls. Throughout the history of European and Islamic intellectual history, the study of the embryo has been intertwined with religion, ethics and natural science.[28]

In this book, it is my contention that the history of embryology and its role in Tibetan scholarly traditions is similarly influential. Discussion of the embryo in Tibetan literature was not restricted to an isolated group of medical traditions; rather, the power of embryological symbolism held sway far beyond Tibet, across the Buddhist world. Tibetan embryological literature provides us with an array of controversial topics. All Tibetan traditions known today agree that conception occurs upon the confluence of three conditions, as described in the account above: the two types of healthy reproductive substance from a copulating man and woman, and a consciousness in the postmortem state awaiting rebirth. When the consciousness finds an appropriate womb, some traditions claim that it takes hold there by means of the three "destructive emotions" (*nyon mongs;* Skt. *kleśa*), attachment, anger, and delusion. Other texts contend that the transmigrating consciousness experiences attraction to one parent and anger toward the other, and that it is due to these emotions that the postmortem period ceases and a new being is conceived. At the moment of conception, some traditions claim that an ordinary transmigrating being loses awareness as it merges into the mixture of reproductive substances. Following conception, full embryological descriptions detail thirty-seven to forty weeks of development, with daily, weekly or monthly records of the process of the psycho-physical body's growth. But the details are debated. How precisely does the consciousness enter the mother's womb? What exactly is the role of the transmigrating being's karma throughout the process of gestation? Which are the primary forces responsible for directing fetal growth? What is the exact sequence of development of the fetus in the womb? Many of these issues are rooted in complex philosophical problems that can also be found debated in other contexts in Buddhist religious and philosophical texts. In chapters to come, I will address some of the contested issues found in Tibetan literature on embryology and consider their place in the wider context of Tibetan religious, philosophical and medical thinking and writing.

This book focuses on stories of human development as they begin to appear in Tibetan texts from the eleventh and twelfth centuries. This includes works authored by Tibetans from this period onwards, works translated into Tibetan from other languages, and earlier works that continued to hold great importance. The centuries preceding these witnessed the break-up of a Tibetan empire that spanned Central Asia over a period of several centuries, the persecution of certain forms of Buddhist culture and scholasticism, and a dramatic range of other social, political and economic transformations across Tibet and surrounding regions. Following these upheavals, a new transmission of Buddhist texts and other forms of intellectual culture arrived in Tibet from India and neighboring regions, and Tibetans themselves began anew to produce a wide variety of literary materials. Over the next several centuries, major monastic sites were transformed into centers for the production, circulation and transmission of scholastic knowledge of various types, including medical knowledge. The concentration of physicians in monastic and other religious centers and the prominent political position of physicians in those centuries points to an important relationship between the politico-religious hierarchy and medical scholars and practitioners of various types. What impact did this relationship have on medical and religious intellectual histories?

Embryology was an important theoretical topic throughout the history of Indian literature, and many shared and conflicting views found there were known to Tibetans of the eleventh and twelfth centuries. During this period, vast amounts of literature poured across the borders of Tibet. As this transmission of intellectual culture arrived from neighboring regions, how did Tibetans evaluate such an eclectic mix of foreign ideas, and how did they adapt these materials to meet their own concerns? As I assess the significance of embryology across religious and medical literature in the chapters to follow, general questions of cultural transmission and adaptation will also surface. As they wrote, how did Tibetans determine when originality was acceptable, and when adherence to tradition was required? Intellectual controversy in twelfth-century Tibet was characterized by a concern to uphold India as the ideal authorizing source. Tibetan scholars at this time possessed numerous sources with which they could easily have maintained connection to India, and yet in embryology this link was broken, as certain embryological concerns – vitally important issues for Indian scholars of all types – were rendered invisible, and other concerns emerged as significant During this tremendously formative period in intellectual history, Tibetans categorized objects of scholarship: some topics required an external legitimating authority, but for other topics Tibetans themselves could exercise individual discretion. During this process, Tibetan disciplines of knowledge were shaped and reshaped.

Caveats and approaches

Before going any further, I must pause to make a few comments about what this book will *not* be. First and foremost, this is not a comprehensive presentation of all instances of, and uses of, Tibetan embryology. It will soon become clear that such a goal would be unattainable, so widely spread are Tibetan embryologies across the vast expanse of Tibetan literature and practice, and so few are the sources that have survived for our examination today. Because it is methodologically more my aim to demonstrate "a style of reading" than to present a comprehensive analysis of the entire range of medical or religious attitudes toward embryology, my sources are selective.[29] The results of this examination, therefore, are not intended to be – and indeed cannot be – a definitive history of Tibetan embryology that attempts to gain a complete vision of the past. Although my conclusions will have social and historical ramifications, this is mainly a study of the development and exchange of scholarly rhetoric within certain literate traditions. As such, I am more concerned with the historicity of *narratives* than the historicity of "reality." As Leslie Kurke expresses it in her work on ancient Greek coinage and games, the discursive structures of the texts are themselves the central "facts" under consideration.[30]

Second, because embryology is written about in the context of many of Buddhism's most esoteric yogic and ritual practices, a detailed analysis of those religious practices might be expected in this book. In the introduction to his *Indian Esoteric Buddhism: A Social History of the Tantric Movement*, Ronald Davidson similarly anticipates his readers' desire for discussion of esoteric Buddhist practice in his book, and he refers such readers to the many excellent ritual and textual studies and translations that address Buddhist ritual, yogic and doctrinal systems in detail.[31] I will refer my readers to these same works, and others as relevant, noting that because this is above all a study of literary expressions of human development, my treatment of Buddhist contemplative or ritual practices themselves is necessarily brief.

Third, I would be remiss in not stating at the outcome that there is properly no such thing as "Tibetan embryology." Embryology, along with physiology and anatomy, are sub-branches of the discipline of biology with specific definition and histories in Euro-American thought, and they have no *direct* terminological or conceptual correlative in Tibetan. What I am calling "embryology" in this book is, in fact, referred to in Tibetan literature simply as "how the body is formed" (*lus kyi chags tshul*), a topic that typically begins with a discussion of conception and typically ends with the moment of birth. There is, likewise, no such thing as a dedicated "Tibetan embryologist," although I may use this designation to refer to Tibetan authors who write about the formation of the body in the womb. Indeed, in Tibetan literature there is properly no single, unambiguous term for "embryo": that which we call in English both the "embryo" and the "fetus" is, in Tibetan literature, variously referred to as the "body (*lus*) forming in the womb," as "that which resides in the womb" (*mngal gnas*), as the "womb" itself (conflating the term for womb, *mngal*, with the embryo), or simply as the "child" (*phru gu*).

A brief comment about what I mean by "literature" is also required here. In this book, I ask that our notion of literature go beyond the everyday, but narrow, sense of its association with fiction alone. Oral narratives aside, the widest, most neutral and value-free sense of the term literature may encompass a full range of written material: philosophical or scientific, fictional or non-fictional, academic or common.[32] This expanded definition may go some way toward acknowledging Cabezón and Jackson's reminder that literature is a Euro-American analytical category that should not be uncritically applied to the Tibetan context, and that, indeed, until the twentieth century there was not a term in Tibetan that clearly correlated to the English term "literature."[33] In this book, however, using the term to refer simply to the wide range of written material available in Tibetan, I need not grapple with this problem.

Finally, while this is in some sense a history of Tibetan medicine, in this work I will not engage in significant description or analysis of Tibetan medicine as a whole, nor will I comprehensively address the content of its sub-disciplines, such as pharmacology (the study of *materia medica*, toxicology, and therapeutics), nosology (the study of the classification of diseases), or etiology (the study of the causes and origins of diseases). As subsequent chapters will show, one central aim of this book is to demonstrate that Tibetan embryology should not be viewed solely within the domain of "medicine" (whatever we may mean by that). We will see, over the course of this work, that embryology defies our expectations in various ways. Where we might anticipate essential connections with gynecology, obstetrics or the experience of pregnancy, for example, Tibetan embryologists will leave us wondering, what are we really talking about here? The key to answering this question will lie, I believe, in the interpretive decisions we make while reading.

Medical epistemology and the embryological narrative

With these caveats in mind, I will suggest now that as we examine Tibetan accounts of human development, we will find that they may be most fruitfully understood through a form of narrative epistemology, rather than what we typically understand to be a scientific epistemology. The term epistemology is sometimes understood in an exclusively scientistic sense; that is, it often describes the belief that the foundation of knowledge rests on *facts* disclosed through observation and argument governed by rules of logical inference. The term is also more widely understood to refer simply to how things are known, focusing on methodological issues involved in the question of what facts are; it is this wider sense of the term that I mean here. As we considered earlier, conventional epistemology has traditionally been, for most contemporary Euro-Americans, grounded in what is characterized as logico-scientific rationality.[34] Logico-scientific discourse functions to demonstrate or prove a statement by linking it to other statements following the principles of formal logic. Such discourse is founded on logical empiricism, the dominant Euro-American philosophy of science until the 1970s and a model of belief about science that still persists in many circles today. According to this view, "reality" exists prior to, and independent of, the effort to understand it or manipulate it, and it is science that most closely approaches the accurate representation of reality. As Charles Leslie and Allen Young note in *Paths to Asian Medical Knowledge*, "This correspondence between reality and the way science represents reality, a match guaranteed by science's epistemology, makes scientific representations not merely useful, but also true."[35] The privileging of the epistemology of modern Euro-American science affects the study of non-modern, non-Euro-American knowledge systems, however, as it is thereby believed that these systems alone "culturalize" reality and are thus "untrue." As discussed above, this attitude is manifest in many Euro-American writings on Asian medical systems.

Narrative epistemology is an alternative to this sort of logico-scientific rationality. The commonplace impression of narrative is conditioned by the prominent role of the novel in literary criticism and also, therefore, by the novel's fictiona truth-status. In the last quarter of the twentieth century, however, many theorists in the humanities and social sciences have come to view narrative not as "just an impressionistic substitute for reliable statistics," but as a valuable way of understanding and explanation in itself.[36] Like the historians described above, philosophers of science have challenged logical empiricism, its ontological privileging of scientific knowledge, and the adequacy of logico-scientific rationality. In its place, some have embraced an understanding of the social and historical contingency of all types of knowledge, including scientific knowledge. Questioning the validity of logico-scientific discourse, many have accepted "narrative rationality." In narrative, principles such as phonetics, rhyme and metaphoric connection can replace rules of formal logic in producing meaningful truths. In *Narrative Knowing and the Human Sciences*, Donald Polkinghorne explains further that narrative is particularly attuned to individual experiences and their meaning by relating them as parts to a whole, and, by noting sequence of action, narrative is sensitive to temporal dimensions of human experience.[37] Rather than relying on general laws, narrative knowing is called for in realms where knowledge is particular and rules emerge from individual instances of action, as in engineering, navigation, common law, meteorology, moral conduct and clinical medicine.[38] As such, narrative knowing is essential to practical reason, the means by which individuals and groups make sense of events and situations and make decisions about how best to act under those conditions. Prominent theorists like Hauerwas, MacIntyre and Nussbaum have also called narrative knowing and expression essential to moral knowing.[39]

What I will focus on in this book is the idea that Tibetan embryology is not most productively approached as "science" or "medicine" in the way that these topics have traditionally been understood in Euro-American thought. Rather, I want to say that embryology – that is, those discussions in Tibetan texts that focus on the development of the human body from conception to birth – may be more fruitfully read as narrative. To call embryology narrative is not to call it fictional, for the narrative form may be used to express information in ways that are fictional or nonfictional, literary or nonliterary. Over the course of this book we will see that Tibetan embryologies are narrativized to a greater or lesser extent, and we will consider why this is so, and what this adds to our understanding of Tibetan writing and interpretation during the centuries in question. We will also see how these embryologies take advantage of narrative's qualities of situated subjectivity and entanglement with time, and its role in practical reason and moral knowing.

In calling embryology narrative, I am suggesting that it partakes of many of the attributes we normally ascribe to a story. Hayden White summarizes fiv such attributes, most of which can be seen to varying degrees in Tibetan accounts of human development: a central subject; a well-marked beginning, middle, and end; peripeteia; an identifiable narrative voice; and the suggestion of a necessary connection between one event and another.[40] In most Tibetan embryologies, the central subject is the developing embryo; in cases where symbolism is explicit, the subject may alternatively be the contemplative who is meant to undergo the spiritual transformation described embryologically. Accounts of fetal development certainly have a well-marked beginning, middle and end: they invariably begin with a description of conception, always present some information about the process of development throughout gestation, and commonly end with the occurrence of birth. The more narrativized embryologies may even possess peripeteia, a sudden or unexpected reversal of circumstances or situation, a common feature in literary works. Many embryologies have an identifiable narrative voice, commonly that of a religious teacher (rarely, as we will see, that of a medical clinician); more rarely, the embryo itself may narrate its experience of conception, gestation or birth. Finally, the details of conception and development are explicitly about the necessary connections between one event and another, an essential feature in the narrative form.

Embryology is a particularly interesting object for study as narrative because, as Daniel Punday has pointed out in "A Corporeal Narratology?", the human body is often forgotten in narratology. Punday explains that narratology has traditionally been interested more in discourse, that is, the manner in which the narrative is expressed, than in focusing on the elements that make up the story – the actual events, actors and places.[41] Looking at these elements involves considering how the objects represented in the story shape the narrative that represents them. Punday does not mean that writers have ignored the human body in individual narratives, but rather that when writers do address the body's role in narratives – for example, to investigate narrative's role in defining gender – they do not generally take the next step and raise fundamentally narratological issues that may affect and be affected by the body itself. Feminist narratology that links gender and narratological concepts, for instance, focuses primarily on women's social position or subjective experience, and not directly on the bodies that the narratives represent. Punday defines the central question of a true corporeal narratology, "How do certain ways of thinking about the body shape the plot, characterization, setting, and other aspects of narrative?"[42]

Hayden White argues that historiography is an especially fruitful ground to think about the nature of narrativity because it is where the imaginative intersects with the real.[43] Like history, embryology is explicitly describing events that are identified as "real," rather than those overtly described as "imaginary." The "real" and the "imaginary" are, of course, complicated concepts in Buddhism, but my claim here suggests loosely that, even in Tibetan literature, both history and embryology are written to express series of events that have actually happened, as opposed to *explicitly* fictional literature, for example, for which there is no such explicit or implicit claim made. Still the question remains what the events described are really meant to indicate. One aim of this book will be to understand what that reality is for Tibetan embryological narratives. We will quickly see that this reality may not be the physical reality of the embryo's development, as is the case in modern biomedical embryology. It may become productive, furthermore, to think of embryology as a kind of historical narrative, an attempt to describe historical events – historical events both at the personal level and at the cosmological level. Another important part of the historical narrative, Hayden agrees with Hegel, are themes of law, legitimacy or, more generally, authority – we will see this to varying degrees in embryology too, drawing the parallel between embryology and historiography even more finely Also part of most historical narratives is the latent or manifest desire to moralize the events it addresses,[44] again a central feature of many Tibetan embryological narratives.

Certainly, not all histories are narratives. White points to annals, which are simply a list of events in chronological sequence, or chronicles, which begin to tell a story but then do not finish it, as examples of historical literature in which the impulse to narrativize events is ignored. Similarly, Tibetan texts narrativize embryology to a greater or lesser extent. The earliest Tibetan-authored medical accounts of human development from the twelfth century follow very closely the *Four Tantras'* spartan account of embryology and have little to add of their own. By contrast, by the fourteenth or fifteenth centuries, embryologies such as those by Longchen Rabjampa, Tsong Khapa or Zurkhar Lodrö Gyelpo are elaborately embellished and take on a variety of narratological features. There are also differences in *what* is narrativized: some writers spend time embellishing the experiences of the embryo in the womb, filling out the embryo's character. In other texts, it is made explicit that gestation is a metaphor for spiritual development, and embryology is thus used to narrativize the experience of spiritual development for the contemplative.

There are two interpretive issues that intertwine throughout this book: one, that of how *I* am understanding traditions of Tibetan embryology, and two, that of how early *Tibetans* understood Indian embryology and developed their own traditions of writing on the topic. On each of these fronts, I am interested in both mimesis, the understanding of how an intellectual model or account of an event is meant to correspond to reality, and hermeneutic, the interpretation of details and their integration into a coherent story. As I consider whether embryological knowing can be more fruitfully viewed as a form of narrative knowing than a form of logico-scientific knowing, embryology appears as a method for truth-telling that expresses religious taxonomies, moral or political reflections, and a variety of other aims. These are true stories, shaped and articulated by physiological concepts. Far from trivial, they use the human body to address some of the most fundamental questions of life: who we are, why we are here, and how we should lead our lives.

Narrative, identity and history

In the next chapter, I will survey the traditions of early human development found in Indian sources that formed the basis for Tibetan writing on the topic. Although embryology was discussed in a wide range of Indian sources for a millennium before reaching Tibet, only a small number of those texts were available to Tibetans by the eleventh century. Those that did make it across the Himalayas represented a fairly disparate range of traditions, however, and Tibetans were thus introduced to Indic embryologies through Āyurvedic medical, Buddhist sūtric, and Buddhist tantric texts. Chinese sources were presumably available to Tibetans as well, and although I will make note of some early Chinese accounts of gestation, I have identified no concrete evidence that these traditions played a role in the development of Tibetan embryological knowledge.

From these origins, Tibetans themselves began composing a wide range of literature that contained discussion of early human development. Chapter three will consider the role of writing on embryology and, more generally, of descriptive presentations of the human body in Tibetan medical literature, beginning with a look at the historiography of medicine in Tibet. This chapter asks how historians grappled with the relationship between medicine and Buddhism prior to the seventeenth century, and how the complex interaction between the two worlds of thought and practice may be seen in how their boundaries are defined What topics were included in the field of "medicine," and how historically contingent is this issue? This discussion begins to problematize the role of knowledge about human development in medical literature, questioning how this may change over time as Buddhist intellectual frameworks pervade Tibetan scholasticism more and more thoroughly.

Chapters four, five and six will illustrate connections between embryology and issues of fundamental importance in Buddhist religious thought and practice, and the ways in which embryology is used as a forum for debating these issues. In chapter four, I will consider how embryology is used to speak about human identity, examining descriptions of the human body in different types of Tibetan literature. Who is the main character in an embryological narrative? Most basically, of course, the embryo is a body. But what is it that embryological narratives in particular allowed Tibetan narrators to say about the body? How did Tibetan understandings of the body shape accounts of early human development? While medical literature focuses on the body's systemic or humoral organization and digestive physiology, these are areas of little concern to religious authors; the body's circulatory system, on the other hand, is a topic of great concern to all. Over several centuries of writing on human development in Tibet, Buddhist models of physiology pervade medical writings, such that knowing about embryology meant knowing about religion. One effect of this is the loss of the pregnant woman as a character in narratives of embryology.

Tibetan accounts of human development can be interpreted on various levels. While on one level the main character is clearly the developing fetus, in some narratives the fetus is a double for the Buddhist practitioner. Who is signified by the character of the fetus, if not the physical body itself? In some texts, the fetus refers to a religious contemplative who wishes to be "spiritually reborn" and who will, therefore, enact the process of embryogenesis through meditation. Chapter five's close examination of the details of gestation will demonstrate that the composition of embryology in early Tibetan literature was far from straightforward. Despite the twelfth-century Tibetan author's impulse to form intellectual alliances with India, certain issues within embryology were clearly left to the discretion of the individual author. Embryological stories depict Buddhist practitioners of morality and meditation who undertake a soteriological process of gestation and rebirth. The stories about these characters are various, however: some tell of the suffering of gestation and agony of birth, and others describe gestation and rebirth positively as opportunities to reach higher spiritual attainments. This chapter will suggest that embryological narratives are related in structure and purpose to literature on the Buddhist path. In examining the relationship between Tibetan narratives of gestation and models of the religious path, I will explore discursive tools used to promote specific religious practices. This chapter tells stories of transformation that situate the seeds of change in the origins of the human body.

There is still more to say about how these stories are composed and what they communicate. In chapter six, I will examine the connections between events in embryological narratives. What causal elements drive those events? Is it solely karma? Or are other causal forces at work during gestation? In this chapter, I suggest that embryology allows Tibetan writers to temporalize doctrinal issues. The "emplotment" of embryological narratives transforms the events of early human development into stories with specific rhetorical functions, and it thereby imbues doctrine with a sense of time. Embryological narratives define certain acceptable paradigms for change and growth. Over the course of this chapter, by examining competing models for causation and human growth, we will see that while karma was vital to some models, others emphasized the power of different psychosomatic forces to effect change. In this discussion we will observe once again that embryology is at the center of a fundamental Buddhist philosophical issue.

At the same time, I will begin to consider the emplotment of the narration of Tibetan embryology itself. How did these narratives interact with each other and with their literary environments during this period of Tibetan history? What might embryology tell us about the historical transformations of medical and religious forms of literature? I will propose that religious traditions did not simply borrow embryology from medical traditions, as is most often assumed – rather, embryology is most fruitfully a *religious* topic. For religious writers, these narratives were a means of embedding doctrinal messages into human identities: such embryologies are religious doctrines that are narrativized into human lives. For medical writers too, at least by the fifteenth century, embryological narratives were a forum for *religious* theorizing – the topic provided a special context for medical scholars to philosophize about issues of vital importance to *Buddhist* thought and practice.

If we continue the thought, we might shift focus from narratives of embryology to historical narratives, arguing that there exists an important parallel between how embryological narratives construct identity and how historical narratives do so. Arguably, if embryology is a narrative that defines individual identity, history is the narrative that defines social or institutional identity. Can we see any parallels between models expressing human identity and models expressing social identity? What are the organizing themes of medical histories in Tibet, for example, and how are their characters described? As is the case in embryological narratives, in historical narratives we see an emphasis on geographic and geometric conceptualization, for instance. The cyclic "moral-temporal structure" that is based on the evolutionary narratives of Buddhist embryology appears as the foundation for the plot of Tibetan historical narratives too. Notions of ethics, causality and identity shape the creative construction of social history through historical narratives just as they do the creative construction of personal history through embryological narratives. Embryological and historical narratives alike appear to be concerned above all with explaining discontinuity as continuity, with making the discontinuous continuous. In the epilogue, therefore, I will gesture toward a new direction of thought, suggesting that just as it is of limited value to read embryological narratives only for information on how embryos grow, there is likewise much more to be understood from a historical narrative than simply what events occurred.

2

THEORIES OF HUMAN DEVELOPMENT

In the Āyurvedic *Compendium* by Caraka (*Carakasaṃhitā*), the chief medical theoretician, Punarvasu Ātreya, advises an assembly of philosophers, "Do not let yourselves become embroiled in complex arguments and counter-arguments nor let yourselves pretend that truth is obvious and easy to attain if one adheres to a single philosophical position."[1] Although Caraka's *Compendium* is one of the most influential medical treatises in South Asia, in this book we will see that Punarvasu's advice to eschew "complex arguments" was rarely heeded. The *Compendium* is generally said to date from the third or second century B.C.E., although it went through several centuries of revision subsequently. During the same period, many primary issues in Indian philosophy were also being debated, including the problems of salvation, selfhood, rebirth and karma. One of these contentious issues was the question of how the human being develops.

In early Indian literature, the development of the human body in the womb is described as a progressive layering of material elements. According to Caraka's *Compendium*, in the first month of gestation the embryo is gelatinous in form, described using the Sanskrit term *kalala*. In the second month, it becomes thicker, or more solid, a state referred to as *ghana*. If it is a male, it is shaped like a tight ball (*piṇḍa*), if it is female, it appears more elliptical (*pesī*), and if its sex is indeterminate or other than male or female, it is like half a sphere (*arbuda*). In the third month the limbs begin to bud and the sense organs appear. In the fourth month, the fetus becomes denser and more compact, and in the fift month it grows larger. The sixth month sees the fetus strengthen, and in the seventh month it is complete. In the eighth month it begins to draw strength or vitality (*ojas*) from the mother, and between the ninth and tenth months it is delivered.[2] Many South Asian embryological accounts are similarly structured, recording primarily which parts of the embryo develop in what order, but Indian writers disagreed about the exact sequence of development. Debates over the embryo's developmental sequence were not held among physicians only, but were spread across the full range of Indian scholarship. With elaborate rationalization, some said the head appears first (because it is the seat of the senses), while others prioritized the heart (as the seat of consciousness), the navel (as the place where food is stored), the intestines (as the seat of air), or the hands and feet (as the principal organs). Some argued – like the preformationists centuries later in Europe – that all parts of the body are perfectly differentiated from the moment of conception, and that they simply grow larger during gestation.[3] In the chapters to follow, we will see that for Tibetan writers, although the divergence of opinion on the issue of sequence of development is less radical than for their Indian predecessors, the question of how the body grows is still of intense interest.

The question of when consciousness emerged was also disputed in Indian literature. Classical Āyurvedic accounts, such as Caraka's *Compendium,* imply that it is active right from the moment of conception, while other traditions suggest that it appears only later in fetal development: in the *Garbha Upaniṣad,* a soul comes to the embryo after a gestation of seven months, and Purāṇic texts locate the time of consciousness entering the fetus in the seventh to ninth month.[4] In many traditions of South Asian embryology and in some Tibetan traditions, as we will see, the fetus is said to have conscious experiences, at least toward the end of its stay in the womb, experiencing feelings of suffering, memories of past lives, and even sentiments of religious devotion.

Sequence of development was but one of many issues central to the study of human development that were of concern not only to biologists, but to philosophers and religious thinkers too. In the context of embryology, philosophers discussed the causes of the formation and development of the fetus, they questioned the precise roles of the natural elements, the soul (Skt. *ātman*) and the mind (Skt. *manas*), and they pondered how transmigration occurred and the role of karma. In thinking about the process of transmigration, Indian scholars were confronted with the problem of the subtle body: what exactly was it that transmigrated? Surendranath Dasgupta summarizes these debates in his *History of Indian Philosophy*. For Sāṃkhya philosophers, the subtle body, necessary as the physical support of an individual's mind during the interval between death and rebirth, travels from life to life, becoming associated with the mind "like an odor is attached to a cloth," until the mind disassociates from it by attaining true knowledge. Caraka's *Compendium* refers to a non-physical factor that connects the soul with the body; Suśruta's *Compendium*, another Āyurvedic classic, also refers to a being that, urged by karma, enters the womb for rebirth. By contrast, according to Vaiśeṣika philosophers, who do not posit a subtle body, the influ ence of uterine heat works on the combination of parental substances, producing successive degeneration and regeneration until a fetal body develops. The mind, which requires a supporting body, enters the fetus only later in gestation. The Nyāya discuss this issue as well, also rejecting the existence of a subtle body and positing an "all-pervading" soul that takes its place in the new fetus.[5]

Inherent in debates over the mechanics of transmigration is also a question about the role of karma – or other causal forces – in propelling a being to a particular womb. Contemporary scholars theorize that early South Asian thinking understood karma mainly as an agent in the realm of sacrificial rituals, which were themselves ultimately responsible for creating a new being.[6] Only with a later "ethicization" of karma, where the quality of a new life was directly determined by the quality of previous actions, did the doctrine of karma come to encompass *all* actions. Steven Collins explains that, "If one's entire life is a sacrificial performance, then every action will have the results which sacrificia performance has – that is, every act will have its effect on the next life."[7] He attributes much of the responsibility for this transformation, a radical move that led to "the internalization of the sacrifice in the life of the renouncer," to the doctrine's interaction with Buddhism.

According to Caraka's *Compendium*, the union of male reproductive substance and female "blood" only produces a fetus when "the *ātman* with its subtle body, constituted of air, fire, water, and earth, and *manas*..., becomes connected with it by means of its karma."[8] The early Indian Buddhist thinker Vasubhandu, likewise, explains that the transmigrating *gandhabba* about to enter the womb is impelled by karma to do so. We will see in the following chapters that in some Buddhist texts karma empowers the energetic "winds" that create the embryo during gestation and then expel the fetus from the womb. In Indian tantric texts, karma is responsible for bringing together the first circulatory channels of the embryo's psycho-physical subtle body. Karma is said by some to determine the sex of the child during gestation. At the same time, however, many texts prescribe rituals to be performed early in development that will overpower this karmic action in the fetus, thereby ensuring the birth of a boy child. The presence of such rites confirms that for the Hindu and Buddhist medical traditions stemming from Caraka, karma is not an immutable force, but rather something that can be affected by human actions. I will return to this issue in Chapter 6.

In early Indian medicine, sequestering a patient in a womb-like cave was prescribed in order to restore a lost equilibrium between the body and the universe. Āyurvedic theory claimed that in the womb the human being experienced the perfect functioning of the three *doṣa* – translated variously as "humors," "faults" or "systemic processes" – and exposure to the outside world and its fluctuating climate of elements was said to throw this balance off, ill-health requiring, therefore, a return to a figurative womb. This medical treatment was applied also to spiritual imbalances: religious initiation practices (Skt. *dikśa*) called for sequestering the initiate in a closed hut, from which he or she is subsequently "reborn."[9] As David White points out eloquently, initiation into a religious order in this manner thus "biologically" links members of the order to each other, as all are reborn of the same womb.[10] Indeed, as far back as the Vedic Brāhmaṇas, sacrificial rites prescribe isolation in preparation for ritual rebirth. We will see in Chapter 5 that detailed religious contemplative practices modeled after the processes of human conception, development and birth are also present in a wide range of Tibetan Buddhist tantric works, no doubt derived from these older Indian traditions and yet articulated in ways that are uniquely Tibetan. In tantric traditions, procreative metaphors are brought to the fore. The study of early human development provides the tantric yogi with an accurate description of the erroneous developmental path of an ordinary being, and this knowledge is the key to learning to repeat this process without committing such error. The womb symbolizes an ultimate enlightened space in tantric Buddhism, although, as we will see, this glorification of female anatomy and physiology has little to do with real women.

Indian medical sources for human development

As Tibet was flooded with aspects of Indian culture in the eleventh and twelfth centuries, it was not only Buddhist texts that captured their attention – a number of Indian medical texts also crossed the Himalayas into Tibet to contribute to the fervor of teaching and writing taking place at the time. In the context of this increase of scholastic activity in Tibet, Indian Āyurveda was established with an unmatched place of influence in the history of Tibetan medicine

Classical Indian Āyurveda is closely related to a range of philosophical systems, the Nyāya-Vaiśeṣika and Sāṃkhya schools playing perhaps the largest roles. Āyurvedic theory is also influenced by yoga traditions concerned with controlling the mind and senses and avoiding excess, and by early tantric principles emphasizing the body and the structural equivalence of macrocosm and microcosm. The conceptual systemization of these philosophical systems into medical theory owes much to medical treatises commonly attributed to three scholars, Caraka, Suśruta, and Vāgbhaṭa, known as the great trio of classical Āyurveda, although the actual identity of these figures is contested.[11] The works ascribed to them are still considered the seminal literature of the Āyurvedic tradition today. Caraka's *Compendium* contains one hundred and twenty chapters divided into eight main sections, or "books": Sūtrasthāna, a general synopsis (thirty chapters); Nidānasthāna, on pathology (eight chapters); Vimānasthāna, on tastes, the systemic processes (Skt. *doṣa*), and classification of patients, physicians, and textbooks (eight chapters); Śārirasthāna, on the human body, including anatomy, reproduction, and midwifery (eight chapters); Indriyasthāna, on prognostic technique (twelve chapters); Cikitāsthāna, on treatment of disease (thirty chapters); Kalpasthāna, pharmaceutical formulae (twelve chapters); and Siddhisthāna, on various therapeutic measures (twelve chapters).[12] We will see that the structure of Caraka's *Compendium* is closely followed by Vāgbhaṭa and, to a degree, by the Tibetan medical text, the *Four Tantras*, as well.

The basic assumptions of classical Āyurvedic thought include the idea of the material constitution of human nature (Skt. *pañcabhūta*) and the notion that human behavior is based on the three "systemic processes" or "humors" (Skt. *doṣa*). The former is closely related theoretically to the Nyāya-Vaiśeṣika philosophical system, and the latter to the Sāṃkhya. The mechanics of transmigration and early human development are discussed in the first chapter of Caraka's fourth major section, the Śārirasthāna, with a cosmological bent that is clearly Sāṃkhyan in inspiration. The chapter begins by outlining the twenty-four Sāṃkhya principles (Skt. *tattvas*), and in his commentary on the Caraka verses,

Cakrapāṇi cites Sāṃkhya texts, the *Sāṃkhyakārikā* in particular, as authoritative sources. The root verses are explicit about their debt to Sāṃkhya; an explanation of the best way to attain salvation, for instance, concludes with the line, "This is what the yogins, the virtuous ones, the followers of the Sāṃkhya system, and the liberated ones say."[13] Even a cursory examination of classical Āyurveda makes clear the overt connections between medical and religio-philosophical traditions in India.

The second author in the trio of classical Āyurvedic authors, Suśruta, is also responsible for a *Compendium* (*Suśrutasaṃhitā*), which is similar in structure to Caraka's treatise.[14] Suśruta's *Compendium* is renowned among Āyurvedic texts for its study of surgery, although it deals comprehensively with all branches of Āyurveda. Despite their fundamental importance in the history of Indian medicine, however, the works of Caraka or Suśruta are not cited in Tibetan literature on early human development prior to modern times.

In Tibet, the most influential Indian medical text with a presentation of early human development is the *Heart of Medicine Compendium* (*Aṣṭāṇgahṛdayasaṃhitā*, Tib. *Yan lag brgyad pa'i snying po bsdus pa*) attributed to the third great author of classical Āyurveda, Vāgbhaṭa. This work is considered the "greatest synthesis of Indian medicine ever produced," and formed the basis of medical education across a wide expanse of South and Central Asia as it was translated into Tibetan, Arabic and other languages.[15] Little is known about the identity of this text's author, although most scholars attribute the text to a seventh-century figure with Buddhist tendencies.[16] His text and its Indian commentaries, along with other medical texts that were not sources for early human development but for other medical topics, were included in the Tibetan Buddhist canon, and they form some of the primary sources for later Tibetan studies of early human development.[17]

Similar in structure to the treatises of Caraka and Suśruta, Vāgbhaṭa's *Heart of Medicine* has 120 chapters. The Śārirasthāna, its section on the human body, addresses conception and fetal development, disorders of pregnancy, parts of the body (anatomy and physiology), classification of vital points, signs of death, and dreams and omens. The first part of this section covers topics such as the formation of the embryo, determination of the embryo's sex, menstruation, the features of healthy reproductive fluids, fertile periods, ceremonies for conception in general and conception of a male child in particular, features of a pregnant woman, the sequence of fetal development, practices of labor and delivery, and postpartum care. As we will see, the structure of this section is loosely replicated by the Tibetan *Four Tantras* and most medical texts on the body in Tibet subsequently. Despite this work being one of the most widely cited sources in Tibetan medical literature, however, and is, in fact, the very basis of much of Tibetan medicine, we will see in that in many respects its authority is disregarded in the study of early human development.

The *Heart of Medicine* reached Tibet by the eleventh century and was translated by the prolific translator Rinchen Zangpo (957–1055). Two Indian commentaries of this work were also quickly made available to Tibetans.[18] Rinchen Zangpo studied and translated the works of Vāgbhaṭa and his commentator Dawa Ngönga, and he taught them to a scholar who carried on this tradition by passing it through a lineage of students.[19] The famous Tibetan physician, Yuthok Yönten Gönpo (1112–1203), is said to have relied on this text especially as a guide in his medical practice for the first part of his life, until he received, edited, and made public the *Four Tantras*.[20]

The *Heart of Medicine* chapter on conception and fetal development is short, and much of its detail is reproduced in the *Four Tantras*, although we will examine in later chapters some significant differences. In the Tibetan canonical version of the *Heart of Medicine*'s account, as in the *Four Tantras*, conception occurs when the transmigrating consciousness is impelled by its own karma into the union of male and female reproductive substances (using the Tibetan terms *khu ba* and *khrag*, respectively). Prefiguring one of several *Four Tantras* theories on sex determination, Vāgbhaṭa notes that when the male substance dominates in volume at the moment of conception, the embryo will be male, when the female substance dominates, the embryo will be female, and when both are equal, the embryo will become a child of indeterminate sex. Defects in the male or female reproductive substances may result in an imperfect fetus or an inability to conceive; medicinal remedies for these problems are suggested, and the characteristics of healthy reproductive substances are also described. The proper time for conception is addressed with an explanation of when menstruation occurs and when a woman is fertile, and the text notes that pregnancy for a woman who is less than the age of sixteen will result in an ill or defective fetus. Certain ceremonial methods of intercourse are also recommended for those who wish to conceive a male child.

Once conception has occurred, the *Heart of Medicine* describes medicinal concoctions to be taken during the first month of pregnancy to ensure the production of a male child, and certain behaviors and foods that are to be avoided by the pregnant woman to ensure the growth of a healthy fetus. As pregnancy progresses, the text details the effects the condition has on the woman, and how she should be treated. Finally, methods for labor, delivery and postpartum care are considered at some length.[21] While there is some discussion of the development of the fetus' body during gestation in the *Heart of Medicine*, the text is more centrally focused on describing the conditions of pregnancy and care of the pregnant woman. Although the *Heart of Medicine* forms the basis of Tibetan medicine for several centuries after its arrival in Tibet, we will see in chapters to come that its emphasis on pregnancy and the experience of the woman is all but lost in later embryological accounts there. This omission becomes more striking over time, as centuries of Buddhist cultural authority replace the concerns of Indian medicine with those of a Buddhist literature in which women are marginalized at best, or, at worst, ostracized or even eliminated.

Early human development in Indian Nikāya and Mahāyāna Buddhism

Discussion of these topics was not limited to Hindu philosophical and medical schools of thought, and the mechanics of conception and the process of fetal development were also of interest to a wide range of early Indian Buddhist writers. Because these sources have been studied elsewhere, here I will only mention a few such issues.[22] It is well known that many Pāli Buddhist works include accounts of fetal development, but the details vary widely. The *Saṃyutta Nikāya*, for instance, outlines five stages of development, using the traditional terms *kalala*, *abbuda*, *pesī*, *ghana* and *pasākha*, each stage lasting a week; the *Visuddhimagga*, by contrast, mentions only four stages. Asanga's *Yogacharyābhūmi* offers yet another arrangement of the stages. While the *Saṃyutta Nikāya* uses the term *pasākha* to describe the fifth stage of embryonic development, accounts in the *Vinaya* use the same term to refer to the embryo's lower body.[23] The question of whether the intermediate being has a body – and what that might mean – was also a topic of contention for Buddhists. Among the so-called Eighteen Schools of early Buddhism, O. Wijesekara comments that Sammatīyas, Pubbaseliyas, Sarvāstivādins and Vaibhāṣikas affirmed the necessity of a corporeal being, while Mahāsāṃghikas, Ekavyavahārikas, Kukkuṭikas and Lokottaravādins did not.[24] Also debated was what exactly this being should be called. For many Buddhists, terminology that might have derived from early South Asian *ātman* theories, implying a permanent and unchanging being or "self," was unacceptable. Some Indian Buddhists settled on the term *vijñāna*, most often translated as "consciousness," to denote the transmigrating factor; Wijesekara points to the use of this term in the *Dīgha Nikāya*'s account of rebirth, for example.[25] He also considers the possibility of another factor in conception, pointing out that the *Mahāṭanhāsaṇkhaya Sutta* of the *Majjhima Nikāya* states that the presence of a being called *gandhabba* is required for conception to take place; Buddhaghosa clearly states that this reference to *gandhabba* is to a being about to enter the womb. As McDermott explains, this is not an "intermediate-state being," which exists in the state between death and rebirth, for Theravādins were opposed to this position. Instead, Theravādins proposed a "rebirth-linking consciousness" (Skt. *paṭisandhi vijñāna*) that arises newly at the moment of conception, linked causally to the previous lifetime "like a sound and its echo," according to Buddhaghosa.[26] Most of these canonical Buddhist texts were well known to Tibetans as they began their own traditions of writing on early human development. How did they resolve these differences? Or did they? If they did not, what may this tell us about embryology as a topic of intellectual discussion?

Among the most influential treatments of human development from early Indian Buddhism are those of Abhidharma literature, presented clearly in the fifth-century work by Vasubhandu, the *Commentary on the Treasury of the Abhidharma* (*Abhidharmakośabhāṣyam*). Abhidharma literature forms the foundation of Buddhist philosophy throughout the Buddhist world, comprising many volumes in Chinese and Tibetan translations of the Buddhist canon. So important is this body of literature that it forms an independent branch of the canon, which is known as the "Three Baskets" (*Tripiṭaka*): the sūtra basket is said to record the words of the Buddha himself, comprising teachings often presented as stories; the vinaya basket describes the code of monastic regulations for monks and nuns; and the abhidharma basket consists of a later collection of scriptures focused on systematizing Buddhist religious and philosophical doctrines.

The *Commentary*'s discussion of human conception and fetal development occurs in its third chapter, "Exposition of the World" (*Lokanirdeśa*), which is a presentation of the physical world, including its various hells and heavens, and its inhabitants. Citing liberally from various sūtras (few of which are identifie by name), Vasubhandu's text is a compilation of early Buddhist views from a range of sources. The "Exposition of the World" begins by introducing the different types of beings and the various realms of rebirth. Here a Buddhist sūtric theory of four modes of birth is presented: beings may be born from eggs (*sgong skyes*, Skt. *aṇḍaja*), from wombs (*mngal skyes*, Skt. *jalābuja*), from heat or moisture (*drod skyes*, Skt. *saṃsedaja*), or from "space" (*rdzus skyes*, Skt. *opapātika*). Beings of this fourth category are also referred to as miraculous births or as apparitional beings, and Vasubhandu defines them as "those beings who arise all at once, with their organs neither lacking nor deficient, with all their major and minor limbs." These beings appear without conception and gestation, and include supernormal entities such as gods, hell creatures and intermediate state beings. Curiously, humans may be born in each of these four manners, and the text cites examples of legendary men of each type.[27]

The next section of the text is a long discussion of the intermediate state, the phase between death and rebirth. Here Vasubhandu defends the existence of the intermediate state and discusses its nature, a contentious topic among early Indian Buddhist schools that has been well studied.[28] Following this topic, the mechanics of reincarnation are addressed. Vasubhandu explains that the male intermediate state being is attracted to the female member of a copulating couple, and a female intermediate state being is attracted to the male member of the couple. The moment of conception is described as follows:

> When the mind is thus troubled by these two erroneous thoughts, it attaches itself through the desire for sex to the place where the organs are joined together, imagining that it is he with whom they unite. Then the impurities of semen and blood are found in the womb; the intermediate being, enjoying its pleasures, installs itself there. Then the *skandhas* harden; the intermediate being perishes; and birth arises that is called "reincarnation" (*pratisaṃdhi*). When the embryo is male, it remains to its right in the womb, with its head leaning forward, crouching; female, to the left of the womb, vagina forward; with no sex, in the attitude in which one finds the intermediate being when it believes it is having sex.[29]

This particular emotional impetus for conception is attributed to beings who are born from wombs or eggs; beings born from moisture, by contrast, are attracted to the odors of a new rebirth site, and apparitional beings are motivated by desire for a particular sort of location.

Next, Vasubhandu explains that, according to sūtric sources, there are four ways to enter into, abide within, and depart from the womb, depending on the level of merit achieved by the transmigrating being. Beings of least merit are unaware of the entire process of conception, gestation and birth. Beings with somewhat more merit are aware of the moment of conception, but are then "unconscious" during gestation and birth; this type of being "has a great outflowing of merit and he is made resplendent through actions" and will become a Cakravartin. The next type of being is aware of conception and gestation but not birth; he or she has "knowledge obtained through instruction, reflection and meditation" and will become a solitary realizer. The final type is aware of all phases of the process, has "both action and knowledge" and will become a Buddha.[30] Robert Kritzer emphasizes this presentation as an important contribution by Vasubhandu. "Vasubandhu's purpose in including the four *garbhāvakrāntis*," or modes of entering the womb, Kritzer writes, "is to complete the account that is left unfinished by the older *abhidharma* descriptions of conception, which only deal with the ordinary, i.e., spiritually unaccomplished, person."[31]

Addressing the suggestion that a transmigrating being must necessarily be a "self" (*ātman*), a notion that is anathema to Buddhist doctrine, Vasubhandu then describes the process of gestation in the context of the Buddhist theory of interdependent arising (*pratītyasamutpāda*). "Growth is gradual," Vasubhandu comments simply, and he cites a scriptural source that lists the five stages of the embryo:

> There is first the *kalala*; the *arbuda* arises from the *kalala*; the *peśin* arises from the *arbuda*; the *ghana* arises from the *peśin*; and from the *ghana* there arises the *praśakhā*, hair, body-hair, the nails, etc., and the material organs with their supports.[32]

After this very brief nod to the issue of fetal development, the text moves to a long and detailed recounting of debates between early Buddhist schools on interdependent arising. The remainder of the chapter addresses such topics as the physical world and hells, the lifespan of different types of beings and the occasions for the appearance of Buddhas and other beings in the world.

Vasubhandu's *Commentary* was a foundational text in Tibet, as in all Buddhist cultures, and Buddhist writers of all sectarian affiliations refer to abhidharma theories as authoritative in matters of embryology. The abhidharma presentation on the topic is succinct, however, serving ultimately as a starting point, or root text, for much more elaborate embryological narratives in Tibetan literature. Vasubhandu's text is a compilation of existing early Indian views on the topics at hand. Its treatment of human conception and fetal development is therefore neither the only, nor the earliest, such account in early Buddhist literature. On the contrary, embryology was of interest in a range of early Buddhist texts, many of which made their way into the languages of China, Central Asia and Tibet to form the basis of new writings on the topic in those regions.

A closely related set of Buddhist sūtras, canonical texts cited as the speech of the Buddha himself, stands out among these as the most widely-cited source in Tibet for topics concerning early human development. This set of texts, now extant only in Tibetan and Chinese, are found with the titles *Sūtra of Teaching Nanda about Entering the Womb* and *Sūtra of Teaching Nanda about Abiding in the Womb*. Although Sanskrit originals for these works are missing, there are several extant Chinese and Tibetan translations, the earliest being a Chinese version from the period of the Western Chin dynasty (CE 265–317).[33] Tibetan versions of the texts are included within the "Jewel Mound" (Dkon brtsegs, Skt. Ratnakūṭa) classification of the Kangyur section of the Tibetan Buddhist canon, and curiously a version of the text is also found as part of the Mūlasarvāstivāda Vinaya. A comparative study of the Tibetan versions by Lalou and several detailed articles comparing Chinese versions by Kritzer address general differences between these works.[34] Both Tibetan "Jewel Mound" texts appear to have been translated into Tibetan from Chinese by the Dunhuang translator Chödrub in the mid-ninth century. Lalou, when comparing the two, concludes that it is unlikely that they derive from the same original,[35] a suggestion that my examination supports as well; additional studies of the Chinese works may clarify this issue. Despite the existence of several translations in the Tibetan canon, interestingly, in later Tibetan discussions of this sūtric tradition, I have not seen acknowledgement of those different versions; they are referred to as if they were a single work. I will, in general, follow this convention myself, therefore, and refer simply to the *Entering the Womb* sūtra, leaving the text critical scholarship of comparing translations to other studies.

In this Mahāyāna sūtra, the Buddha is asked by his younger brother Nanda to explain the factors necessary for conception and the entire developmental process. The Buddha begins by explaining the suitable conditions for conception:

> If a father and mother have intercourse with desirous intention, and the mother's womb is totally healthy and she menstruates regularly, and the aggregates of the intermediate state being are present, at that time it is possible [for the transmigrator] to enter the mother's womb.[36]

The Buddha next describes what the intermediate being may look like, followed by a discussion of what it means to menstruate regularly. Several reasons for failure to conceive are outlined. The health of the mother's womb is important to successful conception, and this topic is elaborated upon at length: conception will not occur if the mother's uterus is afflicted by any of a long list of conditions, such as possessing defects of wind, bile, phlegm, or blood; being filled with fleshy growths or medicines; being shaped like an ant's waist, the mouth of a camel, the axel or hub of a chariot; and so forth.[37] This discussion is followed by a description of the moment of conception that is similar to that of abhidharmic and other sūtric traditions:

> If the womb of the mother is totally healthy, if the intermediate state being sees the act of intercourse, if the [disease] conditions described above are absent, and if the father, mother and child have the karma to come together, then the intermediate state being will enter the womb. When that intermediate state being enters the womb, moreover, mental distortions (*sems phyin ci log*) will arise [in that being]: if it is a male, desire for the mother and anger toward the father will arise; if it is female, it will desire the father and feel anger toward the mother.[38]

The sūtra explains that intermediate state beings will experience the moment of entering the womb in different ways according to their karmic inheritance, with some feeling as if they are entering a splendorous mansion and others feeling as if they are slipping through a hole in a wall. The Buddha then describes the initial embryonic mixture of the male reproductive substance, the female reproductive substance and the transmigrating consciousness, as well as the importance and particular roles of the natural elements on the embryo. After a detailed week-by-week account of fetal development, the Buddha discusses the physical and mental suffering of the new child that begins right after birth and the importance of religious practice as the means to escape suffering. The sūtra addresses the length of life, the inevitability of disease, the basis of suffering and the importance of renouncing mundane pleasures in favor of religious practice. Again similar to Vasubhandu's account, the experiences felt by four types of beings when entering, abiding and exiting the womb are presented, followed by a discussion of the superiority of a human life, the suffering of other life forms and, again, the importance of religious practice. The Buddha's discourse closes with the instruction to seek liberation from rebirth by understanding the impermanence of human existence.

It is clear that the details of conception and gestation in this text are presented in the context of a Buddhist soteriology. As in Vasubandhu's account, but unlike Āyurvedic presentations, the experience of the pregnant woman is all but ignored here. While the sūtric tradition of gestation is more densely descriptive than the fairly terse abhidharmic version, still the framing context for these accounts – or the purpose of these stories – is the presentation of a Buddhist teaching on impermanence and suffering. As we will see in subsequent chapters, the *Entering the Womb* sūtra is extensively quoted by nearly every Tibetan author who writes about early human development in both medical and religious traditions. During debates on embryological topics, other sūtras are referred to as well as authorities on the process of transmigration, the nature of the transmigrating entity, the workings of karma and the four (or sometimes five) elements of nature, the relationship between the mind and the body, and other topics relevant to human development. It is plain that while Indian medicine was the basis for much early medical scholarship in Tibet, the works of Indian Nikāya Buddhism and Mahāyāna Buddhism that made it across the Himalayas formed the basis of knowledge about early human development in later Tibetan medical and non-medical literature.

Practicing gestation in Indian Vajrayāna Buddhism

Another significant class of Indian texts utilized by Tibetan authors discussing early human development is the tantras of Vajrayāna Buddhism. Detailed contemplative practices overtly modeled after the processes of human conception, development and birth – to be considered further in chapter five – are present in a wide range of Indian Buddhist tantras, such as the *Kālacakra*, *Vajrabhairava*, *Guhyasamāja*, *Cakrasaṃvara*, *Saṃvarodaya* and *Hevajra* tantras, as well as in numerous exegetical works. Indeed, esoteric Buddhism is renowned as a site for the prolific narration of human development, expressing a particular interest in the soteriological capabilities of the human body.

For Tibetans, an especially important tantric source for human development and knowledge of the body in general is the *Kalacakra* tantra. Classified within the esoteric highest yoga tantra category of such texts, this work is dated to the early decades of the eleventh century, making it possibly one of the last of the major Buddhist tantras to be authored in India. The *Kālacakra* is well known for its comprehensive presentation of human psycho-physiology and is thus the basis for much writing on the close interactions of psycho-physiological mechanics and esoteric religious practice. The text is also celebrated for its complex yogic system and teachings on topics as wide ranging as medical therapeutics, botany, alchemy, astronomy and cosmology. The "most significan goal" of the *Kālacakra* religious system, however, Vesna Wallace writes in a comprehensive study of this work, "is the transformation of one's own gross physical body into a luminous form devoid of both gross matter and the subtle body of *prāṇas*,"[39] or energetic "winds." Thus, the elaborate presentation of human physiology found in the text is ultimately offered for the purpose of advanced contemplative practices, a goal, we shall see, that is central to most Tibetan tantric presentations of embryology and physiology as well.

The *Kālacakra* tantra is divided into five chapters addressing the world system, the individual, initiation, religious practice and gnosis (*ye shes*, Skt. *jñāna*). Human psycho-physiology is included within the second of these divisions. The starting point of the *Kālacakra* world-view is the notion that the individual and its environment, i.e. the cosmos, both share the same material basis, energetic nature, and manner of origination and destruction. This means that to know fully the individual and understand its path to salvation, knowledge of the cosmos is essential. Presentations of human origination are thus preceded, in the

Kālacakra and other tantras modeled similarly, by a description of the origination and destruction of the various Buddha-fields and world-systems of the cosmos. These worlds arise, initially, on the basis of the collective karma of sentient beings – that is, the good and bad actions of sentient beings cause the creation and dissolution of the various world-systems in the Buddhist universe. The tantra explains the role of the energetic karmic winds in activating this process, an explanation that is then mirrored in the discussion of the winds in the creation of an individual human in the womb.[40] The other natural elements, water, fir and earth, play specified roles in these creation stories as well

In *Kālacakra* embryology, the newly conceived embryo develops due to the actions of the energetic winds. The fetus is also said to consume substances with six flavors (bitter, sour, salty, pungent, sweet and astringent) that are derived from the six elements (earth, water, fire, wind, space and gnosis). This enables the fetal body to develop in the same way as does the cosmos. The father's reproductive substance generates the fetus' marrow, bones, channels and sinews, and the mother's reproductive substance generates its skin, blood and flesh Earth, water, fire, wind and space also play specific roles in the creation and development of the fetus' body. A month after conception, ten subtle channels (*nāḍī*) emerge in the fetus' heart, and seventy six channels emerge from its navel, traveling throughout the body. Arms, legs and head begin to protrude after the second month, and by the end of the third month they are clearly developed. Subtle channels continue to proliferate and in the fifth month the fetus has three hundred and sixty bones and joints. By the end of the sixth month, it has flesh and blood and can feel pain and pleasure. The seventh month sees the development of hair, the apertures of the body and more channels, and by the end of the eighth month, joints, bones, marrow, the tongue, urine and feces are fully formed. In the ninth month, "the fetus experiences pain as if it were being baked in a potter's oven" and when it is born at the end of that month, it experiences pain as if "being crushed by an anvil and hammer."[41] Wallace points out that many of the details of *Kālacakra* embryology closely mirror earlier Buddhist texts, and, indeed, we will see some of these similarities in chapters to come. The *Entering the Womb* sūtra, for instance, appears to be the source for its explanation of the conditions required for conception and the nature and development of the embryo. As in Vasubhandu's *Commentary*, the *Kālacakra* embeds human gestation in the context of the notion of interdependent arising (*rten cing 'brel bar 'byung ba*; Skt. *pratītyasamutpāda*). Other aspects of its presentation, however, seem more closely linked to Indian medical treatises.[42]

The *Kālacakra*'s account of gestation demonstrates explicitly the intricate correspondences between human and cosmos, as Wallace's study of the tantra describes in detail. Knowledge of embryology is an essential part of the path to liberation because it facilitates a full understanding of ordinary reality, which is then the basis for understanding ultimate reality.[43] Knowing the structure and functions of the human body intricately is thus a key step on the path to escaping the cycle of death and rebirth, which is effected by completely extinguishing one's own mental and physiological processes and replacing them with purifie Buddha bodies.[44] The *Kālacakra* path of practice is organized like other advanced tantric systems into three stages: the initiation, the generation stage and the completion stage, aspects of which are similarly likened to the development of the body in the womb, only now in a ritually purified way. These too are described thoroughly by Wallace, and so I will not go into greater detail here; in later chapters, however, we will return to other examples of these tantric modes of practice.

Chinese traditions of "nurturing the fetus"

Before proceeding in the next chapter to discuss indigenous developments in medical knowledge within Tibet and how these were affected by the influx of Indian cultural artifacts, we should note that India was not, of course, the only source for medical knowledge in Tibet. While we might assume significan influence from Chinese sources, however, direct contact is difficult to confirm In medical treatises, just as in religious texts, Tibetan authors do not credit Chinese traditions with contributing knowledge on human development. Certainly, more research is needed to begin to address the nature and effect of direct connections between the traditions.

Although not overtly acknowledged by Tibetans, the topic of human gestation is, in fact, treated extensively in Chinese literature. Sabine Wilms discusses early and medieval Chinese texts on "nurturing the fetus" (Ch. *yang tai*) in which the development of the fetus is described, together with how that development affects the mother's body, recommendations on maternal diet and behaviors, and medicinal treatments for various symptoms of pregnancy.[45] The earliest example of such a work is a manuscript from the Mawangdui tombs, which were closed in BCE 168. Entitled, by modern Chinese editors, the *Book of Gestation and Birth* (*Taichanshu*), this work includes a month-by-month account of gestation, as well as guidelines on maternal health, on burying the placenta, on conception, on manipulating the embryo's sex, and on easing delivery.[46] As we will see to be the case with Tibetan literature, Chinese texts vary on the details of gestation. The Mawangdui manuscript claims that fetal sex is determined at the time of conception, but that it can still be changed magically during the firs month of pregnancy, a period during which the fetal form remains malleable. The *Book of Gestation and Birth* records magical acts and medicinal recipes for this transformation based on a principle of "inner visualization to complete the child" (*neixing chenzi*), a notion that what the mother sees can influence the form of the fetus.[47] Chen Ming has traced the continuity and transformations, from the Han to Tang periods in Chinese medical writing, of this tradition of first trimester malleability and the techniques for changing fetal sex. His research argues for a strong influence on Chinese embryological writing from India, suggesting that texts such as the *Ekottarāgama* sūtra, which was translated into Chinese in CE 397 and which includes a typical Indian Buddhist account of conception, and also the several translations of the *Entering the Womb* sūtra, had an impact on Chinese traditions of human development.[48] Beyond indicating common topics of interest across texts and traditions, however, Ming's work does not demonstrate direct lines of knowledge transmission between them.

Several authors have studied links between Chinese writing on human development and philosophical or religious traditions. Wilms suggests that several centuries of "nurturing the fetus" literature display a changing body of knowledge that links gestation and pregnancy with philosophical and religious accounts of cosmogenesis. She notes that in the Han period,

> male interest in the female body was rather limited when it came to medical treatment. In the context of pregnancy, it consisted of a theoretical understanding of gestation, significant primarily as a model for cosmic processes of creation and transformation. Thus a close textual parallel of this account of gestation is found for example in the *Huainanzi*, a syncretic compilation of philosophy and cosmology representative of early Han philosophical Daoism.[49]

In *Representations of Childhood and Youth in Early China*, Anne Kinney also reports a rise in interest in theories that correlated fetal development with cosmogony during the late Warring States and Han periods. She notes that the earliest known forms of embryology were, in fact, most centrally concerned with expressing political or spiritual aims. "By describing the unfolding of both the cosmos and human life as guided by one power," she writes,

> these texts reinforced the view that one who understands how the Dao orders nature will understand how to govern the world. Additionally, texts such as the *Wenzi* and the *Huainanzi* enjoin the man who desires all-penetrating wisdom to acquire knowledge of cosmogonic origins and principles by casting off the burdens of civilization, that is, by reversing human development so that it proceeds backwards in time to infancy, the prenatal state, and finally to its origin in undifferentiated chaos. The goal of this meditative strategy is to enable the practitioner to perceive the Dao at its purest and most fundamental and then to act in accordance with it.[50]

Kinney sees embryology as playing a role in the transition from the authority of the ancestors and civic bureaucracy to the authority of natural law, a shift that takes place in philosophical and political theory. She notes a related transformation in health care practices, which viewed conception, birth, and child development as governed by the more predictable laws of nature.[51] Charlotte Furth's work also records an increasing interest in a clinical knowledge of birth with the linking of gestation to philosophical or religious traditions. Song period medical writings, she explains, were attracted to theories of gestation and birth primarily as microcosmic enactments of the processes of creativity and change that characterized all the universe's phenomena. "Concern with birth as a clinical problem gained dignity," she notes further, only "when birth was considered as a replication of cosmogenesis according to the teachings of philosophical and religious classics."[52]

While we will see in chapters to come that these general aims and connections are strikingly similar in Tibetan literature, the structure and detail of early Chinese accounts of gestation appear to be quite different than their Tibetan counterparts and, more significantly, Tibetan texts never cite Chinese sources as authoritative. While connections of some type, theoretical or methodological connections for instance, may indeed exist between Chinese and Tibetan embryological thinking, there are also major differences. Given the lack of acknowledged connections by Tibetans themselves, and given that the subject is vast enough to require a research project of its own, the possible links between Chinese and Tibetan traditions will not be the focus of the present work.

Cultural inheritance and adaptation

As intellectual culture poured into Tibet from neighboring regions, Tibetans had available to them a range of sources from which to study foreign views on religious and medical practice and theory. The history of religion and medicine in India indicates that these were indeed separate disciplines of study and practice and yet, at the same time, the bond between them was profound and pervasive, ranging across the depths of theory and the breadth of practice. According to Kenneth Zysk, the earliest Indian medical knowledge was part of an ascetic religious movement, a portion of which became known as Buddhism.[53] Much of the medical knowledge of early Buddhist monasteries was presented in the vinaya chapters of the *Mahāvagga*, within the corpus of texts on the Buddhist monastic code of conduct. In Mahāyāna Buddhism, the obligation to heal the sick was stipulated in disciplinary codes, and the followers of the *bodhisattva* path were said to be able to heal both spiritual and physical afflictions. It was thus explicitly understood that the healing of the body permitted the calming of the mind and the cultivation of awakening. Developing alongside the Buddhist monasteries and supporting communities in India, medical knowledge was a regular component of Buddhist scriptures, eventually producing monk-healers and Buddhist monastic hospices and infirmaries, until finally becoming part of the standard curriculum in monastic universities. As a tradition where soteriology is defined as relief from suffering, it is indeed not surprising that Buddhism should share concepts and terminology with medicine.

What it was that "medicine" consisted of during these centuries, and how this may have changed over time, however, has been little studied. While the close connections between medical and Buddhist traditions are unambiguous in general terms, certainly the nature of this relationship will vary by topic; a nuanced understanding of the multifarious complexity of the relationship between medicine and Buddhism should, therefore, be gained through multiple studies of granular nodes of connection. In this book, the subject of human development is just such a case study for an investigation of this relationship. Thinkers of all religious traditions philosophized about the origins of life, and questions about how humans are generated in the womb, what happens after death, why individuals appear different from each other and a host of other issues, were keys to philosophic inquiry. Early human development is thus a topic that spans the borders of religious and medical literature, and yet its various iterations are different in structure, aim and content, depending on context. The literature of Indian Nikāya and Mahāyāna Buddhism located embryology in the context of Buddhist teachings on suffering and ethical behavior. The contemplative practices and rituals in the tantras of Indian Vajrayāna Buddhism taught human development as a model for spiritual development. The Indian medical tradition represented by Vāgbhaṭa's treatise placed embryology in the context of the study of human anatomy and physiology and focused largely on obstetrical care. Finally, we notice that Chinese knowledge of the body and its development is curiously absent in Tibetan presentations of these topics. How these various embryological narratives are interpreted at the beginning of the thirteenth to sixteenth-century Tibetan renaissance, how these interpretive choices are made, and how those choices dictate the future of medical and religious writing, are questions that shape this book. Tibetans inherited various presentations on the origins of the human being. Each articulated an understanding of the body that displayed both its embeddedness within an internal system of meaning and its interconnectedness to external realms of thought and action. In the next chapter, I will consider how best to situate indigenous Tibetan writing on embryology. As Tibetans themselves began to think about human development, into what larger historical and literary narratives did it fit

3

INTERACTIONS BETWEEN MEDICINE AND RELIGION IN TIBET

In this chapter, we begin to consider the role of writing on human development and, more generally, of descriptive presentations of the human body in Tibetan literature itself. In so doing, we will also reflect on some key historical questions: what topics are included in the categories of "medicine" and "religion" according to Tibetan literature, and how might this change over time? What is the role of the human body in medical and religious literature, and does this change as Buddhist intellectual frameworks pervade Tibetan scholasticism more and more thoroughly? Looking at literary sources and historical events that may illuminate these issues, the interactions between medical and religious traditions will be organized here into three main historical periods. First, an early period, consisting of the centuries prior to the eleventh-century "later propagation of the doctrine" in Tibet, is characterized by most medical historians as an internationally cosmopolitan age when scholars flocked to Central Tibet from regions around Eurasia to collaborate on the building of knowledge about medicine and other topics. Second, the eleventh to early thirteenth centuries comprises a period when the flood of scholarship from India forced Tibetans to engage in a monumental project of assimilating these works and creating traditions of their own. Finally, the third is a period sometimes referred to as the Tibetan renaissance, roughly the thirteenth to sixteenth centuries, when an earlier focus on organizing and synthesizing incoming works from India turned to a flowering of indigenous composition by Tibetan intellectuals in all fields of scholarship. We will consider for each period how medicine is historicized by later Tibetan writers, and how its interactions with Buddhism are characterized. Along the way, we will also take note of writings on physiology and early human development – that is, organized expositions dedicated to describing the human body – and look at the changing roles these topics may play in medical and religious literatures.

Eurasian cosmopolitanism versus Indian Buddhism: a historiographical conflict

As are many scholars today, Tibetan historians looking back on the early period were troubled by the relationship between medicine and Buddhism. The existence of two historical narratives about the origins of Tibetan medicine suggest that historians felt conflicted about the relationship between medicine and Buddhism. Most Tibetan historians emphasize the cosmopolitan nature of the early period of medical learning and development, as we will see in the next few pages. But another strain of historiography, by contrast, emphasizes the contextualization of Tibetan medical knowledge within the history of Buddhism in India. As Buddhism increasingly dominated Tibetan intellectual and institutional domains, a pressure to make medicine Buddhist is seen not only in the historiography of medicine but also in the way medical scholars wrote about topics such as the structure and origins of the human body.

Little is known about medical practices or medical knowledge in the earliest periods of recorded Tibetan history. Details on medical history prior to the reign of the seventh-century Tibetan king Songtsen Gampo are especially unclear, although some records suggest that Tibetan medical practice at that time involved dietary prescriptions, healing rituals, a pharmacopoeia and, possibly, minor surgery. Contemporary historian Kalsang Trinley describes very early healing rituals using the Tibetan Zi (*gzi*) stone and fire, and the practice of trepanation.[1] Systematic accounts of human development or human physiology, however, are absent in these sources. While little is known about the actual practice or scholarship of medicine during this period, later historians emphasize the close connections between medical practitioners and the royal court. One of the first links between India and Tibet in the context of medical history is said to have occurred during the reign of the fifth-century Tibetan king Lha Totori Nyentsen, said by Buddhist historians to be the first Buddhist king of Tibet.[2] Historians report that during his reign two doctors, Biji Gajé and Bilha Gadzé, came from India to teach medicine in Tibet. The king offered his daughter to Bilha Gadzé, and their son, Dungi Torchak, is known as the first Tibetan doctor.[3] His sons were appointed chief physicians in the royal court, a relationship that continued for generations.[4] Contacts between the medical traditions of the two great cultures are reported sporadically throughout the next generations of kings. The act of placing the historical origins of the Tibetan medical tradition with an Indian doctor may serve a historian's need to ensure the centrality of India as the epistemological authority. Nevertheless, historians assert that various systems of medicine and astrology were brought from China as well, beginning with the reign of Namri Songtsen, made king of Tibet in the Yarlung Valley at around AD 600.[5]

Knowledge of medical practices is said to have grown in Tibet in an internationally collaborative manner. King Songtsen Gampo (d. 649) was closely involved with scholars and intellectual traditions from China and Nepal through his two foreign wives, and from India through various scholars commissioned by the king to travel to that land. Accounts of his reign describe contact between Tibetan and Chinese medical traditions, with Chinese medical texts carried to Tibet by the king's Chinese wife. Songtsen Gampo is said to have convened a meeting at his court of three physicians, from India, China and a region to the

West.[6] Pasang Yönten and others speculate that it is the Greek medical system represented by Galenö, the physician from the West, trade-inspired travel having brought him, or at least the tradition he represented, to Turkistan, and from there to Tibet.[7] Galen was an extremely influential physician from the Greek medical tradition who lived from AD 129–199; obviously it is not he, but rather simply a representative of the Greek tradition generally, that is meant by this figure active in Tibet. Unani medicine was also at this time a prominent system of medicine in Baghdad, however, so it is not entirely clear that it is Greek medicine represented by the figure known as Galenö. These three visiting doctors are said to have translated texts from their own traditions into Tibetan and collaborated on the authorship of new texts, none of which are known to be extant today.

The cosmopolitan nature of Tibetan medical development continued with subsequent monarchs. Over several centuries, the historical record of Tibet depicts it as a place where scholars from (to use modern-day terms) Iran, Iraq, Afghanistan, Pakistan, India, Nepal, Uzbekistan, Tajikistan, Mongolia, China and Russia gathered and shared knowledge about medicine and healing. Under the control of king Tri Songdetsen (reigned 756–797), during which time the Tibetan empire reached its zenith, medical connections to India, China and elsewhere continued to flourish through royal support, and teams of physicians continued to produce medical texts and translations.[8]

The royal interest in Buddhism, said to have been initiated by Songtsen Gampo, intensified during the reign of Tri Songdetsen, and thus this was a fertile period not only for the development of medical knowledge, but also for the growth of Buddhism in Tibet. It is during this period that the tantric master, Padmasambhava, and the Bengali scholar, Santarakṣita, invited to Tibet by Tri Songdetsen, laid the foundations for Tibetan Buddhist tantric and monastic traditions. Notably, many of these early Buddhist figures are also known for their contributions to medical knowledge. Recognized as the founder of tantric traditions in Tibet, Padmasambhava is credited with initiating Tibetan lineages of the *Vajrakila*, *Hayagriva*, *Guhyagarbha* and other tantras, with composing texts on a wide range of subjects, including medicine, and with concealing many "treasure" texts (*gter ma*), discovered centuries later in various locations around Tibet. Padmasambhava, known as a manifestation of the Buddhas Amitabha and Avalokiteśvara, is thus considered the ultimate "author" of thousands of treasure texts later taken from rocks, bodies of water, temples, architectural elements such as columns, or the minds of visionaries. While nearly all forms of Tibetan Buddhism acknowledge the importance of certain treasure texts, which span a full range of subject matter, including historical, doctrinal, liturgical and medical treatises, the Nyingma or "Ancient" traditions in particular – that is, the earliest of Tibetan Buddhist traditions – rely on treasure texts as authoritative.

Another influential figure in Buddhist Nyingma history, Vairocana, joined scholarship of Buddhism with that of medicine: he is said to have studied medical texts in India with Dawa Ngönga, the chief student of the Indian

Āyurvedic master Vāgbhaṭa, whose work formed the basis of much of Tibetan medicine. Vairocana is credited with the translation and composition of numerous medical texts, sometimes under the pseudonym Chöbar.[9] Historian Sanggyé Gyatso explains that Vairocana himself presented the *Four Tantras* to the king and to Padmasambhava, but on Padmasambhava's advice the text was then hidden in a pillar at Samyé for later rediscovery.[10]

The final decades of the eighth century and the beginning of the ninth century saw a rise in Tibetan Buddhist writing that continued through the two subsequent reigning kings. Indian and Tibetan scholars, including influential intellectuals such as Vimalamitra, Buddhaguhya and Śāntigarbha, worked together to translate Buddhist sūtras, śastras and medical texts from Sanskrit into Tibetan. The intellectual exchange across the Himalayas crossed both ways, as Indian masters were invited to Tibet and Tibetans, such as Vimalamitra of Great Perfection (*rdzogs chen*) fame, and the legendary eighth-century medical scholar Yuthok Yönten Gönpo himself, are said to have traveled to India to study.[11] This was an extremely productive period in Tibetan scholarship: the ninth-century Tibetan Denkar catalog documents over seven hundred translated works, a count that does not include a great many tantric texts and Tibetan authored texts on non-canonical topics such as medicine.[12]

In Buddhist and medical histories alike, this era is represented as richly creative; in the field of medicine in particular, however, the period is characterized by an intense level of international collaboration. Medical histories report that during the reign of Tri Songdetsen, a medical congress was convened at Samyé, led by the legendary eighth-century Yuthok Yönten Gönpo. Tri Songdetsen's meeting brought together scholars from various neighboring regions, and they were asked to translate medical texts from their own languages into Tibetan. This effort is said to have resulted in the translation of scores of medical texts from Sogdia (*kha che*), Turkistan (*stag gzig*), Drugu (*gru gu*), Nepal (*bal bo*), Dolpo (*dol bo*), and India.[13] In addition to this rich geographic collaboration, however, historians also emphasize substantial contributions to medical knowledge by many of the main figures known primarily for their role in the development of Buddhism. Thus, from the earliest period of recorded history, authors of religious and medical texts were joined in the same individual; texts classified as medical in content were considered to be naturally within the domain of expertise of prominent religious figures

With the reign of King Lang Darma (d. 847), a persecution of Buddhism in Tibet resulted in the defrocking of monks and the destruction of Buddhist temples and monasteries. The great Yarlung Empire fell and for the next century Buddhism in Tibet lacked centralized royal or state support, surviving only in local family lineages until the Buddhist revival period beginning at the end of the tenth century. While this period marks a break between two eras that are referred to in the Buddhist tradition as the "early propagation of the doctrine" (*snga dar*) and the "later propagation of the doctrine" (*phyi dar*), Sanggyé Gyatso argues that the medical tradition, by contrast, continued without interruption. Characterizing Tibetan medicine as a system developed collaboratively by ten international and indigenous traditions, he claims that it grew gradually and continually in Tibet from the time of Songtsen Gampo and that the Buddhist periodization scheme is, therefore, inappropriate for the medical tradition.[14]

Despite a historical record of intense literary production in the field of medicine during these centuries, today we have access to relatively little textual evidence of such prolific scholarship. Of the few early texts that survived for our examination and are classified now as medical literature, however, none of them appear to include discussions of human conception, the mechanics of transmigration or the manner of early human development. Discussion of these topics does, however, exist in Buddhist literary sources circulating among Tibetans of this period. Tantric traditions that formed the foundations of the Nyingma school, later to be systematized by the great fourteenth-century scholar-poet Longchen Rabjampa, were flourishing through the literary and pedagogical activities of masters who combined religious with medically-oriented thought, such as Padmasambhava and Vairocana, and by Mahāyoga masters such as Vimalamitra, Buddhaguhya, and Śāntigarbha. This matrix of early Nyingma thinkers disseminated a range of tantric practices that focused on the subtle intricacies of human psycho-physiology, a topic which therefore received great attention in their works. From the earliest period of Tibetan history, therefore, we see that systematic consideration of the origins, structures and processes of the human body falls within the context of religious, and not medical, practice.

Linking medical history with Buddhism

In 1702, Sanggyé Gyatso completed a substantial history of medicine that has served as a foundational text on the topic ever since. As does the account we have just reviewed, his narrative portrays the early period of Tibetan medicine – from the "pre-historical" period to the eleventh century – as a cosmopolitan age in which medical knowledge was collaboratively generated by scholars from regions across Asia. At the same time, however, and paradoxically, he also links Tibetan medical history to Buddhist history. This historiographical impulse – seemingly at conflict with a portrait of medicine as internationally collaborative – situates the origins of Tibetan medicine not with Indian Āyurveda but with the Buddha himself, noting that Sakyamuni taught a medical text called the *Vimalagotra* at his first sermon at Sarnath, and that the Vinaya contained instructions to monks on practicing medicinal healing techniques. Various sūtras are said to include instructions on healing, and the bodhisattvas Mañjuśri, Avalokiteśvara, Vajrapaṇi and Tāra are recognized to have composed treatises on various medical topics as well.

Sanggyé Gyatso's history of medicine is largely a compilation of earlier histories, many of which can be identified, and thus while his is a late work, it does give voice to historical perspectives of an earlier era. The impulse to link the origins of Tibetan medicine with the Buddha in India can be traced to the very earliest extant Tibetan histories of medicine. I have written elsewhere about the thirteenth-century collection, the *Eighteen Additional Practices* (*Cha lag bco brgyad*), which contains one of the earliest known histories of medicine to emphasize a presentation of medicine as an essential and original component of Buddhism. That work, the *Great Garuda Soars* (*Khyung chen lding ba*), subsumes the practice of medicine under the practice of Buddhism, and places medicine using cosmogonical, historical and bibliographical arguments in the highest class of Buddhist knowledge, that which was spoken by the Buddha himself. The *Four Tantras* itself is given this authoritative status as Buddha-voiced, making the foundation of Tibetan literary traditions of medicine from the thirteenth-century onwards essentially Indian, and essentially Buddhist.[15]

Not all Tibetan historians agree with this view of the *Four Tantras*, as I will discuss shortly. However, once it is introduced in the thirteenth century, the view of Tibetan medicine's connection to Buddhism is pervasive and recurring for historians, despite its apparent conflict with the presentation of medical knowledge as resulting from a polyphony of Indian, Nepali, Chinese, Turkic, Arab-Persian, Greek and other voices.

Striking the path: organizing the influx of Indian culture

The period known in Buddhist historiography as the later propagation of the doctrine from India saw a dramatic growth of literature of all forms in Tibet, including both religious and medical writings on human development. This movement began in western Tibet with the king Yeshé Ö, who sent a group of Tibetans to India to become translators of Buddhist texts; this mission produced Rinchen Zangpo and Ngog Legpé Sherab. These two figures and their immediate students traveled extensively, produced many Buddhist as well as medical texts, and spawned several generations of scholars of religious and medical practice and theory. Rinchen Zangpo studied and translated the works of the Indian Āyurvedic scholar Vāgbhaṭa and his commentator, including the *Heart of Medicine*, discussed in the last chapter, passing this knowledge as a (retroactively appointed) lineage founder to many students. Sanggyé Gyatso records the names of numerous individuals who studied medical texts with Rinchen Zangpo; his four most famous students were known as the "four great Ngari doctors." From the lineage of one of these, for instance, emerged Darma Gönpo, who wrote two nosological texts said to have been central in a distinctive Bodong (*bo dong*) medical tradition.[16] After studying briefly with the translator Ngog Legpé Sherab, a scholar named Zhang Zijibar traveled to India to study at Nalanda, returning to Tibet to author numerous medical texts, in particular, and instruct scores of students.[17] Many other intellectuals active at this time authored and revealed medical literature as well as Buddhist works.[18]

The intellectual energy of this period produced scholars known as organizers of the great Sarma or "New" schools of Tibetan Buddhism, such as Marpa

(1012–1096), whose students founded the Kagyü tradition, Khyungpo Nenjor, founder of the Shangpa Kagyü tradition, and Drogmi (992–1072), founder of the Sakya tradition. The trajectory of the newly developing Sarma schools was influenced by Yeshé Ö's outspoken rejection of certain tantric Buddhist practices, particularly those derived from the *Guhyagarbha* tantra, which was of special importance to the Nyingma traditions. Yeshé Ö commanded his translators to follow Mahāyāna doctrine and in 1042, he invited Atiśa (987–1054) from Bengal to strengthen in Tibet a form of monasticism that would complement tantric practice.

During this period in history, many prominent scholars addressed the topic of human development, following Nikāya, Mahāyāna or Vajrayāna approaches to the topic evident in the Indian sources available to them. Gampopa (1079–1153), for instance, a founder of the Kagyü tradition known for combining the early Tibetan Buddhist Kadam teachings with tantric teachings of the Indian *mahāsiddhas*, wrote on conception and early human development in his *Jewel Ornament of Liberation*. Although Gampopa is known to have been a doctor in his younger years, thus combining religious and medical expertise, interestingly, as we will see, he does not acknowledge medical models of human development at all in the *Jewel Ornament*. As a doctor, could he not have known the *Heart of Medicine*, which addresses human development explicitly? Or, did he simply consider Buddhist sūtras to be more authoritative on this subject? This period also saw a proliferation of commentarial literature, some of which was concentrated into the literary genre known as the "stages of the (Buddhist spiritual) path" (*lam rim*). Human development became an important topic in this genre of literature. Stages of the path texts, which became extremely important in the history of Tibetan literature over the centuries, is particularly associated with Atiśa and the Tibetan Buddhist Kadam sect founded by his main disciple. These types of texts outline a sequential path of Buddhist practice, arranging the main traditions of thought and practice along a graded path. For most such texts, tantric practices are placed at the highest stage of the path. In chapter five, I will suggest that one reason Tibetan authors found the embryological narrative compelling may have to do with its easy affiliation with the structure and purpose of this increasingly popular literary genre on the Buddhist path.

An early example of such a text, the *Great Jeweled Wishing Tree*, is by the Sakya scholar Drakpa Gyeltsen (1147–1216), a contemporary of the medical figure Yuthok Yönten Gönpo. Drakpa Gyeltsen, a prominent scholar from the influential 'Khön family and a Sakya throne holder, was the author of many texts on numerous subjects, including at least one medical text, and thus like many of his time, he combined religious and medical authority.[19] As was the case with Gampopa, when Drakpa Gyeltsen wrote about human development, however, it was in the context of religious practice, not medicine, and he looked to Buddhist tantras, not medical texts, as sources of information on the topic. The *Great Jeweled Wishing Tree* is one of his most important religious texts, and it is one of the longest early Sakya esoteric texts. Drakpa Gyeltsen's embryological narrative in that work begins with a traditional summary of the Buddhist four types of rebirth – miraculous, egg-born, moisture-born and womb-born – and an explanation of the causes of conception. His account of fetal development addresses both coarse and subtle body aspects, and it precedes a detailed explanation of the psychosomatic tantric anatomy of maṇdalas, circulatory channels and winds. In chapters to come, we will see that Drakpa Gyeltsen's account of early human development differs greatly from medical or sūtric models: his presentation of conception ignores the role of the natural elements; his descriptions of gestation and adult physiology do not mention the three systemic processes (*nyes pa*, Skt. *doṣa*); and he disregards the role of many of the energetic winds considered so essential by other writers to the growth of the body.

During this period, many prolific scholars who authored works on Buddhist practices, paths of spiritual progress, or tenet systems also wrote the occasional text on medical topics such as pharmacology or nosology. It appears, therefore, to have been fairly common for an educated scholar of Buddhism also to be trained in such medical topics, to the extent even that they would feel authorized to write on them. What is distinctive about this period is the rise of scholars who focused primarily on medical topics. Beginning with Rinchen Zangpo's dissemination of the Indian medical traditions through the translation of the *Heart of Medicine* and other Indian medical texts, lineages of medical scholars began to transmit these traditions throughout Tibet. These Indian works thus formed the basis for a literary tradition of medicine in Tibet that lasted for several centuries, eventually being replaced almost entirely by the *Four Tantras* and its own commentarial traditions.

If the early period of Tibetan medicine is characterized by its internationally collaborative nature, the picture is drawn differently for the centuries in question here. It was into a thirteenth-century context of growing sectarianism and intellectual allegiance to India that the *Four Tantras* emerged, a work that is still today considered the principal medical text in Tibetan medicine. While its origins are uncertain, the work seems to have been arranged in the form we know today toward the end of the twelfth century by the famous Tibetan physician Yuthok Yönten Gönpo.[20] Like his legendary eighth-century namesake, Yuthok is remembered as having begun his study of medicine as a child and traveled to India numerous times as a young adult. In addition to revising or enhancing the *Four Tantras*, he is considered the author of portions of the *Eighteen Additional Practices*, as well as numerous other texts no longer extant. Yuthok's many students continued his teachings, and it is said that the texts produced by these physicians, including those of the *Eighteen Additional Practices* collection and the several texts produced by Yuthok's famous twelfth-century student Sumtön Yeshé Zung, dominated medical scholarship for several generations.[21]

The *Four Tantras*, written in verse and presented in a format similar to that of many Buddhist tantras, is structured as a dialog between an emanation of the

Buddha named Rikpé Yeshé and a student, Yilekyé. The Buddha is said to have taught the text appearing as a Medicine Buddha in a place called Tanaduk, possibly identified as Mount Meru or a "medicine jungle" in Uddiyana.[22] This mythical history is presented in the *Root Tantra* of the work. At Tanaduk, surrounded by his disciples, the Medicine Buddha falls into a meditative state called "expelling four hundred and four diseases." Colored light rays radiating out from his chest eliminate diseases from all beings in all directions around him. The sage called Rikpé Yeshé then emerges from his chest and says,

> Friends, know this! Those beings who wish to stay healthy and cure disease should learn the oral teaching of medicine (*gso ba rig pa*). Those who wish for long life should learn the oral teaching of medicine. Those who wish to receive religious teachings, wealth and happiness should learn the oral teaching of medicine. Those who wish to liberate beings from the suffering of illness and who wish for the esteem of others should learn the oral teaching of medicine.[23]

The sage Yilekyé then asks Rikpé Yeshé to teach medicine to the audience, and Rikpé Yeshé transmits the text.

The *Four Tantras* consists of one hundred and fifty six chapters arranged in four units, or "books": the *Root Tantra* (*rtsa rgyud*), cryptically summarizing the entire text; the *Explanatory Tantra* (*bshad rgyud)*, with a description of the human body and general information about the causes of disease and the principles of therapeutics; the *Secret Oral Tantra* (*man ngag rgyud*), containing specific instructions and methods of diagnosis; and the *Concluding Tantra* (*phyi ma rgyud*), containing specific information about various types of treatments. The primary sources for the *Four Tantras'* view of the human physical structure and processes from conception through death (topics we may call embryology, anatomy and physiology) are found in the first seven chapters of the *Explanatory Tantra*. Chapters two through six of that book consider how the body is formed (*grub pa lus gnas*); similes of the body (*'dra dpe phung po'i gnas lugs*); the structure of the body, somewhat analogous to what we call anatomy (*lus kyi gnas lugs*); characteristics of the body, somewhat like what we call physiology (*lus kyi mtshan nyid*); and actions and classifications of the body (*lus kyi las* and *lus kyi dbye ba*), also roughly equivalent to physiology. Generally following the structure of the classical Indian medical texts, the seventh chapter then discusses signs of death (*lus kyi 'jig ltas*). After this point, the remainder of the book consists of a general explication of causes and symptoms of disease, and classifica tions and methods of therapeutics. The chapter on early human development – the *Explanatory Tantra's* second chapter – considers four main topics: the causes of formation of the body, the conditions that aid in the body's development, the sequence of the body's development and the signs of impending birth. It is this chapter, and subsequent commentaries on it, that forms the basis for much of our understanding of Tibetan medical embryology.

The historical origins of this text were controversial in Tibet for centuries, beginning almost immediately after its dissemination at the time of Yuthok Yönten Gönpo; these debates have been addressed elsewhere.[24] While according to some historical traditions the *Four Tantras* is the translation of an Indian text, and according to others it is an indigenously Tibetan text, most scholars today agree that it must be largely Tibetan, but heavily influenced by Indian, Chinese and other medical traditions. Historically, however, arguments have taken opposing views: on the one hand were those who asserted that the work had divine origins, following the claim of the text itself, and on the other hand were those who maintained that the work was of human authorship. The first source to attribute divine origins to the *Four Tantras* is a text by Sumtön Yeshé Zung, a student of the twelfth-century Yuthok Yönten Gönpo.[25] Written in verse, it is a history of the *Four Tantras* lineage up to Yuthok which states that Vairocana received the text from Dawa Ngönga in Kashmir, and that the text was indeed originally spoken by the Buddha Rikpé Yeshé in Uddiyana. It states further that Vairocana presented the work to king Tri Songdetsen, who hid it in a pillar at Samyé until, one hundred and fifty years later, it was recovered by Drapa Ngönshé, an eleventh-century treasure revealer. The account from this text subsequently became the orthodox view of the *Four Tantras'* origins, despite the fact that Drapa Ngönshé's involvement with the *Four Tantras* is questionable historically: the comprehensive fifteenth-century Tibetan history, the *Blue Annals*, for example, does not mention his discovery of the *Four Tantras* or any other texts, nor is this event mentioned in a (no longer extant) early biography of Drapa Ngönshé himself, as reported by the Nyingma author Sodokpa Lodrö Gyeltsen (1552–1624).[26] According to this tradition, however, the *Four Tantras* was an early translation of a Buddha-voiced Sanskrit original, hidden in Tibet, to be discovered later by Drapa Ngönshé. Drapa Ngönshé is said to have passed the text to Üpa Dardrak, purportedly born in 1126, the same year as the famous twelfth-century physician, Yuthok Yönten Gönpo. Üpa Dardrak passed the text on to a figure named Könchok Kyab, who was responsible for giving it to Yuthok Yönten Gönpo.[27]

This view of the dissemination, via India, of the *Four Tantras* has been supported by some Tibetan scholars and rejected by others.[28] The thesis of the text's Indian origins, known as the "establishment of the *Four Tantras* as a canonical work" (*rgyud bzhi bka' ru bsgrub pa*, or simply, *bka' sgrubs)*, is part of most medical histories known by the title "Interior Analysis" (*khog 'bubs*). Another group of early historians, by contrast, emphasized the role of a Tibetan author – the twelfth-century Yuthok Yönten Gönpo – in the creation of the *Four Tantras*, attributing to him editorial or authorial agency to varying degrees. Karmay explains that the tradition of attributing authorship to Yuthok originates with the text entitled *History of Yuthok Lineage Masters* (*g.yu thog bla brgyud lo rgyus*), likely authored by a student of Yuthok.[29] Early texts promoting the thesis of the *Four Tantras'* human authorship, a genre of medical history designated "Responding to Controversies" (*rtsod yig*), are now very rare, existing primarily only as citations in other works. Karmay summarizes a fifteenth-centur "Responding to Controversies" argument that provides sixteen points proving that the *Four Tantras* is a Tibetan work, taking into account issues of "religion, history, linguistics, popular beliefs, customs, habits, diets, botany as well as utensils, medical or otherwise."[30] Sumpa Khenpo Yeshé Penjor (1704–1788), likewise, completely rejects the notion of the *Four Tantras* as a revealed work, asserting that it is an originally Tibetan text composed on the basis of Indian and Chinese medical knowledge by Yuthok Yönten Gönpo.[31]

Some historians straddled these opposing views, however, proposing a compromise. In this view, Yuthok merely edited, and perhaps expanded, the original *Four Tantras* core he had received. Sanggyé Gyatso claims in his *Blue Beryl*, for instance, that Yuthok Yönten Gönpo took an Indian Buddha-voiced core text and simply adapted it to Tibetan needs.[32] The mid-sixteenth-century medical history in the *Feast for the Learned* (*mkhas pa'i dga' ston*) is silent on the issue of the translation of the *Four Tantras*, but it states that the twelfth-century Yuthok Yönten Gönpo compiled the work himself "as Yilekyé,"[33] thus preserving *both* the view of the divine origins of the text and that of its Tibetan "authorship."

With the twelfth- and thirteenth-century writings of Yuthok's students – at least one of whom is known to promote the notion of divine authorship, and another believed to promote human authorship – distinct schools formed immediately around disparate commentarial traditions on the *Four Tantras*. While the debate was contentious, those who claimed the *Four Tantras* to be a largely Tibetan work proved most influential ultimately, although this view is commonly tempered with the assertion that Yuthok authored the text having taken on the divine form of Yilekyé. Text critical evidence suggests that the version now extant began with early core elements that were inherited from India around which additional segments grew over time in Tibet. Despite the text's self-identification as divine revelation, and the acceptance of many prominent scholars of this view, the question of the origins of the *Four Tantras* comes to light as one of the most controversial topics through centuries of writing on Tibetan medical history. It is another example of the conflict over what extent medicine should be Buddhist, arising at a time in history when to be Buddhist was to be influential at the most politically powerful levels of society

The heyday of medical scholasticism

José Cabezón labels the extremely prolific period of the thirteenth to sixteenth centuries "the heyday of Tibetan scholasticism,"[34] and this was as much the case for medical traditions as for other schools of thought and practice. During this period Buddhist ideals and theoretical structures began penetrating medical scholasticism. Although Tibetans had previously dominated surrounding lands and cultures, these centuries saw them fall under the rule of a series of powerfully hegemonic leaders. Despite the efforts of Sakya dignitaries to appease warring Central Asian Mongols led by Genghis Khan, in the thirteenth century Mongol raids penetrated Tibetan regions. With the Buddhist influence of Sakya Pandita (1182–1251) on the Mongol ruler, Godan Khan, however, a wary peace settled between the two leaders, and although the Mongols maintained nominal control over the region, Tibetans themselves were allowed administrative rule. For several generations after the deaths of Sakya Pandita and Godan Khan, the Buddhist "patron-priest" relationship continued between the rulers of the two regions. Infighting raged between large monastic institutions in Tibet during the thirteenth century, and after Mongol rule subsided at the beginning of the fourteenth century, Tibetan rival factions finally managed to dislodge Sakya hegemony.

While during these centuries Tibetans were looking northward toward Mongol regions politically, it was southward to India that they looked for intellectual authority, and Indian Buddhism took on an unprecedented power. The connections between medical and religious traditions grew more intricate during this period, as sectarian and disciplinary differences were more carefully articulated. Prominent physicians were high-level attending physicians for the Sakya leadership.[35] Over the period of the next couple of centuries, the politico-religious leadership grew closer to the hierarchy of medical scholars and leaders, a relationship that also had an impact on the nature of medical scholarship. The growing interest among medical scholars in the topic of human development is a reflection of this increasingly close connection to Buddhism. As the *Four Tantras* slowly became known after the twelfth century, it began to amass a vast commentarial literature, with such compositions continuing to the present date. The nineteenth-century literature index by Akhu Rinpoche mentions sixteen commentaries on the entire *Four Tantras*, plus eight devoted solely to the *Root Tantra*, nine to the second tantra, two to the third tantra and twelve to the fourth.[36] The earliest commentaries on the *Four Tantras*, dating to the time of Yuthok himself and likely authored by his students, are quite sparse and add little to the *Four Tantras'* account of human development or physiology.[37] A commentary on the *Explanatory Tantra* authored by Yuthok's student, Sumtön Yeshé Zung, for instance, addresses the causes of conception, the conditions for fetal growth, and the signs of birth. His commentary on these topics, however, is terse, adding little significant detail.[38] As we will see in later chapters, what these early texts on human development do not say may be more interesting than what they do say, and over the centuries, commentaries on human development become increasingly complex and gradually more Buddhist in nature.

If early medical commentators were uninspired by the topic of the origins of the human body, however, it appears to have been a domain of great interest for authors of religious texts. The *Six Doctrines of Naropa* (*Naro chos drug*), a text widely studied during the eleventh and twelfth centuries, became an influentia source for those from all Buddhist traditions who studied and wrote on human physiology for centuries to come. In the Nyingma tradition, the eleventh-twelfth-century *Seventeen Tantras* (*Rgyud bcu bdun*), and the eighth-twelfth-century *Collected Tantras of Vairocana* (*Vairo rgyud 'bum*), two chief collections of the Nyingma Heart Essence (*Snying thig*) tradition, were also prominent sources for later Tibetan formulations of the body and contemplative and healing practices that focused on the body. Another important resource from this period for later thinkers, religious and medical alike, was a work on yogic physiology and practice by the Kagyü author Rangjung Dorjé (1284–1339). His *Profound Inner Meaning* (*Zab mo nang don*), for instance, presents Buddhist views on the tantric body, including topics such as the conception and formation of the body; explanations of the locations, functions and movements of the channels, winds and quintessential essences; the relationship of these to the consciousness; the link between the inner body and the external world; and the use of the subtle body features in contemplative practice. Rangjung Dorjé's writings were influential for later medical thinkers, in particular the important sixteenth-century *Four Tantras* commentator Zurkhar Lodrö Gyelpo.

Among Buddhist writers, therefore, this period was a fertile one for the systematization of knowledge on human physiology and its significance for contemplative practice. The influential Nyingma thinker, Longchen Rabjampa (1308–1364), and the charismatic figure, Tsong Khapa (1357–1419), founder of the Geluk school, both wrote extensively on early human development. Longchenpa, for instance, ties extensive accounts of human development to the foundations of a distinctive religious practice. His *Treasury of Precious Words and Meanings* (*Tshig don mdzod*) involves a presentation of Tantric paradigms of Buddhist enlightenment that relies on rhetorical and poetic uses of language and traditional Buddhist symbols.[39] This text ignores completely the structure of the *Four Tantras*, the *Heart of Medicine*, or other early medical sources on human development, however, nor does it consider any of the most important physiological or embryological topics in those works. Moreover, the structure of his presentation bears only a faint resemblance to other tantric Buddhist texts. Longchenpa organizes this work into eleven main headings, an organizational structure later adopted by others in his tradition. The eleven headings include an explanation of the origins of the universe (topic one), an account of the origin of the human individual (topic two), a detailed description of human psychophysiology (topics three through six), discussion of a series of yogic practices and signs that these are being performed successfully (topics seven through nine), analysis of the phases of death and postmortem existence (topic ten), and, finally, a study of enlightened experience (topic eleven). Chapters that focus on human physiology and development describe the individual's enlightened essence, or "Buddha-nature," the tantric physiological structure by which this enlightened essence circulates throughout the body, and the four "lamps" that allow this essence to exit the body through the eyes into external space. The enlightened essence that has left the body in this way is the object of a series of contemplative practices prescribed in subsequent chapters of his work, and I will discuss later in this book how elements of this distinctive contemplative system are reflected in Longchenpa's presentation of fetal development. Over several centuries of the Tibetan renaissance, therefore, knowledge of human physiology and development continued to play an important role in philosophical and religious literature, often forming the very basis of advanced religious practices. Although at the beginning of this period few medical writers focused attention on the organized exposition of human physiology and development, by the end of this period it had become a topic of great interest to the most influentia medical commentators.

Institutionally, the thirteenth to sixteenth centuries saw the organization of distinct sectarian or disciplinary traditions in both medical and Buddhist traditions. In the fifteenth century, two prominent schools of Tibetan medicine arose, the Northern tradition (*byang lugs*) and the Southern tradition (*zur lugs*), which dominated the organization of medical teachings for the next two centuries until the time of the Fifth Dalai Lama. The leaders of these traditions exemplified the interpenetration of medicine and Buddhism, being well trained in both bodies of scholarship and highly placed in both administrative hierarchies. The founder of the Northern tradition was Jangdak Namgyel Drakzang (1395–1475), known simply as Jangpa. Said to have had medical talents since childhood, Jangpa was the author of numerous medical texts; prominent also in the religious hierarchy, he was a friend of the second Dalai Lama, Gendün Gyatso (1475–1543). Ordained as a Buddhist monk, he is said to have been a skilled religious scholar, authoring religious texts and teaching religion.[40] The Northern tradition flour ished until the time of Sanggyé Gyatso, who was critical of the school and effectively terminated its further development, writing it out of history.[41] Indeed, the seventeenth-century medical history by Jaya Pandita does not mention the Northern tradition or its scholars, and the nineteenth-century medical history by Akhu Rinpoche lists the works of Northern school founder, Namgyel Drakzang, under the category of "rare literature."[42]

The founder of the Southern tradition was Zurkhar Nyamnyi Dorjé (b. 1439). Like the founder of the Northern school, Nyamnyi Dorjé is known for his religious as well as medical scholarship. He is said to have been heavily influence by the *Heart Essence of Yuthok* (*G.yu thog snying thig*) teachings and is credited with authorship of several chapters of that collection as it exists today. He also relied a great deal on the Buddhist tantras in his medical writings. Nyamnyi Dorjé is known especially for furthering the advancement of Tibetan pharmacology through convening a pan-regional medical conference devoted to the topic, after which he composed numerous texts on pharmacy and *materia medica*, including the work for which he is today the most famous, the still-used *Ten Million Relics* (*Bye ba ring bsrel*).[43] Among the many students of this tradition is Kyempa Tsewang, the major *Four Tantras* commentator mentioned in the firs pages of this book.

In the fifteenth and sixteenth centuries, several major commentaries on the *Four Tantras* were composed by some of the chief figures in medical history: two of these are the central commentarial sources in the present study. Authored by prominent medical scholars also known for religious erudition, these works show an extensive influence of Buddhism on medical scholarship. The *Four Tantras Commentary,* written in 1479 by the famous physician Kyempa Tsewang, is a text still used by Tibetan medical students today. Kyempa Tsewang begins his discussion of the formation of the body with a presentation of "the support," the mind, and "the supported," the body. He summarizes a Buddhist description of mind, and then moves to a commentary on the *Four Tantras* exchange between Yilekyé and Rikpé Yeshé, beginning, as the *Four Tantras* does, with a summary of the seven topics discussed in the context of the teaching on the body. Contemporary editions of his commentary are structured by the *Four Tantras'* seven chapters: the manner of formation, similes of the body, anatomy, physiology, classifications and actions, and signs of death. The section on how the body is formed is subdivided into teachings on the manner of conception, the causes of fetal growth and signs of birth. As we will discuss in chapters to come, topics that arise in this commentary include the role of karma and the natural elements in successful conception and fetal development; disorders of the reproductive substances that may prevent conception; the mechanics of menstruation; sexual definition of the embryo; the sequence of fetal growth; rituals that ensure the generation of a male fetus; brief mention of recommended behavior for the pregnant woman; and a summary of tantric Buddhist accounts of fetal development. The text displays a powerful knowledge of Buddhist literature, and its eloquent and lengthy discussions are in sharp contrast to the terse *Four Tantras* commentaries of two hundred years earlier.

Composed nearly a century later, the *Transmission of the Elders* by Zurkhar Lodrö Gyelpo (1509–1579) is the most influential commentarial work of the Southern tradition of Tibetan medicine.[44] This text is also widely used by medical students today. Said to be the nephew of Zurkhar Nyamnyi Dorjé,[45] Zurkhar Lodrö Gyelpo is generally considered part of the Southern school, although he received training in both traditions. Lodrö Gyelpo spent his life as a monk at Tsurpu and was a serious scholar of religion, authoring numerous (no longer extant) religious texts and studying widely with various contemporary experts, including the eighth Karmapa in Gampopa's Kagyü school, Mikyö Dorjé (1504–1554), among others.[46] He also spent time in residence at Sakya monastery, a site renowned for medical education as well as for political influence, receiving teachings on several important medical treatises there. Lodrö Gyelpo is famous for having discovered a hidden edition of the *Four Tantras* penned by Yuthok himself, and on the basis of this he created a revised edition of the classic text subsequently known as the Dratang edition of the *Four Tantras* (*Gra thang rgyud bzhi*), published posthumously in 1640.[47] Lodrö Gyelpo's *Transmission of the Elders* was the last text to be clearly identified as part of the Southern medical school.

Lodrö Gyelpo's sophisticated commentary draws on medical knowledge and philosophical debates from a variety of schools of Tibetan medical and religious thought, using Tibetan and Indian sources widely. Like Kyempa Tsewang, Lodrö Gyelpo's presentation of human development organizes the discussion into three large sections on conception, fetal development and growth, and signs of birth. He addresses many of the same topics as Kyempa Tsewang, although generally with a much more detailed and critical attention to other traditions and their similar or variant views. Many of the opposing positions noted in this text are references to a commentary by Jangdak Namgyel Drakzang, the founder of the Northern school, placing the two texts in direct dialogue. Lodrö Gyelpo is also said to have drawn heavily on the *Heart Essence of Yuthok*, a collection that integrates theoretical medical studies with religious meditation practices.

Not all commentaries on the *Four Tantras* were composed by individuals known primarily as physicians, as are those figures described above. The prolifi sixteenth-century Kagyü author Pema Karpo (1527–1592), the regent Tenpé Gönpo (1760–1810), and Mipam (1846–1912) – all renowned authors of Buddhist philosophical texts – wrote commentaries on the *Four Tantras* as well. One of the most influential seventeenth-century commentaries is Sanggyé Gyatso's *Blue Beryl*, completed in 1688. As noted earlier, Sanggyé Gyatso was the regent of the Fifth Dalai Lama, as well as the founder of the Chakpori medical college in Lhasa and commissioner of a famous series of medical illustrations (*thang ka*). He was also a prolific writer on many subjects in addition to medicine, including religion, history and astrology. It is clear that throughout Tibetan history, medicine was a topic about which many religious thinkers felt not only competent but also authorized to write about, sometimes in a cursory way but often at great length. Medicine was a central component of training in the great monastic universities of Tibet, and as these institutions became increasingly powerful in the educational structure of the Tibetan intellectual elite, the connections between medical and religious scholarship grew ever closer and ever more complex.

After the period of the twelfth-century Yuthok Yönten Gönpo, emphasis in medical histories such as that of Sanggyé Gyatso shifted from a focus on the internationally collaborative nature of medical knowledge to a highlighting of the prolific scholarship produced by great doctors. Such histories report that these doctors were famous not only for their medical talents but for religious sophistication as well: many were monks, residing at the prominent monastic institutions of the day and studying with leading Buddhist teachers. Many were also members of politically influential families, or otherwise closely connected to the political leadership. As Buddhist monastic institutions formed cohesive, powerful identities around the charisma of significant religious leaders, medical institutions were created similarly, their identities defined by politically shrewd, scholarly men and their textual accomplishments. The medical history written by Sanggyé Gyatso in the seventeenth century thus defines medicine in much the same way that certain politically dominant forms of religion were defined at the time. Emphasizing the centrality of monastic institutions and the valorization of Indian models of authority, Sanggyé Gyatso paints the history of the medical tradition in a way acceptable to the political and intellectual authority of his own era. What we cannot know by this account, of course, is what types of localized and popularly-oriented activities may have been conducted by physicians during these centuries.

While the specific doctrines and teachings of the various medical and religious traditions are obviously different, what is of note here is that many of the prominent historical narratives of these traditions are stylized in remarkably similar ways. What the stylized structure of historiography conveys is not superficial: history defines the past, and the past is the core of one's identity in the present. By presenting the history of medicine in a similar manner as the history of Buddhism, therefore, medical knowledge was effectively and fully claimed, according to the medical histories available to us today at least, as part of the Buddhist religious hegemony of Tibet. If histories of Tibetan medicine convey the increasingly close connections between medical and religious traditions in Tibet politically and institutionally, what remains to be addressed is what the *content* of medical and religious texts may tell us about these connections. What counts as "medical knowledge" is not static over time. The question of how the content of medical texts shifts to reflect changing political and institutional situations will be considered in chapters to come. First, however, in the remainder of this chapter, I will examine further the general intellectual and literary contexts for narratives of human development in Tibet.

Locating human development in the narrative of Tibetan history

Medicine and religion in Tibet, despite a close interaction throughout history, are – or became at some point – disciplines and genres of literature with separate identities. Thus, for instance, there are Tibetan histories of medicine (*khog dbub* or *khog 'bugs*), defined as such in contrast to historical genres like royal succession (*rgyal rabs*), monastic chronicles (*gdan rabs*), or religious histories (*chos 'byung*). According to the influential enumeration of ten "arts and sciences" (*rig gnas*, Skt. *vidyā sthāna*), an Indic taxonomy codified in Tibet by the thirteenth-century scholar Sakya Pandita but in use for some time before then, the study of religion (*nang don rig pa*) and the study of medicine (*gso ba rig pa*) are two distinct members of the five major arts and sciences. Organized in the fourteenth century, the Tibetan Buddhist canon places medical texts under a category of technical treatises and, until the seventeenth century, medicine was taught in monasteries as one of the worldly arts and sciences.[48]

The enumeration of ten arts and sciences was an import from India overlaid upon the Tibetan context, with varying levels of suitability, sometimes disregarding indigenously Tibetan methods of classifying learning and knowledge. Of course, the concepts of literature and literary genre are of Euro-American origins, and so their applicability to the Tibetan context must also be questioned. Nonetheless, there *are* Tibetan means of subdividing knowledge that can, at least loosely, correspond to forms of Tibetan textual output. The classification of the ten major and minor arts and sciences is one such taxonomy, used by

Tibetans for centuries, although Indic in origin. Other modes of classifying Tibetan literature can be found in the Tibetan Buddhist canon of translated Indian texts, which includes a distinct category for medical texts, or in the collections of Tibetan texts by specific authors (*gsung 'bum*), which also possess internal taxonomies in the form of tables of contents (*dkar chag*).[49] What can be observed here is that in all of these schemes, "medicine" (*gso rig*) as a category unambiguously receives a place of its own in Tibetan taxonomies of literature and knowledge. Whatever "medicine" is, we know that by some standard or in some way it is *not* "religion" (an equally problematic category, if not more so), just as it also is not "logic" nor "grammar," two other primary classificatory categories. What we will think about in this book is what counts as "medicine." Before approaching the details, however, first let us consider how texts are classified *within* the broad category of medicine. According to contemporary Tibetan medical scholars, there is no clearly articulated, standardized indigenous Tibetan scheme for classifying types of medical literature.[50] We can nevertheless describe several general types of writing, considered by subject matter, associated with the category of "medicine," although certainly some texts cover several topics and do not fit easily into one of these categories

One genre of medical writing is, of course, the history, and there are a number of Tibetan works still extant, ranging from the thirteenth century to the present date, on the history of medicine. The history of medicine is also occasionally discussed as a discrete topic within general Tibetan histories. The most famous medical history today remains Sanggyé Gyatso's 1702 *Interior Analysis*, which details the development of medicine in India and in Tibet, with biographies of many important medical practitioners and descriptions of numerous texts. Sanggyé Gyatso's *Interior Analysis* lists many hundreds of medical texts translated into Tibetan, or composed in Tibetan, prior to the eighteenth century. Although the vast majority of these works are now believed not to have survived, Sanggyé Gyatso frequently describes the contents of the texts he mentions, either briefly, such as by stating that a text is, for example, "on treating the eighteen infectious diseases," or more fully, by providing a table of contents for the work. Most medical texts listed in this history – perhaps ninety percent of those mentioned – are about the diagnosis, classification or treatment of diseases, or about the preparation of medicines; speculation on the contents of these types of texts is possible using the example of surviving texts of similar types.

Texts on nosology, pharmacy and *materia medica* form the bulk of Tibetan writing considered medical in most historical periods. Nosological texts are listings, descriptions and classifications of specific diseases, typically composed more in the manner of a reference than as a work of extended prose. Early examples include several texts of the *Eighteen Additional Practices* collections;[51] the third section of the *Four Tantras*, the *Oral Secret Tantra*, is another example of this type of work. This type of writing can also be found in the *Storehouse of Precious Treasures* (*rin chen gter mdzod*), a collection of texts revealed by Padmasambhava, Vimalamitra, Vairocana and others.[52] Such texts continue to be written and published today, and are important references for practicing physicians.

Texts on pharmacy and *materia medica* describe therapeutic prescriptions that involve the combination of medicinal substances, including the identification, collection methods and preparation of those substances. Still today considered the fundamental works on the topic, two reference guides by Tendzin Püntsok composed in 1727, for instance, describe over 2,200 substances, the former containing information on raw materials and the latter focusing on pharmacological and pharmacognostic details.[53] The fourth unit of the *Four Tantras*, the *Concluding Tantra*, is also an example of this type of text, and other extant early examples include the *Eighteen Additional Practices'* eleventh, thirteenth and seventeenth texts, about which I have written elsewhere. Early publications describing therapeutic techniques make various recommendations, some largely pharmacological in nature, and others more focused on ritual, meditation and mantra recitation. Examples of the latter include, for example, portions of the *Eighteen Additional Practices'* twelfth text, which discuss meditation practices and mantras to be used by doctors as healing strategies, and mantras and other ritual practices to be used for the protection of babies and children. Text fourteen from that collection addresses rituals, meditations and mantras for the treatment of lymph disorders, leprosy and dermatological disorders, and the collection's eighteenth work describes mantras for healing wounds, head injuries, eye problems and other ailments. These examples remind us that distinguishing between medical and religious therapies is not a simple matter.[54]

What is interesting for our purposes here is that a dedicated disciplinary structure to accommodate discussion of the human body – subjects we know as anatomy and physiology – does not exist within medical literature. Several chapters of the *Four Tantras' Explanatory Tantra*, which form the basis for much of this book's study, are the primary examples of this type of medical writing. Significantly, although there are hundreds, if not thousands, of works devoted to pharmacy or nosology, there appear to be very few texts in the medical canon devoted exclusively to discussion of the structure or function of the human body itself. Surveys of dynastic period medical literature in Sanggyé Gyatso's medical history include some texts that *appear*, from their titles, to focus on an explication of the human body from the perspective of human dissection. Pictorial illustrations of the human body and illustrations of disease states and therapeutic activities could also be said to comprise an independent category of medical documentation that focuses on the structure of the body. Fernand Meyer notes, however, that today only one medical painting predating the famous series of seventeenth-century medical paintings is known to exist, a fragmentary Dunhuang document depicting moxibustion points on a human figure. He points also to references in medical histories to early texts or documents that appear to include medical drawings, in the works of Yuthok Yönten Gönpo in the twelfth century, Drangti Penden Tsojé in the thirteenth century, and Zurkhar Nyamnyi Dorjé in the fifteenth century[55]

While much is said about human development by medical writers over the centuries, in fact, the subject occupies a fairly small corner of medical literature as a whole, existing primarily in a single chapter of the *Heart of Medicine*, a single chapter of the *Four Tantras* and, then, in subsequent commentarial works. In Tibetan religious texts, by contrast, narratives of human development are plentiful and found in various contexts, sometimes even playing a central role in a given Buddhist philosophical and contemplative system.

In this chapter, we have seen medicine and religion in Tibetan history interact in various ways. At times, there is conflict. Was the *Four Tantras* spoken by the Buddha, or composed by Tibetans? Should the early history of Tibetan medicine be characterized as internationally collaborative, or as essentially Buddhist? At times there is convergence, as learned scholars trained in a wide range of subjects composed works classified as religious and as medical, the two disciplines existing in the body of a single individual. And there is complementarity, with well-read authors drawing equally from the classics of medicine and from the Buddhist canon as needed to support discussions that ranged beyond the confines of either. In different contexts and from different perspectives, each of these modes of relationship may be observed. What the historical survey of the last two chapters suggests, however, is that organized writing about the human body's development and structure is not as plainly a part of medicine as we might have assumed, reading these traditions from our contexts, our own perspectives. It may instead be the case that the domain of religion provided Tibetans with richer potential when thinking about the human body and its development. In the following chapters, we will consider in greater detail how this is so. We will think about narratives of early human development as vital and creative venues for addressing fundamental questions about identity, responsibility and personal creativity. Each of the next three chapters will thus demonstrate how human development is linked to issues of fundamental importance in Buddhism: to the Buddhist concern with corporeal taxonomies, to central topics in Buddhist cosmology and astrology, to Buddhist soteriology, to the centrality of karma and Buddhist ethics, and to the complexities of Buddhist doctrine and practice. At the same time, we will continue to explore the changing intellectual and literary context for human development, a discussion that will investigate the nature of medical and religious interactions over a period of several centuries in Tibet.

4

THE FETAL BODY, GENDER AND THE NORMAL

In an obvious way, medical systems are naturally about human bodies. In the previous chapter, however, we wondered whether the organized presentation of the human body's structure and functional features may, in fact, play less of a role in the history of Tibetan medical literature than we might have assumed. Indeed, strange as it may sound to the modern ear, it will serve us to note that the inclusion of the study of the body in the field of medicine in Europe – in the form of physiology, anatomy, or embryology for example – is a particular historical occurrence in our own intellectual history.[1] Even a cursory look at Buddhism, on the other hand, tells us that systematic presentations of the body are of vital importance for religious thinkers of that tradition. It is well known that Buddhist theorists have generated tomes of scholarship on the classificatio and functions of various aspects of mind or mentality – a topic clearly separate in Buddhism from the study of the body. But narratives of gestation are, on the most literal level, explicitly focused on the development of the body, not the mind. What it is that this topic allowed Tibetan writers to say about the body?

The primary question for this chapter and the next is, who are the main characters in narratives of embryology? Tibetan accounts of human development can be interpreted on various levels, and such narratives may be addressed to assorted fictional and real audiences. While on one level the main character is clearly the developing human being, in some narratives the embryo is a stand-in for the Buddhist practitioner. Before addressing this symbolic main character – the topic of chapter five – we will first consider, in this chapter, how the literal main character, the embryo itself, is described. Most simply, of course, the embryo is a body, or at least at some point mid-way along the gestational process, it is a body with limbs, skin, facial features, sexual characteristics and so forth. It is more than this, however, if we begin with the presupposition that the human body, in a particular literary or social context, works as a vehicle for the organization and expression of beliefs about the nature of human beings and their place in the social and cosmic order.

Studies of Buddhist or Āyurvedic theories of embodiment sometimes see the body as a material entity in need of treatment that can be understood no differently than bodies of the twentieth-century medicalized Western world. By this account, physical bodies exist across the world and throughout history exactly as Euro-American scientists know them to exist today. This view understands bodies to exist independently of culture, language, history or lived experience, seeing the skin as the absolute boundary of the body.

But skin is permeable. A more contexualized understanding of the body thus allows us to see that Buddhist authors throughout history have creatively used the vocabulary of embodiment to convey subtle philosophical and psychological messages about Buddhist doctrine and the possibility for enlightenment. In the latter part of this century, some academic disciplines have questioned our own understanding of the body, pointing to the historical and social specificity of notions of embodiment and calling for a revision of the mechanization of the body. For cultural theorists if not scientists, what is meant by the term "body" is no longer a given, as thinkers struggle to identify the philosophical, social and political influences governing the relationship between bodies and minds and their particular contexts. Buddhist authors in Asia have been grappling with similar questions for centuries. Buddhist philosophical texts explicate the multi-dimensional experience of embodiment using myriad terms – ordinary body, gross temporary body, subtle fundamental body, illusory body, pure illusory body, truth body, form body, rainbow body and vajra body, to name only a few. These traditions enjoy a rich vocabulary for conceptualizing modes of embodiment, and they use various images, symbols, metaphors and representations of the body to construct various forms of subjectivity and relationship.

Early Indian Buddhism, for example, advocates numerous practices aimed at generating a sense of aversion toward impermanent phenomena as a means of gaining insight into the nature of saṃsāra. The ordinary human body is a common object of meditation in this effort, and meditative techniques promote an awareness of the body's defiled nature. Many of the Buddha's earliest teachings involve instruction on the foulness of the human body and, to this end, monks were sent to burial grounds to contemplate rotting corpses. For each of thirty-two parts of the body, for instance, Buddhaghosa outlines five forms of loathsomeness for contemplation. The human body in these early texts is graphically described as a putrid, leaking boil with nine openings:

> This boil, monks, is an apt metaphor for the body which is made up of the four great elements, begotten of mother and father, formed from a heap of boiled rice and sour gruel, subject to impermanence, concealment, abrasion, dissolution, and disintegration, with nine gaping wounds, nine natural openings, and whatever might ooze out from this, foulness would certainly ooze out. Therefore, monks, you should be disgusted with this body.[2]

Such instructions are presented to meditators combating the negative emotion of desire. Ubiquitous in early Indian writings, such views of the ordinary human body are also offered by later Mahāyāna thinkers. In the *Way of the Bodhisattva*

(Skt. *bodhisattvacaryāvatāra*), for instance, Śāntideva advocates recognition of the likeness of the ordinary body to a corpse:

> Seeing a skeleton that does not even move, you are terrified
> Why aren't you frightened by a walking corpse animated by a vetāla?
> You are disgusted by skeletons in the cremation ground,
> But you enjoy yourself in the cremation ground that is the village fille
> with walking crowds of skeletons![3]

Embodiment is not viewed negatively in all forms of Buddhism, however, and theories of embodiment proliferated as Buddhism diversified across Asia. Prominent among these is the doctrine of the spiritual bodies of the Buddha, a scheme in which the Buddha manifests as either a "Form Body" (*gzugs sku*, Skt. *rūpa kāya*) or a "Reality Body" (*chos sku*, Skt. *dharma kāya*), where the former is metaphysically the Buddha's profound realization, and the latter is the Buddha's manifested physical and verbal existence in the world of sentient beings. This doctrine is also configured as three bodies: the Form Body is subdivided into an Enjoyment Body (*longs sku*, Skt. *sambhoga kāya*), an idealized manifestation of the Reality Body as a teacher in a Pure Land, and the Emanation Body (*sprul sku*, Skt. *nirmāṇa kāya*), which appears in the flesh in the ordinary world of sentient beings. With Mahāyāna and tantric traditions, the ineffable reality of the Buddha's enlightened realization was internalized within every sentient being; according to this doctrine, all sentient beings possess a Buddha's body, referred to as an individual's enlightened "Buddha nature."

The taxonomy of embodiment, as an intellectual practice, is a central feature of Buddhist doctrine throughout history and across Asia. In Buddhist traditions, some beings are materially embodied, and others are embodied as mind or as light. Bodies are gross or subtle; male, female or "other"; physically normal or abnormal. The Buddhist three-body theory describes three aspects of enlightened embodiment: the Reality Body is formless and abstract, and it is the source of the Emanation and Enjoyment Bodies; the Emanation Body is a Buddha in human form; and enlightened bodhisattvas, often residents of a Pure Land, possess Enjoyment Bodies. Even deities take on bodies that are semantically coded as good or evil: bodhisattvas have distinctively superior bodies, often of exceptional beauty and supernatural physical and mental ability. Buddhist cosmology, defining six realms of rebirth according to what type of body one receives, describes the bodies of hell beings, hungry spirits, animals, humans, demigods, and gods. And always, Buddhist embodiment is wholly moralized: there are bad bodies (animals, hungry ghosts, or women), good bodies (male humans, bodhisattvas), and best bodies (a Buddha's body). This chapter will consider how the study of early human development participated in the taxonomy of embodiment.

Scholars of Buddhism commonly contrast the focus on negative depictions of the human body characteristic of early Buddhist practices, with the comparatively valued status of the human body in tantric meditation practices. Some have further pinpointed attitudes toward the body as the locus of the intersection of medical theory and Buddhist doctrine. In this chapter, I will ask what Tibetan writers said about embodiment through the medium of embryology, considering how stories of early human development are used by Tibetan medical and religious authors to describe, or prescribe, models of human identity, and to question how individuals differentiate themselves from one another. This chapter will outline some general features of two theories of physiology, that of Tibetan medicine and that of Buddhist tantra, both inherited from Indian models, and it will focus on two aspects of physiology. The first, which describes the body's systemic and digestive physiology, is a functional and interactive presentation of the body that is emphasized in medical texts and rarely discussed in religious ones. The second, which depicts the intricate circulatory system of fluids and energies throughout the body, is of importance to both medical and religious literature, particularly as medical traditions become more deeply embedded in Buddhist frameworks. I will then look at how embryological narratives contribute to these theories of embodiment. Finally, returning to the question of who the main characters of these narratives are, I will consider another individual, the pregnant woman.

Functional physiologies: humoral and digestive systems

In Chapter 2, I described a textual inheritance that provided Tibetan authors with Indian medical theory. Āyurvedic writers regarded the human body as a conglomeration of bodily constituents (Skt. *dhātu*) that are made up of the fiv natural elements: water, fire, air, earth and space. The body functions properly when the bodily constituents are correctly proportioned. The bodily constituents are created from the food one consumes: the purified component of food yields the constituent of nutritive "food-juice" (Skt. *rasa*, sometimes also translated as chyle or plasma), producing, subsequently, the constituents of blood, flesh, fat, bones, marrow and reproductive substance (in Sanskrit, *rakta, māmsa, medas, asthi, majjā* and *śukra*, respectively). The impure component of food forms waste products (Skt. *malas*) that are excreted from the body in the form of urine, sweat and feces. Other bodily waste products include the threesome of *vāta*, *pitta* and *kapha*, typically translated into English as wind, bile or gall, and phlegm or mucus, respectively, following the humoral terminology used in the study of ancient Greek thought. These three, the *doṣa*, are perceived to be primarily responsible for bodily morbidity and are regarded as the most essential factors in the determination of a human's constitution. The correlation with Greek humors is a loose one at best, and some theorists who have examined this terminology closely have been led to reject the term "humor" to represent these three forces or processes of the body. Loizzo and Blackhall, for instance, describe the three *doṣa* as "three aspects of self-organization [that] may best be conceived as systemic aspects of activity, vitality, and stability."[4] The doctrine of the three "humors," or, as I will more often refer to them in this book, "systemic processes" (Skt. *doṣa*), is the basis of Āyurvedic pathology and therapeutic technique, and it is a doctrine that is also the foundation of Tibetan medicine. Despite the inadequacy of referring to the three *doṣa* as wind, bile and phlegm, however, I will use these terms here.

With a few exceptions, a human's constitution is dominated by one of the three systemic processes from the moment of conception. While the exceptions include rare individuals in perfect health exhibiting a systemic equipoise, more common is the categorization of individuals according to a continual predominance of one or the other processes. Significantly, then, the doctrine of the three *doṣa* – whether in Āyurvedic or Tibetan medicine – is valid in understanding good health as well as pathology. In good health, the *doṣa* remain in balance with each other and with one's environment and food consumption. When some aspect of a certain process is provoked, however, and the equilibrium is tipped, disease results. The physician's role, therefore, is to identify which aspect has increased or decreased to the detriment of the whole system. Treatment consists of returning the systemic processes to their normal state, taking into consideration the patient's diet, behavior, stage in life and seasonal factors.

Tibetan medical presentations of the body are similar to classical Āyurvedic presentations.[5] Tibetan medical systems in the tradition of the *Four Tantras* describe the body as composed of two principal components: one, the substances of the body, or the bodily constituents (*lus zungs*, equivalent to the Āyurvedic *dhātu*), and two, the functional processes (*'du ba*, meaning literally "gathering together") that activate the body's substances. The latter are the "faults" or "systemic processes" (*nyes pa*, equivalent to the Āyurvedic *dośa*). Together, these two – the substances and the forces that act upon them – comprise the "aggregates" (*phungs po*) of the ordinary human body. The bodily constituents and systemic processes are related as object and subject, Tibetan medical texts calling the constituents the "objects of disturbance" (*gnod bya'i khams*) and the *nyes pa*, or systemic processes, the "agents of disturbance" (*gnod bya*).[6]

As in the Āyurvedic model, the bodily constituents in Tibetan medicine are the seven substances of the body: the nutritive essences of food and drink (*dwangs ma*), blood (*khrag*), flesh (*sha*), fat (*tshil*), bone (*rus ba*), marrow (*rkang*), and the reproductive substances (*khu ba*). Each of these has specifie functions in maintaining bodily structure and processes. After food has been digested it takes one of two forms, nutrients (*dwangs*) and wastes (*snyigs*). This separation of nutrients from wastes occurs in the lower stomach area. Waste products are then further separated into liquids and solids and excreted as urine and feces. Nutrients pass to the liver and are metabolized to form the basic substances of the body's physical constituents. In the liver, the physiological processes of decomposing phlegm (*tshim byed bad kan*), digestive heat (*me drod*), and the fire-accompanying wind (*me dang mnyam pa'i rlung*) act to transform the nutrients into blood, which is sent throughout the body and then transformed into the next bodily constituent, flesh. Flesh is transformed by additional metabolic factors into bone tissue, which in turn produces bone marrow. The nutritive aspects of marrow, when utilized by the reproductive system, produce the reproductive substances in males and females. The digestive system of separation and transformation is precise, each substance providing direct nourishment for specific functions or organs of the body. The end point of the entire digestive process, which is said to take six days, is the creation of the reproductive substances, which are therefore considered to be the quintessential distillation of all the physical constituents. The quality of one's general health, as well as one's life span and complexion, are ultimately said to be determined by the quality of the distilled reproductive substances. It is thus the human body's finest quintessence that is involved in the creation of a new human body at the time of conception.[7]

The bodily substances and digestive processes are presented in the fourth and fifth chapters of the *Four Tantras' Explanatory Tantra*. The fifth chapter explains that the three systemic processes – wind (*rlung*, equivalent to the Āyurvedic *vāta*), bile (*mkhris pa*, equivalent to the Āyurvedic *pitta*), and phlegm (*bad kan*, equivalent to the Āyurvedic *kapha*) – are united in an individual from the moment of conception. While these three processes can disturb health and even cause death, it is important to note they are not the sole causes of ill health. As in Āyurveda, they are only the causes of ill health when they are displaced; when operating in their natural location and serving their natural function, they are sources of bodily health and well-being.

The three systemic processes are numerologically qualified in various ways. Each is first divided into five types according to individual function. Thus, as explained above, during digestion a form of the phlegm-process is responsible for breaking down consumed food, a form of the bile-process then digests the food, and a form of the wind-process separates the fully metabolized foodstuff into wastes and essential nutrients. Each of the three systemic processes also possesses six qualifying characteristics that further describe the specific effects or qualities these processes express as bodily experiences. So, for instance, the wind-process is characterized by six qualities: rough, light, active, subtle, cold and hard. Roughness, experienced as a rough tongue or rough skin, is an expression of the presence of the wind-process in the body. The wind-process' quality of coldness is likewise what causes an individual to shiver or desire hot drinks. Each of the five types of the three processes is also assigned a particular set of five functions and five locations in the body. The wind-process is responsible for sensation, including the workings of consciousness, as well as for the movement of substances and qualities around the body, and it is located in the vessels linked to the sense organs in and around the head, chest, heart, stomach and anus. The bile-process is responsible for bodily color and heat, including the digestion of food, and is found in the stomach, intestines, liver, heart, eyes and skin. The phlegm-process is affiliated with psycho-physical qualities such as stability, smoothness, and connectivity, and it is located around the chest, stomach, tongue, head and joints.

As physiological agents that functionally organize the body's activity, vitality, and stability (using Loizzo and Blackhall's expression), the wind, bile and phlegm processes affect embodied experience from before the time of conception until one's death. Tibetan medical texts claim that an appropriately balanced systemic make-up in the male and female reproductive substances is one of the necessary conditions for successful conception and formation of the embryo. The *Four Tantras* carefully explains why systemic or other defects in these factors will result in the failure to conceive, or in the conception of a child that is in some way abnormal.[8] The text describes how systemic imbalances will damage the reproductive substances and affect the likelihood of successful conception: a wind disorder will make them rough, dark and astringent; a bile disorder will turn them sour, yellow and bad smelling; a blood disorder will cause the reproductive substances to decay, and so forth.

Although their balanced presence in the male and female reproductive fluid is said to be required for successful conception, however, the three processes as a set are typically given no role in the development and growth of the body during gestation, according to Tibetan embryological narratives. The *nyes pa*, or the set of three systemic processes of wind, bile and phlegm, are rarely even mentioned in accounts of gestation. (As I will discuss in chapter six, the role of the winds is important for some embryological accounts, but these cases rely on Buddhist sūtras and tantras, not medical theory.) This neglect of the set of the three systemic processes in the growth of the fetus is remarkable given the importance of understanding these physiological agents in the etiological, diagnostic and therapeutic practices of Tibetan medicine.

Also central to Tibetan medical physiology is the concept of bodily heat (*me drod*). Heat is causally responsible both for digestion and for the separation of substances into wastes and essential nutrients. Heat is a necessary part of each of the seven constituents, three systemic processes, and three excretory substances. Many chronic diseases are caused by an insufficiently strong power of bodily heat, and many therapeutic techniques are therefore aimed at improving heat. The modern Tibetan medical scholar, Tubten Püntsok (b. 1955), explains that when consumed foodstuffs have entered the stomach, they are digested by heat:

> By being blown on by the fire-accompanying wind that abides in the stomach, the potency of heat, which is fire-like in nature, blazes greater, and by that means the food and drink are digested in the region of the stomach. For example, it is like putting medicine and herbs into a vessel and boiling them into *khanta*, [a hard, dried type of medicine that can be preserved for a long time].[9]

Again, however, despite the centrality of the concept of heat to Tibetan medical physiology, it is given no role in medical embryologies. The key features of Tibetan medical physiology, the *nyes pa* or systemic processes and bodily heat, are both neglected in medical accounts of early human development. Could it be that these essential aspects of the body are not operative in the developing fetus?

This seems unlikely and, indeed, it is never stated that those aspects of physiology are unique to adults. As we explore this odd fact, consider this: the disconnect between the fetal physiology of embryological narratives and the adult physiology of other aspects of medical theory may indicate not that fetuses and adults have different physiologies. Rather, it may suggest that embryology was a subject that even medical writers came to think of as more essentially "religious" in nature. If the source for information about fetal physiology comes ultimately from religious, not medical, traditions, this may account for the difference in content, emphasis, or tone observed here. Let us turn now to a component of physiology, the circulatory system, that is important to both religious and medical traditions.

The circulatory system

In Indian and Tibetan Buddhist tantric contemplative systems, the basis of human physiology is the subtle architecture of channels, winds, and quintessential essences (respectively, *rtsa*, equivalent to the Sanskrit *nāḍī; rlung*, equivalent to the Sanskrit *prāṇa* or *vāyu;* and *thig le*, equivalent to the Sanskrit *bindu, tilaka*, or *śukra*) and the four, five or six channel nexus or "wheels" (*'khor lo*, Skt. *cakra*). Tantric physiology begins with a vertical spinal column in which, or along which – this is debated – are three primary channels. While tantric systems vary to some degree, in general, the locations and functions of the three primary channels are agreed upon. In brief, the central channel (*dbu ma*, Skt. *suṣumṇā*) runs vertically through the center of the wheels from the genitals to the crown of the head. Control over the entry of the winds into the central channel and their maintenance within that channel, which is ordinarily empty, is the objective of many of the most advanced tantric contemplative practices. Running vertically through the center of the body to the left and right of the central channel are the solitary channel (*rkyang ma*, Skt. *piṅgalā* or *lalanā*) and the flavor channel (*ro ma*, Skt. *iḍā* or *rasanā*), respectively. The white-colored solitary channel, along the left, is said to face downward, and the red-colored flavor channel, on the right, is said to face upward. The upper tips of these two channels connect at the nostrils, and it is through these channels that ordinary respiration travels. The bottom ends of these two channels approach the lower tip of the central channel, but ordinarily they do not touch the central channel. It is the aim of many advanced tantric practices to cause the ends of the right and left channels to touch the central channel so that the respiration may enter the central channel during the course of contemplative practice. The lower tips of the right and left channels are also associated with expelling waste matter from the body: in men and women of good health, urine emerges from the solitary channel and, for women, menstrual blood from the flavor channel. The central channel is associated with the release of reproductive fluids, at least for men.[10] While in general this presentation is agreed upon in tantric Buddhist texts, there are variations in detail. One such variation, of particular relevance to the embryological narratives studied in this book, is that of the Nyingma scholar Longchenpa; I will return to his account of the channels and their role in embryology in chapter five. Another variation explains that below the navel, the solitary and flavor channels split, making four, two forking to the right and left, and two reaching to the front and back. The twelfth-century *Explication of the Treatise for Nyak* by Sachen Künga Nyingpo (1092–1158), for example, explains that the channel running to the right holds and discharges the reproductive constituent originally received from one's mother (referred to by Künga Nyingpo in tantric code language as frankincense), the channel running to the left holds and discharges the reproductive constituent originally received from one's father (referred to as camphor), the channel running to the front holds and discharges urine (referred to as musk), and the channel to the back holds and discharges feces. Each of these channels exist in this way for both men and women. Emphasizing the importance of these channels to the creation of the human individual, Künga Nyingpo notes that "these are known as samsara channels because they produce the body that is generated by karma, as well as the mind of subject and object."[11]

Many volumes in Indian and Tibetan literature are occupied by discussion of the three channels, their functions, their relationship to other aspects of the body psychologically and physiologically, and the techniques for controlling their functions during meditative practice; the intricacy of this fascinating topic precludes its full discussion here. Despite the complexity of the subject and its importance throughout centuries of literature, in the dialogue between Tibetan medical and religious traditions the very existence of these three channels is questioned. The sixteenth-century medical commentator Lodrö Gyelpo cites an unidentified Vajrayāna scholar to assert that the tantric presentation of three channels is a trope developed to enhance contemplative practice, and that, in fact, the three channels do not exist in the body. Lodrö Gyelpo asks in response how a soteriologically transformative effect could possibly occur as a result of completing such tantric practices if the three channels did not even exist.[12] Other scholars assert that if these three channels really exist, they ought to be clearly visible in a corpse. Commenting on this debate, the contemporary Sakya scholar Tsultrim Gyeltsen (d. 2001) points out that many elements of the body, such as aspects of the bodily constituents or forces of illness, are invisible and yet their effects prove their existence.[13]

Also important in tantric physiological accounts are elaborate descriptions of the winds and the quintessential essences. The twelfth-century Sakya scholar Drakpa Gyeltsen, for instance, explains that when discussing winds functionally, tantric traditions generally describe five primary winds, often called the fiv "outer" winds (*phyi'i rlung lnga*), and five subsidiary winds. The life-sustaining (*srog 'dzin*) wind is located at the heart and is generally responsible for the integrated relationship between mind and body. In many cases, the life-sustaining wind is differentiated from the other nine winds as being either associated with, or synonymous with, the innate wisdom (*ye shes*) wind. Disturbance of this wind can thus result in insanity or death. This is an important wind in many embryological narratives, as we will see shortly. The downward-clearing (*thur sel*) wind is located near the anus and responsible for waste elimination. The fire-accompanying (*me mnyam*) wind is at the navel, aiding in the digestive process, as mentioned earlier. The upward-upholding (*gyen rgyu*) wind is at the throat, enabling speech, laughter or vomiting. The all-pervasive (*khyab byed*) wind, finally, pervades the entire body. While the names of these winds can vary slightly by tradition, Drakpa Gyeltsen also describes five subsidiary winds, located at the sense organs and the joints and responsible for interacting with external objects: the serpent (*klu*) wind, located at the eyes; the tortoise (*ru sbal*) wind at the ears; the chameleon (*rtsangs pa*) wind at the nose; the Devadatta (*lhas byin*) wind at the tongue; and the bow-victor (*gzhu las rgyal*) wind in the joints. Each of the ten winds is also associated with the elements and with colors.[14] While in some embryological narratives the winds are essential causes of fetal growth, the winds described in those accounts are not – with the exception of the life-sustaining wind – the ten winds of Buddhist Tantra listed above. (I will return to this issue in Chapter 6.)

Some Buddhist systems also categorize winds according to how they circulate in the body. Using this type of organizational scheme, Drakpa Gyeltsen presents a twofold arrangement of winds: the karmic (*las*) wind, which is by nature continually moving in and out of the body during ordinary respiration, and the innate wisdom (*ye shes*) wind, most of which is generally said to remain stationary in an ordinary person's body. This too is debated, however; Drakpa Gyeltsen claims that in the *Kālacakra* tradition part of the innate wisdom wind does move, spreading to various parts of the body at certain times of the day, seemingly equivalent to the "life force" (*bla*) described below.[15]

The third aspect of traditional tantric physiologies, the quintessential essences (*thig le*), are figured both physiologically, as the red and white forms of female and male reproductive substance, and metaphysically, as agents closely involved in the process of spiritual enlightenment. Also correlated in some accounts with the "life force" (*bla*) type of vitality "channel," these substances are generally said to travel around the body serving various functions throughout the day at certain locations. For example, one often feels dull or sleepy at noon because the quintessential essences are located in the area of the heart at that time of day and therefore interfere with the clarity of one's consciousness. The route of these substances throughout the body over the waxing and waning of the moon and over the course of a year is also recorded, dictating optimally effective dates and seasons for both meditative and medicinal behaviors.[16] Buddhist contemplative literature describes processes for purifying the white-colored and red-colored quintessential essences and directing their activities toward certain key points of the body. To be discussed further in chapter five such complex advanced contemplative practices, sometimes performed during controlled sexual intercourse, aim to purify the body and the mind and generate experiences of enlightenment.

This simplified overview of tantric physiology, which is an intricate subject that deserves a book-length study of its own, indicates broad outlines of concern for Buddhist scholars focusing on human physiology. Considered primarily an object of study in Tibetan medical traditions, the theory of the human body's systemic and digestive physiology sketched out earlier, on the other hand, plays little if any role in most Tibetan religious traditions. While religious systems that teach yogic practices do draw on notions of inner heat that are related to the physiology of digestive heat described in medical texts, the technicalities of digestive physiology and its relation to the maintenance of the bodily constituents are rarely addressed in religious literature. When we turn to the circulatory system, however, we see a much closer interaction between medical and religious systems. Significantly various aspects of the circulatory system also play a large role in both medical and religious presentations of the growth of the fetus.

The general model of the circulatory system portrayed in early Tibetan medical literature is derived from classical Indian Āyurveda. Āyurvedic medicine describes a network of hundreds of large and small ducts, or channels, variously named *nāḍī, śirā, srota* or *dhamanī* in Sanskrit, that transport nutrients, wastes, respiration and other substances throughout the body. By connecting internal organs, these channels are responsible for digestive and other physiological processes. They also facilitate the movement of joints and limbs, and they carry sensory information that allows sense organs to function. The precise enumeration of various types of channels and their functions is a contested topic, and debates among Indian medical scholars concerning the circulatory system are common. The structure of the circulatory system in medical texts, moreover, is different than the circulatory system described in Indian tantric texts.[17] Although over the centuries some Tibetan writers have tried to unite medical and tantric accounts of anatomy and physiology, descriptions of the body in South Asian literature are so numerous and complex that few differences are fully reconciled.

In Tibetan medical literature of the *Four Tantras* tradition, descriptions of the human circulatory system focus on the circulatory channels (*rtsa*). These are sometimes translated into English as "veins," "arteries" or "nerves," although the term *rtsa* in Tibetan is not directly equivalent to any of these. These channels are the basis of the circulatory system of winds, blood, and other energies and fluids that connect all aspects of the body. The contemporary scholar Tubten Püntsok explains that in Tibetan medicine, channels are classified in several ways.[18] According to one taxonomy, there are black channels (*nag rtsa*), also called blood channels (*khrag rtsa*), and white channels (*dkar rtsa*), also called water channels (*chu rtsa*). Blood channels are further divided into "pulsating" channels (*'phar rtsa*) and "staying" channels (*sdod rtsa*), which are sometimes today translated as arteries and veins, respectively. Tibetan medical texts also classify channels functionally, in which case there are four types: channels of embryonic formation (*chags*), channels of existence (*srid*), connecting (*'brel*) channels, and vitality (*tshe*) channels.

The development of the circulatory system is an important event in most Tibetan embryological narratives. The fourth chapter of the *Explanatory Tantra* presents the fourfold functional division of channels just mentioned, beginning with three channels of embryonic formation (*chags rtsa*). Called the water or white channel, the blood or black channel, and the wind channel, these three are said to extend from the navel of the embryo. The water or white channel travels vertically along the left side of the body, and the *Four Tantras* tradition states that it forms the brain; its functions and activities are thus primarily focused in the upper part of the torso and head. The blood or black channel travels vertically along the right side of the body and is related to liver function, as well as to the emotion of anger and the bile-process; its activities are concentrated in the central part of the torso. The third channel of formation is associated with the emotions of desire and attachment and the region of the sexual organs, as well as with the activities of the winds.[19] Although the issue is contested, some religious and medical scholars, including Lodrö Gyelpo, Sanggyé Gyatso, and the eminent twentieth-century Sakya scholar Tsultrim Gyeltsen, identify these three channels in the *Four Tantras* with the three channels of tantric physiology.

The second of the fourfold functional division of channels, the existence (*srid*) channels, are themselves of four types. They are said to be responsible for sensory engagement with the external world, what we would call emotional feelings, and nourishment of the bodily constituents. Tubten Püntsok explains that in the *Four Tantras* tradition, once the channels of formation have been completely produced in the embryo, the existence channels develop in four locations in the body and branch out into hundreds of surrounding auxiliary channels. Situated in the head, the first existence channel is responsible for the function of the sense organs. The second existence channel, in the heart region, is the basis of memory, conceptuality, and awareness of the self or ego. The third channel is located at the navel and, in this tradition, is considered responsible for the embryonic body's growth. The fourth channel, in the area of the genitals, is referred to as the source of one's family lineage.[20] Although the *Four Tantras* does not use the term "wheels" (*'khor lo*) in this context, Tsultrim Gyeltsen argues that the four existence channels and the surrounding auxiliary channels described in the *Explanatory Tantra* are the four wheels referred to in Buddhist tantric systems.[21]

The circulatory channels are also divided into white and black, or water and blood, channels. The sixteenth-century medical scholar Lodrö Gyelpo associates the white existence channel with the tantric solitary channel (*rkyang ma*) running vertically along the left side of the body, and the black existence channel with the tantric flavor channel (*ro ma*) running along the right side of the body.[22] In the adult, hundreds of subsidiary channels branch off from these two main channels, acting as "connecting" (*'brel*) channels that interlink the limbs and organs throughout the entire body. As in the Āyurvedic tradition, Tibetan medical texts debate the precise pathways of these hundreds of channels. The black channels are said to be filled exclusively with blood and, passing through the liver, are involved in the sustenance and development of the seven bodily constituents; a subset of these are the channels used in the medical practice of blood-letting. The main white channel, also traveling from the head to the tail bone, is so called because it is white in color. It and its branch channels, sometimes glossed in English as "ligaments," "tendons," or "nerves," are responsible for many of the functions also attributed to the existence channels, such as regulating emotions, enabling physical movement, and allowing speech and mental functions.

Finally, the *Explanatory Tantra* states that there are three types of vitality (*tshe*) channel: one type that works throughout the entire body, a second type that accompanies respiration, and a third that also pervades the entire body acting as a sort of "life force."[23] According to the interpretation of Lodrö Gyelpo's sixteenth-century *Transmission of the Elders*, the vitality channels are not "real" (*dngos*) channels; rather, they refer simply to forces within the body that maintain life.[24] Human life is by definition dependent upon the continuation of three physiological functions: the radiance (*gzi mdangs*) of the body caused by the metabolized essence of the reproductive substance, the movement of the breath, and the digestive heat of the body.[25] When these functions are discontinued, death results. The vitality channels, therefore, refer to the activity of these three functions in sustaining life. Pervading the entire body, the first of the three vitality channels is the body's digestive heat (*me drod*), which separates and refines the essential nutrients and wastes during the digestive process, thereby maintaining the function of all the bodily constituents that ultimately produce the body's "radiance" or vitality. The second vitality channel is the "innate wisdom" (*ye shes*) wind that accompanies respiration. The innate wisdom wind is distinguished from the karmic (*las*) wind; the *Transmission of the Elders* explains that the karmic winds are those breaths that move in and out of the nostrils regularly, whereas the innate wisdom wind is the special type of wind that is only controlled through advanced yogic manipulations.[26] If the totality of innate wisdom wind is incorrectly circulated through the respiratory system, a person may become severely ill or die; for this reason, these yogic practices are considered dangerous and are restricted to advanced contemplatives. The third type of vitality channel is the body's "life force" (*bla*), which is physiologically defined as the distilled essence of the body's reproductive substance, the refine substance that results from the total metabolic system that creates each of the bodily constituents. This life force is said to migrate throughout the body along a predictable track over the duration of a month, although the precise course of this track differs according to the various tantras, medical texts, and astrological texts in which this subject is discussed in detail.

Another important channel described in the *Four Tantras* tradition is the life channel (*srog rtsa*). This channel is not named in the *Explanatory Tantra*'s fourfold functional division of channels, enumerated in that book's fourth chapter as described above, but it is mentioned in the context of embryology in the *Explanatory Tantra*'s second chapter. That chapter states that the life channel develops from the navel during the sixth week of gestation. The identification of this life channel in relation to the other circulatory channels operative in adult physiology was, and still is, hotly contested among medical and religious scholars. Some medical scholars claimed that this life channel corresponds to the black blood channel; still others claimed it was the white channel or the spine itself.[27] Summarizing Lodrö Gyelpo's position on this issue, the Sakya scholar Tsultrim Gyeltsen posits that the life channel that initiates embryonic growth is to be identified as the central channel (*dbu ma*) of the tantric traditions; that is, these scholars, both of whom are eminent for their medical as well as religious scholarship and practice, argue that the two terms are synonymous for the same circulatory function.

Although the *Four Tantras* did not organize its presentation of the circulatory system in the same manner as the religious tantras did, it is clear that many Tibetan medical scholars over the centuries have been concerned with reconciling the two systems, and that the discrepancies bothered them. The human circulatory system is one of the most complex and heavily theorized topics in Buddhist medical and religious scholasticism: this aspect of human physiology was important to everyone, and yet it is in religious contexts that the topic is most richly considered. In the twelfth century, the Sakya master Drakpa Gyeltsen wrote that it is vitally important for religious practitioners to know about the body's circulatory physiology because the body is the basis for meditation practice. He cites the *Saṃpuṭi* tantra to say that, "[Even if you knew all] the rituals of the 84,000 divisions of the dharma, without knowing the nature of the body none of those [practices] would have any effect."[28] Attempting contemplative practices without a clear understanding of the body, Drakpa Gyeltsen continues, is like trying to milk an animal by tugging at its horns. Taking reverence for the body to an extreme, some tantric traditions focused the very heart of enlightened essence in the clarifie reproductive substance: for males, the semen. All other aspects of the esoteric body were likewise given divine import. "Our own body is primodially spontaneously present as the maṇḍala of the Victorious Ones," intones the *Heart-Essence of the Dakinis*, "and all the channel constitutents and quintessential essences are actually Buddhas, Heroes, and Sky Dancers." Only through recognition of the purity of our bodies is enlightenment possible, this tantra proclaims:

> Should you not recognize your own body as the maṇḍala of the Buddhas, and thus abandon the quintessential essences, meditate on your tutelar deity externally, make offerings externally, search for primodial gnosis externally, and meditate (on it externally), it is impossible that you can become free from cyclic existence even should you amass these spiritual accomplishments for three zillion eons.[29]

In Chapter 5, we will further consider how knowledge of the body was so critical to religious practitioners and what impact this may have had on medical traditions.

Characterizing embodiment: gendered, defective and "normal" bodies

Tibetan religious and medical writers clearly found themselves amid numerous competing models of the psychosomatic body. In many works, adult physiology is a subject that directly follows embryology, clearly linking the two topics; in some cases, physiological details are presented in the context of embryology itself. To return to the central question at hand for this chapter, then, what have we learned so far about how Tibetan writers identified the main character of their embryological narratives? First, remember that here we are not addressing the symbolic level on which the embryological narrative may depict a fictional or idealized Buddhist religious practitioner (the topic of the next chapter), but rather the portrayal of a more literal character, the embryo itself. Beginning with the obvious, then, we could presume that the embryo is something that will grow into an ordinary adult body – the term "ordinary" implying that this adult is assumed not to possess the extraordinary body of a Buddha. We would expect, therefore, that the embryo shares a physiology with the adult body (or that if this is not the case, it would be noted). And yet we noted earlier that although medical physiology, and indeed medical theory overall, is dominated by the theories of systemic processes and digestive heat, these physiological components play little or no role in medical accounts of fetal development. We will see in chapters to come that to the extent that medical embryologies are concerned with the developing physiological function of the fetus, it is only the circulatory system of channels and winds that are addressed. And these, we recall, are the matters of physiology in which religious and medical thinkers *share* an interest. Let us save this thought for now, however, and think about some of the other aspects of embodiment that are addressed in embryological accounts.

What type of body it is that embryology describes is far from straightforward, and narratives of human development turn out to be sites for working out some of the more difficult issues in medical and religious physiology. For example, most such Tibetan narratives educate their readers about gendered bodies. Although in common parlance today the terms sex and gender are used interchangeably, the distinction between the terms has been debated. For some theorists, sex refers to fixed biological aspects of being male or female, and gender to certain behavioral, social, and/or psychological features of individuals. Sex emphasizes the fixed and objective marker of a particular set of genitalia on the body, in other words, whereas gender is a more malleable and interpretive quality of a person's social status and behavior. Other theorists, however, such as Judith Butler, object to this dichotomy, arguing that sex is objective or natural only in the context of discursive practices that deem it so; sex is thus as culturally constructed as gender. Assuming male and female sex to be fixed, objective and natural this arguments goes, obscures the fact that different cultures may categorize sexual difference differently. Indeed, in the case of Indian and Tibetan literature, a third category is added to the male/female pair for individuals whose genital presentation is not clearly identified as male or female. This third category in Buddhist and medical texts, a category most commonly termed *ma ning* in Tibetan and *paṇḍaka* in Sanskrit, although other terms are used too, has been carefully examined by Janet Gyatso.[30] As in the materials Gyatso examines, it is largely physical characteristics that are addressed in the case of Tibetan embryological accounts. But because the texts go beyond an objective assignation of genitalia to a valuing of one set of genitalia over the others, there are clear social or ideological aspects to the discussion as well.

The topic of sex determination is not an insignificant one in Tibetan medical commentaries. In fact, if one judges by page length, no other topic during their commentaries on the *Explanatory Tantra*'s second chapter rates higher in importance to medical writers such as Kyempa Tsewang or Lodrö Gyelpo. In this corpus there are several theories on how the developing embryo acquires a particular set of sexual characteristics. One verse in the *Explanatory Tantra* states that conception occurring on the odd days (the first, third, fifth and so on) following the completion of a woman's menstrual cycle will likely result in the generation of a boy fetus, while conception occurring on the even days will result in a girl.[31] In this scheme, which also appears in the Āyurvedic *Heart of Medicine* tradition, the third sex (*ma ning*) is not mentioned. Only a few verses later, paradoxically, the *Explanatory Tantra* states that sex determination is made on the basis of the ratio of male and female reproductive substances present during conception. The *Explanatory Tantra* notes,

> More [male] reproductive substance (*khu ba*) will produce a boy, and more [female] blood (*khrag*) will produce a girl;
> even [amounts] will produce a child of indeterminate sex (*ma ning*), and if [the mixture] splits, twins will be born.[32]

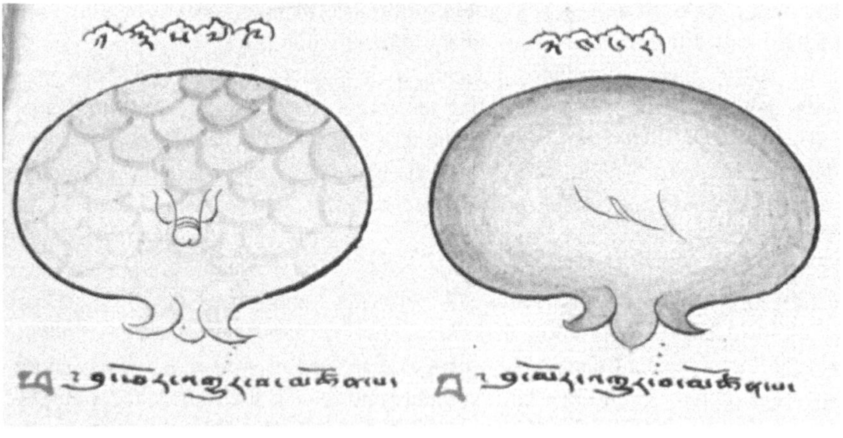

Figure 4.1 The medical painting explains that conception on odd days will bring about a boy, and conception on even days, a girl.

Interestingly, not only is this scheme found in the *Heart of Medicine*, as we saw earlier, but it may also be compared to a Middle Persian tradition described by Bruce Lincoln; that texts posits, "whenever the man's seed is more powerful, then there is a son. When the woman's seed is more powerful, there is a daughter. And when the two seeds are equal, then twins and triplets come into being."[33] While documentation of connections to regions outside India would be fascinating, such notions are found also within the Indian traditions on the topic, such as in Cakara's *Compendium* and the *Niruktopaniṣad*, in addition to the *Heart of Medicine*, and so connections beyond South Asia would be difficult to prove.[34] Going into more detail, the *Garbha Upaniṣad*, for example, claims that, "An excess of the father's semen produces a male, an excess of the mother's semen a girl, and an equal amount of the two semens, a eunuch (or, rather, a hermaphrodite, *na-puṃsaka*). A troubled spirit produces the blind, the lame, hunchback and dwarfs. When the sperm is crushed by the wind and splits into two, twins are born."[35]

So far, we have two models of how the embryo becomes sexually differentiated. But there are more. Another theory on the origins of sex identification, a model that we have seen in Indian Buddhist Abhidharma texts, is presented also in the sūtra tradition of embryology and those who follow it.[36] Lodrö Gyelpo summarizes,

> Alternatively, when the intermediate state being enters the reproductive substances of the parents, it will think "that is mine" – whatever child is born as a male is repelled by the father and is attracted to the mother; whatever child is born as a female is attracted to the father and repelled by the mother. Through recognizing this, it is conceived and enters the womb.[37]

Here it is essential to conception itself that sex identification be made – without sexual characteristics, an ordinary being is not conceived. Many Tibetan embryological accounts repeat the notion that emotions of aversion and attraction toward the two parents are central to the success of conception and the formation of a sexually defined and gendered human.[38]

Despite these statements, albeit contradictory, that fetal sex may be predetermined, after the third week of gestation the *Explanatory Tantra* and its commentaries recommend a series of ritual and medicinal means, which are derived from the Indic *Heart of Medicine* tradition (and before that perhaps from the *Ṛgveda* and *Atharvaveda*) to ensure the development of a male child.[39] While in Tibetan literature no such rituals are recommended to promote the growth of female or indeterminate sexual characteristics, the *Heart of Medicine* itself does offer advice for those wishing to conceive girls. Kyempa Tsewang and Lodrö Gyelpo claim that rituals to ensure the birth of a boy must be performed at this point because in the third week the embryo's sex is still indeterminate.[40] The first page of this book described several such techniques and, while abandoned by many today, these approaches are not only artifacts of the past: contemporary Tibetan doctor, Yeshé Dönden, described various methods in a 1980 article, insisting that religious rituals can overpower the karmic destiny of the fetus. "In other words," he writes, "even if the foetus has the karma to be born a female, religious rites can postpone the karmic action for this lifetime." Dönden describes several ritual options.[41] In chapter six, I will consider the power of religious and medical procedures, such as rituals and other behaviors, to overwrite karmic destiny. Here, our attention is drawn merely to the multitude of notions about sex determination in accounts of early human development.

The *Explanatory Tantra*, despite having earlier claimed that sex was determined at conception, states that the sexual characteristics are presented definit ively in the fourth week of gestation, at which time the embryo will be rounded (*gor gor po*), oval (*mer mer po*) or elongated (*nar nar po*) according to whether it will be born as a boy, girl or child of indeterminate sex, respectively.[42] Finally, the issue emerges again at the end of gestation: the *Explanatory Tantra* notes that when a boy is about to be born, the right side of the woman's belly is fir and higher up, her body is light, she sees men in her dreams, and her right breast expresses milk first. A girl baby will be born, conversely, if the left side of her belly is higher, her body heavy, she sees women in her dreams, and milk appears first in her left breast, additional indictors being an urge to be around men and a sudden pleasure in singing, dancing and jewelry.[43]

What is interesting about these conflicting views is their untroubled presence side by side in a single chapter of the *Four Tantras*. Rather than resolving conflict by compromise or by choosing one theory over others, all available theories have been offered, leaving later commentators to cope with the contradictions. However, most commentators seem equally untroubled by the multiple views,

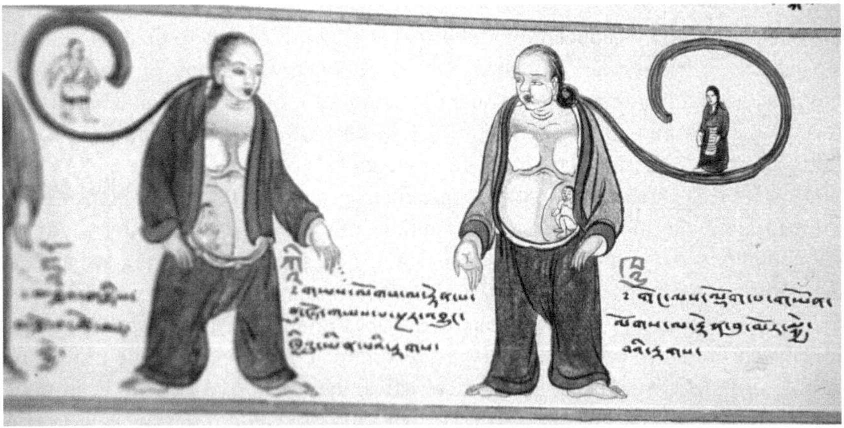

Figure 4.2 The *Four Tantras* tradition also states that the child will be a boy if the woman's belly is heavy on the right side and a girl if she is heavy on the left side.

content to repeat them without worrying about reconciliation or adjudication. Why would this be so? After noting a contradiction in the mechanics of conception in a Middle Persian embryological treatise, Lincoln comments that "The very fact of such a contradiction is itself instructive, however, revealing as it does, how little concerned this passage is with the physiology of reproduction in the last analysis."[44] In the chapters to come, I will propose a similar interpretation, suggesting that we will learn more from embryology in Tibetan literature if we see it as a story of something other than the empirically verifiable physical embryo.

Fetal bodies as a whole are not the only thing gendered by embryological narratives: individual fetal body parts are also assigned male or female origins. The *Explanatory Tantra* explains that, "From the father's reproductive substance the bones, brain and spine are generated; from the mother's menstrual blood (*zla mtshan*) the flesh, blood and vital and vessel organs are generated."[45] Subsequent Tibetan commentators find little to say about this verse. It appears to be a mainly tantric tradition: it is not present in the Indic medical tradition represented by the *Heart of Medicine*, nor in the exoteric Buddhist tradition represented by texts such as Vasubhandu's *Commentary* or the *Entering the Womb* sūtra. Structurally similar correlations are, however, found in Buddhist tantric texts, such as the *Saṃvarodaya* tantra, which attributes the embryo's sinew, marrow and reproductive essence (*khu ba*) to the father's contribution and its skin, flesh and blood to the mother's contribution; or the *Kālacakra* tantra, which claims marrow, bones, circulatory channels (*nāḍī*) are created by the father's reproductive substance, and skin, flesh and blood by the mother's; or Longchenpa's corpus, which links brain, marrow, bone, fat and muscle to the father's "white" contribution and the skin, flesh, blood, hair and lymph to the mother's "red" contribution.[46] In an East Asian context, Bernard Faure connects the tradition of attributing soft and red components (skin, blood, flesh, fat, heart and internal organs) to women, and hard and white components (hair, nails, teeth, bones, ligaments) to Chinese funerary rituals, noting also a parallel with Greek and Egyptian notions of conception.[47]

The assignation of sexual characteristics is not a morally neutral issue, and thus the characterization of the embryo goes beyond a description of genitalia to a socio-cultural and ideological statement about gendered bodies and their relative value. While women's bodies are clearly inferior, embryological narratives in the medical tradition also discuss varieties of "defective" bodies. Impurities in the male or female reproductive substances are generally said to lead to failure to conceive, as mentioned above. In some cases, however, conception may occur, but these impurities will result in a child with physical deformities, such as a cleft lip, extremely short stature, or too many or too few limbs or sense organs. Kyempa Tsewang states that such abnormalities may also be caused by a poorly proportioned accumulation of the natural elements, the bad karma of the transmigrating consciousness, the parents having focused on such an object during intercourse, or evil spirits.[48] Such statements provide interesting evidence of Tibetan notions of physical imperfection and normalcy. Note, for example, that birth as a person of ambiguous sex is not typically considered physically defective; nor is the female form explicitly labeled a defective male, as in early Greek literature.[49] By contrast, Indian Buddhist texts list physical characteristics that disqualify one from monastic ordination, such as dwarfism, missing limbs, blindness, deafness, or leprosy, sometimes including the atypical configuration of sexual organs.[50] Nevertheless, boy children are clearly considered more desirable than girl children and in medical texts in general, women's bodies are considered different enough from men to warrant special nosologies: certain chapters in medical texts are specifically devoted to "female diseases," the bulk of medical literature thus oriented specifically toward the male as the human exemplar. "Normal" bodies are without question typically configured male bodies

Female physiology

I began this chapter with a plan to identify the main character in the story of embryogenesis and I have focused on the developing embryo, doubtless for most readers the natural protagonist. Some may ask, however, what about the pregnant woman? Is she not an important figure in the story of gestation? In this chapter so far, we have focused on male bodies, which are, indeed, the focus of nearly all Buddhist and medical descriptions of physiology in Tibet. In Tibetan medicine generally, female bodies are discussed only in isolated contexts, the default body being male. In this section, we will examine how embryological narratives present the female body, a character whose role in these stories is curiously neglected.

Many early Indian Buddhist texts depict female bodies in graphic detail as objects of revulsion for a monastic audience. Such passages, luridly presenting the repugnance of the female body, have been well documented in studies such as Liz Wilson's *Charming Cadavers: Horrific Figurations of the Feminine in Indian Buddhist Hagiographic Literature*. Robert Kritzer has also studied misogynist presentations of female bodies, particularly those found in the accounts of gestation in Vasubhandu's *Commentary* and the *Entering the Womb* sūtra. These passages emphasize the disgusting, malodorous qualities of the vagina and the womb. Vasubhandu's *Commentary*, for instance, characterizes the vagina as,

> like an excrement-hole, a cruelly foul-smelling, dark pool of ordure, the home of many thousands of families of worms, permanently oozing, constantly in need of cleansing, hot, slimy, and drenched in semen, blood, mucus, and impurities, terrifying to behold, covered by a thin, perforated skin, the great ulcer-like wound in the body, produced from the result of previous karma...[51]

The *Entering the Womb* sūtra's view, upon which Vasubhandu's presentation is apparently based, is similarly colorful, although offered in the sad context of describing the removal of a dead fetus in the thirty-eighth week of gestation:

> Nanda, if that [fetus] residing in the womb performed many negative and non-virtuous actions in previous lifetimes and then enters another womb, due to such causes and conditions, when it is about to emerge from the womb its hands and feet will be upside down and crossed; unable to turn around, it will die. At that time a knowledgable woman or a skilled doctor, smearing his or her hands with soft butter or oil, or the melted oil of a Shalmali tree or another soft substance, will pick up a sharp knife in his or her hands. [The vagina] is a nauseating swamp hole, extremely foul-smelling like a pack animal's excrement, inhabited by countless hundreds of thousands of worms and dripping with unclean substances, putrid and rotting with reproductive substances, blood and fumes – if you see it, you will be repulsed. Into that unclean place ... his or her fingers will be inserted, and with a sharp knife the body of the [fetus] residing in the womb will be cut into pieces and removed from the mother's womb. As a result, in the experience of miserable suffering that is intolerable and harsh, that mother will face death. Even if she does not die, it will be no different than death.[52]

Some of the disgusting features of the vagina seen in these passages may also be found as descriptive of other aspects of the human body – any human body – in meditation manuals for monastic audiences, as discussed at the beginning of this chapter. Here, they have simply been adopted to describe female anatomy in particular. Significantly, Kritzer points out that while Indian medical texts such as the *Heart of Medicine* may admit the vagina to be unpleasant when diseased, it is not characterized as such in general in that tradition. Thus, a negative orientation to the female body may be traced to early Indian Buddhist presentations, he argues, not to Indic medical traditions which, although still considering the male to be the default body in most contexts, nonetheless lack the stridently derogatory language of the Buddhist text.

In the Tibetan embryological narratives that are the focus of this book, the female body is addressed in several contexts. First, to describe how conception occurs, medical writers must reflect on reproductive substances and fertility. Recognizing that female fertility was periodic and related to monthly cycles, they discussed the mechanics of menstruation in some detail – why it occurs, when it occurs, and how it occurs – requiring a foray into female reproductive physiology. Medical commentators drew on both Indian medical sources and Buddhist tantric sources for these matters.

According to general Tibetan medical physiology, male and female reproductive substances are created at the end of the metabolic processing of food and drink that creates each of the bodily constituents, as outlined above. Contemporary scholar Tubten Püntsok explains that at the end of the metabolic process,

> Marrow (*rkang*) divides into essence and waste: the essence becomes *khu ba*, with white and red elements, and the waste becomes the oiliness of skin and feces. That *khu ba* again divides into essence and waste: the essence becomes the ultimate radiance of the physical constituents, and the waste becomes the white and red elements, the seeds that will be caught in the womb.[53]

Thus, the purified essence of the sixth bodily constituent, marrow, is *khu ba*, a generic term for male and female reproductive substances. The *khu ba* that is the purified essence of marrow goes through another metabolic process, resulting in a further purified essence known as "ultimate radiance" (*mtha' thug pa'i mdangs*). The waste matter of that process is the reproductive substance – the "white element" (*khams dkar*) or "red element"(*khams dmar*) – also called a "seed" (*sa bon*), for it is what is caught in the womb at the moment of conception. While the "white element" is another name for the male reproductive substance, and the "red element" is another name for the female reproductive substance, both males and females generate red and white elements. In the female, the white element creates breast milk.[54] The term *khu ba* is thus used on two levels: first, it is the general term for the last of the seven bodily constituents, which is the reproductive substance of males and females; second, when the metabolic process is examined in closer detail, we see that the seventh constituent also undergoes metabolic transformation, resulting in a waste product, sometimes called *khu ba* and sometimes *khams* that is, itself, the "seed" of conception. Tubten Püntsok explains further that the "ultimate radiance," which is the most purified essence of the constituents, combines with an essence (*dwangs ma*) of blood inside the existence channel and this becomes the potent force abiding at the heart that pervades the entire body, ensuring a long life, clarifying the senses, and causing overall bodily brightness and radiance.[55] In discussing when conception can occur, Kyempa Tsewang explains that it is the female "red element" that is periodically expelled as menstrual blood:

> The waste [that has been separated from] the radiance (*mdangs*) has two parts, the white and red elements. From those, the red part passes from the reproductive vesicles (*bsam se'u*) to the womb (*mngal*), and that very blood [i.e., the red element] that is gathered there every month [is the menstrual blood].[56]

While Tubten Püntsok's description of this process is fairly clear, the various and sometimes overlapping uses of the terms *khu ba*, *dwangs ma*, *khams*, and *mdangs* in descriptions of digestive and reproductive physiology generate some ambiguity. To complicate matters, tantric physiologies also address these processes using different terminology. Kyempa Tsewang seems untroubled by this, however, citing the *Hevajra* tantra to explain how menstrual substances are emitted from the body given the tantric three channel physiology: menstrual blood, which is itself the woman's reproductive substance, falls from the lower tip of the right side, red-colored flavor (*ro ma*) channel in women.[57] As to how these tantric channels may be understood in relation to the channels of medical physiology, this has been a thorny and well debated issue for many centuries of Tibetan writers, as discussed above. In this context, Zurkhar Lodrö Gyelpo posits, for instance, that the black existence channel connects to the flavo channel and the white existence channel connects to the solitary channel, and that the white and red elements may thus travel between them.[58]

Exactly how the menstrual emission leaves the woman's body is not entirely straightforward either. In addressing the conditions making conception possible, the *Four Tantras* describes the period of life when a woman is fertile:

> In a woman between the ages of twelve and fifty
> blood that accumulates from the clarified essence (*dwangs ma*) each month
> flows, dark and odorless, from two large channels and
> drawn to the door of the womb by the winds, it falls for three days.[59]

Here, the clarified essence is that substance collected in the reproductive vesicles (*bsam se'u*) at the end of the metabolic process. The term *dwangs ma* sometimes refers to the nutritive essences that are the first of the bodily constituents to develop from a person's intake of food and drink into the stomach, as we have seen. The term may also refer to the substance created at the *end* of the metabolic process, namely the seventh constituent of *khu ba*. In the context of menstruation, it is this substance that accumulates in the reproductive vesicles of a woman and is then emitted from the womb at certain times of the month as waste. How the substance makes this journey, however, is a topic of some debate. Kyempa Tsewang takes recourse to citing early medical works in Tibetan, the *Heart of Medicine* and Sumtön Yeshé Zung's *Four Tantras* commentary, explaining that according to those traditions, two channels lead to the "mouth" of the uterus or womb (*bu snod* or *mngal*, two terms often used interchangeably) from the right and left of the reproductive vesicles, and those channels further connect to the vagina, allowing the menstrual blood to leave the woman's body.[60] This may seem straightforward, but Zurkhar Lodrö Gyelpo takes issue with the description. "If the two channels that run from the reproductive vesicles are connected with the mouth of the womb," he complains, "it's illogical to say that blood goes inside the womb, because the mouth of the womb faces downwards!"[61] Although Lodrö Gyelpo disagrees that the reproductive vesicles connect to the *mouth* of the womb, he does not dispute connection of another sort. Thus, he explains,

> For most women from age twelve to age fifty, the red substance (*khu ba dmar po*), which has gradually been processed out from the nutrients (*dangs ma*) of food, abides in the reproductive vesicles, and it itself is

> the blood (*khrag*) that collects in the reproductive vesicles each month. That blood also ... passes from that connection of the two great channels at the left and right of the reproductive vesicles and womb, and it enters into the womb. At that point, that very blood, its color a little dark and odorless, is made to exit the door of the womb (*mngal*) by the downward-voiding wind; for up to three days a little bit of it drips, and then it stops.[62]

Worth noting here, is the equation of the reproductive substance or "red element" with the substance that is emitted during menstruation. Menstrual emission is not the same substance as the blood in the rest of the body, therefore, although it is often simply called "blood" (*khrag*); in the context of discussing menstruation, the emitted substance is also called *zla mtshan*, or "monthly sign." To distinguish male and female reproductive substances in the context of conception, medical texts will most often refer to the former as *khu ba*, and the latter as *khrag*, although there is a sense in which both are technically *khu ba* (and indeed on some occasions they are designated as such). Controversies over the precise definition, origins and behaviors of the female and male reproductive substances in Indian medical literature have been thoroughly studied by Rahul Peter Das in his *Origin of the Life of a Human Being*.[63] These issues are intriguing and deserving of a deeper analysis in the case of Tibetan traditions too. While the embryological literature discussed in this book does not go into much greater detail than is addressed here, a broader study of Tibetan literature on such matters would no doubt shed further light on the complexities of female physiology.

While female reproductive physiology is central to this technical discussion, notice that these authors are not, in fact, saying much about the woman herself – about her experience of pregnancy, or about how to best care for her during this period. This subject, for the most part, is of little interest to medical commentators, and of even less interest to religious writers when considering the subject of early human development. In the context of embryology, the *Four Tantras* and its commentarial tradition make no more than a handful of comments about women as persons beyond their reproductive physiologies. How to recognize that a woman is menstruating is discussed in a few words, written for the benefi of men wishing to plan fruitful sexual activity (the woman herself would, of course, know that she is menstruating). Kyempa Tsewang explains, for instance, that when menstruating, the woman

> is weak without there being any other disorders, her facial appearance is thin and poor, her breasts and waist quiver, and her eyes and belly shake and tremble. Healthy women will not conceive a child [at this time]. Every month blood emerges, and she exhibits the signs of the womb opening. Desire for a man is also regarded as a sign of a woman who is menstruating.[64]

After a woman has conceived, brief mention is made of how she feels: the *Four Tantras* states that a woman's "desire has been satisfied and her body becomes weary and heavy."[65] Kyempa Tsewang's commentary contributes nothing to expand on this verse, however. Zurkhar Lodrö Gyelpo also has nothing of his own to add; he merely cites the Indian medical tradition to add that the woman's "heart flutters a little, she is lazy and tired, and her hair falls out."[66] Similarly, and remarkably, very little is said of the woman's nine month experience of pregnancy. Medical literature is silent on the topic until the end of gestation. When it is time to deliver the baby, the *Four Tantras* comments,

> The signs that the birth is imminent are sluggishness,
> relaxing of the womb, heaviness in the lower body, pain in the pelvis and waist,
> and pain in the abdomen and bladder;
> the vagina opens, much urine [passes] and pain rises uncontrollably.[67]

Here too, however, Kyempa Tsewang's commentary does nothing but summarize the verse, and Lodrö Gyelpo again finds no inspiration to offer comments of his own, providing little more than additional citations from the Indian medical tradition. For these medical commentators, what is interesting about embryology is most certainly not the woman carrying the baby.

The absence of the woman in Tibetan accounts of embryology is all the more notable when compared to the Indian medical tradition of Vāgbhaṭa, whose work was so influential on Tibetan medicine in other respects. In the *Heart of Medicine*, a woman is said to be fertile between the ages of twelve and fifty, in a verse nearly identical to that of the *Four Tantras.* Similar, also, is the verse on the signs of conception. In addition to these passages, however, the *Heart of*

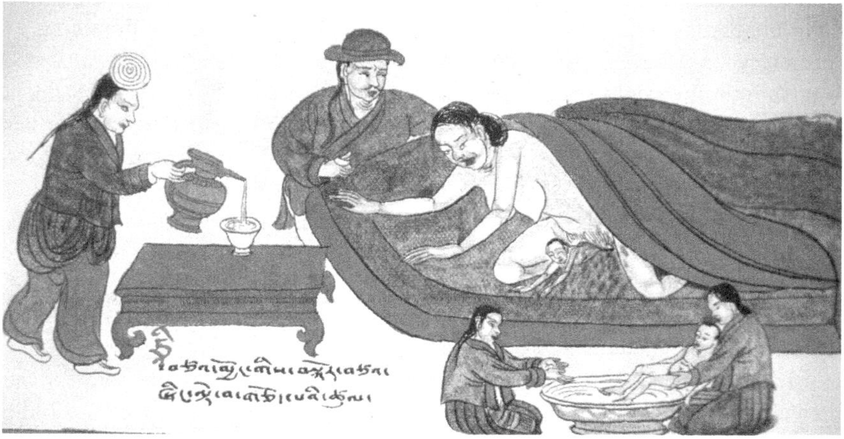

Figure 4.3 A woman gives birth.

Medicine has much to say about the condition and care of the pregnant woman.[68] It describes specific methods of sexual intercourse that will ensure a male child and offers behavioral recommendations for menstruating women, pregnant women and women in labor. The text explains, for instance, that,

> She who has conceived
> should be waited upon by husband and attendants
> who are agreeable and helpful;
> she should always consume
> fresh butter, clarified butter and milk [69]

To address the woman's discomfort in the seventh month, moreover, the text recommends special foods and ointments:

> In that case fresh butter, the syrup of a juniper tree (*rgya shug*),
> sweet tasting medicines, and infusions are helpful.
> Feed her foods that are sweet and light,
> a little salty and oily.
> Rub her chest, breasts and belly
> with an ointment of Sandalwood and orchid.
> Smear in a mixture of Tellicherry bark and rabbit's blood
> with the "three fruits" [concoction] or *Eneya*.
> Rubbing her with an infusion of sesame oil
> and the leaves of Oleander, massage it in.
> She should be anointed with orchid, Neem, Indian madder, and basil.
> She should be attended to with bathing and rubbing
> in the water of a sweet Barberry tree.[70]

Numerous additional prescriptions of special foods, ointments, enemas and baths are recommended to relieve discomfort in the eighth and ninth months of pregnancy. As the end of pregnancy approaches, the text suggests that the woman retire to a delivery room attended by midwives, and ointments, baths, a thin gruel, specific postures and other techniques are prescribed to care for her during labor and delivery. These passages are then followed by another long section on one and a half months of postpartum care, thus ending the *Heart of Medicine* chapter on "the entry of the body into the womb" (*lus kyi rum du zhugs pa*).

While in many ways the *Heart of Medicine* and *Four Tantras* are similar, and while *Four Tantras* commentators often cite the *Heart of Medicine* as an authority on medical matters, here, by contrast, in the discussion of the *woman's* experience of pregnancy, a striking difference is observed. While care for the pregnant woman and scrutiny of her experience is a central part of the Indic medical tradition, in Tibet very little of this is retained as part of embryology. These issues are not ignored by Tibetan medical scholars entirely. Methods and rituals to induce birth in a long or difficult labor are discussed in chapters on pediatric disorders (*byis pa'i nad*), found in chapters seventy-one through seventy-three of the third book of the *Four Tantras*. Here, there are practices and rituals described for ensuring a safe and auspicious birth, caring for the woman after birth and for the new infant, disposing of the placenta, nursing, and cutting the umbilical cord, plus ceremonies to perform after birth, rituals to ensure that male babies stay male, and rituals for naming the child. The chapters on women's disorders (*mo nad*), chapters seventy-four through seventy-six of the *Secret Oral Tantra*, the third book of the *Four Tantras*, also contain information on gynecological and obstetric problems, including amenorrhea or menorrhagia (*khrag tshabs*), various uterine diseases and tumors, and eight obstetric problems: disorders of pregnancy (*mtshan ma'i nad*), various uterine diseases and protracted labor (*bu ma phyin pa*), breech birth (*mgo mjug log pa*), adherent placenta (*rog ma phyin pa*), uterine prolapse (*bu snod lug pa*), postnatal hemorrhage (*khrag ma chod pa*), postnatal ailments (*nad gzhug las pa*) and postnatal infections (*dug thabs*). Another source for specifically female disorders is chapter forty-three, which describes diseases of the female genitalia (*mo mtshan nad*) caused by excessive sexual activity, unsuitable diet, or certain behaviors during menstruation or after childbirth. (Disorders of the male genitalia are described in the topic on sexual diseases (*gsang ba'i nad*), in the forty-second chapter, also caused by excessive sexual activity and including painful sensations, urethral obstructions, ulceration and rashes.) Other sources for similar types of information are texts on pharmacology in which prescriptions for contraceptives or abortifacients, or remedies for menstrual disorders and so forth are described.

What is notable here is that ordinary care for the woman during pregnancy and delivery, and even any significant observation of her experience of pregnancy, is simply not a part of Tibetan medical accounts of fetal development. How might we explain this? Perhaps it is that here, too, we see evidence that embryology, for medical scholars of the renaissance period, was more essentially a religious topic than a medical topic. Conception and gestation were matters that first brought to mind the authority of the religious canon, with its focus on the physiology of the circulatory system and its neglect of female experience. The early period of Tibetan medical history, which was dominated by the Indic *Heart of Medicine* as the first respected exemplar of medical literature, was slowly overshadowed by the *Four Tantras'* rise to fame. Giving way to the renaissance flurry of scholasticism with its increasing emphasis on Buddhist paradigms of thought and authority, embryology, as a topic of thought and writing, slipped quietly under the authority of Buddhism, even for medical writers. One effect of this shift was the loss of the woman in the official stories of gestation. In the context of embryology, women's reproductive physiologies were simply the raw material in which humans were incubated, and while the pathological experience of problematic pregnancies were addressed elsewhere in medical literature, the liberative motifs that were part of many Tibetan embryological narratives did not exist for the pregnant woman.

Encountering the narrative's central subject

Embryology in Tibetan literature tells a story that identifies and defines a particular type of human being. In this chapter, I have considered some of the ways that Tibetan medical and religious authors characterize the adult body, and I have asked how embryological narratives played a role in this characterization. While medical models focus heavily on the body's digestive physiology and its systemic (humoral) organization, these are areas of little concern to religious authors. The geometric semantics of the body's circulatory system, on the other hand, is a topic of great concern in religious *and* medical literature, although the details are contested. While Tibetan physiological theories are diverse and often contradictory, they all depict a male body characterized by features originating in the womb. Embryological narratives give human bodies gender, morally charging the fetus on the basis of its sexual organs. During gestation, human bodies are defined as defective or normal, again shaping the body in ways that are not neutral in significance. In many texts, as we will see further in chapter six, the story of embryogenesis is itself embedded in a narrative of cosmic proportions: it is not solely about the birth of a new human being, but also about the enfolding of that being into a wider, universal context that is constitutionally identical to it. In other words, embryology tells us that humans are made up of the same stuff as the universe. The fetus is literally created by food, which constitutes and sustains the very substances of the human body; by the natural elements, which make possible its structure and activity; and by its own self-organizing processes. The identity of this narrative's character, an idealized male human, is formed by a set of adaptive interactions, and the border between individual and context is not physical, as would be marked by skin, for example; rather, it is deeply interactive and contextualized.

In this chapter, I have discussed a fictionalized fetus as the main character in the stories at hand. We have noted that the pregnant woman does not make much of an appearance in this story; we will again argue in chapters to come that, in Tibet, embryology is not centrally about that potential mother. Indeed, perhaps it is not about her at all. There is another character in these Tibetan narratives, however: the one who is represented symbolically by the embryo, the practitioner of meditation. That character will be the topic of the next chapter.

5

GESTATION AND THE RELIGIOUS PATH

In the real lives of religious practitioners in Asia, ritual actions modeled after embryogenesis are enacted in public and private ways. Complementing the complex contemplative practices that are formed around embryological theory, there are various popularly accessible religious practices that are modeled after human conception, fetal development and birth. From initiation rites that prescribe "incubation" in womb-like huts, to rejuvenation therapies, to preparations by alchemists, yogis and other contemplatives, Asian religious traditions describe methods for bodily transformation that are expressed in terms of gestation and birth. Such practices are ancient: in Vedic ideas of rebirth through sacrificial initiation, the sacrificer tossed himself, as a seed, into the sacrificial fire the womb, in the hope of being reborn into a new self-created reality. Internalizing the sacrifice, later yogic practices modeled after human fetal development are a complex extension of these rites, a literal re-enactment of the most primordial of bodily transformations, that of embryogenesis.

These are not isolated practices restricted to remote groups of specialists; rather, the power of embryological symbolism prevails across Asia. There are numerous "womb-caves," sacred to Hindus, Buddhists and Taoists, where the connections are explicit. The entrance to southeastern Tibet's Cari, for instance, revered as the home of both Hindu and Buddhist deities, is a narrow fissure called the goddess' vagina, and it holds a lake of red mercuric oxide, identifie as the sexual fluids of the resident divinities.[1] Francois Bizot examines Buddhist cave rituals in Cambodia, where the theme is rebirth as a new being who will not experience rebirth again; the body is symbolically re-formed by returning to the womb. These rites are performed by lay Buddhists and have a more esoteric component for monks. Rituals are performed in multi-chambered caves with pools of mineral-colored water and glistening stalactites. Participants are told explicitly that they are entering a womb, and the geological features of caves are given appropriate names: stalactites are called "umbilical cords" and practitioners are instructed to cleanse their faces in pools of colored water referred to as "amniotic wells." During their stay in the cave, contemplatives practice specifi breathing exercises. Cambodian rites such as these are modeled after creation texts describing the development of a primal "dhamma being" fashioned embryologically from the five elements; it is this primal experience that meditators attempt to create for themselves upon entering the womb-cave.[2] The Japanese Buddhist Shugendo cult of sacred mountains also features similar rituals.[3]

In this book, I do not examine the numerous contemporary and historical popular ceremonies using embryological symbolism as the basis for ritual action, as in the case of such practices described above where individuals enter physical spaces representing wombs. Because I am looking at literary expressions and uses of embryology, and not at the real-life activities of religious agents or medical practitioners today or in the past, I will forego the fascinating question of how people really acted or still do act, using their knowledge of human development. Rather, in this chapter I will ask, who is it that is signifie by the character of the embryo, if not the physical embryo itself? What are the stories told about fetal growth, and who are the stories about? The embryo characterized in Tibetan narratives does not necessarily refer to a literal (even if fic tional) embryo. In some esoteric texts, it is clear that the embryo is meant to signify a religious contemplative who wishes to be "spiritually reborn" and will therefore enact the process of gestation through meditation (or so the story goes). In this chapter, I will consider how this symbolic character is portrayed.

This chapter will also look at the story being told about such a character. Although the processes of gestation and birth form a conceptual basis for a variety of rituals across Asia, I will focus primarily on embryological rhetoric in Tibetan Buddhist presentations of religious contemplative practices and models of the religious path to liberation. Embryological stories depict exemplary Buddhist practitioners of morality and meditation who, beginning with spiritual qualities that are embryonic in achievement, undergo the soteriologically charged, metaphysical activity of gestation and rebirth. The stories about these characters are conflicting however: in one model, the suffering of gestation and the agony of birth are used to encourage religious practice; in another model, gestation and rebirth are viewed positively as opportunities to reach new spiritual attainments. In examining the relationship between Tibetan embryologies and models of the religious path, I will thus also be considering the *discourse* of the many stories of human development. A narrative's story, or that which is narrated, is not the same as *how* the story is narrated, or its discourse. Stories are often told in such a way as to express a moral, teach a lesson or present an interesting experience, for example.[4] We will find narratives of gestation that use various discursive tools to promote specifi religious practices: some are poetic, some are highly structured, and many offer particular representations of space that are integrally related to the story's underlying message. As it turns out, *how* stories of gestation are told is controversial, and we will see that although the discourse of gestation affords an opportunity for creativity for many Tibetan writers, structural commonalities between embryological narratives suggest an interesting point of interaction between religious and medical literary and conceptual traditions in Tibet.

Also associated with each story is a plot. The plot of a story is its logical and causal structure; as Ricoeur tells us, it is "the intelligible whole that governs a succession of events" in the story.[5] In other words, emplotment is the process that transforms events, which simply happen, into a unified, singular story.[6] We might assume that the plot of an embryological narrative is straightforward: a man and woman copulate, and the embryo that is conceived grows until it is sufficiently developed to leave the womb. In a literal sense this is what Tibetan embryologies describe, and yet a closer examination of the details of gestation indicates that the composition of these narratives in early Tibetan literature was far from straightforward. Tibetan writers made numerous choices about how to portray the growth of the embryo. Despite an author's impulse to form intellectual alliances with India through his writings, it seems that certain issues within embryology were left to the discretion of the individual, regardless of the availability of Indian source materials. In this chapter, I will suggest that we may reconcile this disconcerting discrepancy by a closer consideration of the plot behind the story of embryology. Is the gestation of a fetus all that embryology is about?

The following pages will consider some of the ways that Tibetans used embryological concepts to express normative religious views on how to follow a religious path. The Buddhist concept of the path (*lam*, Skt. *mārga*) is roughly comparable to the Western notion of soteriology, the theory of salvation.[7] The path, in Buddhist literature, is a description of a process during which the religious practitioner embodies Buddhist truth. It is the plot of one's spiritual progress, weaving together a complex set of events into a single story. The path integrates a complex of ethical and ritual experiences and doctrines into a description of recommended religious practices leading to a goal. The Buddhist practitioner thus alters his or her world-view, character and behavior in the effort to make forward progress along the path. Significantly, Buswell and Gimello note that some paths of practice prescribed in Buddhist accounts may never have been performed: "some seem designed actually to be followed by real practitioners," they write, while "others appear to be merely inspirational in intention, mārgas of myth in which the path is presented as one or another kind of heroic quest."[8]

In Tibetan Buddhist writings, the structure of the path was the focus of a specific class of text: "grounds and paths" literature, associated with the "stages of the path" literature mentioned briefly in chapter two. This genre is devoted explicitly to describing paths that are graded by spiritual levels of accomplishment, or grounds (*sa*, Skt. *bhūmi*). These manuals provide instructions on religious practices, information on the obstructions that impede one's progress toward liberation, and description of landmarks to be encountered along the way to liberation. They also explain the nature of the enlightenment experiences to be attained, the characteristics required of a practitioner, and the different paths that may be taken by practitioners of different skills. In this chapter, I will propose that one of the reasons Tibetan religious writers found embryological narratives particularly compelling has to do with their easy affiliation with the structure and purpose of this increasingly popular form of literature on the Buddhist path.

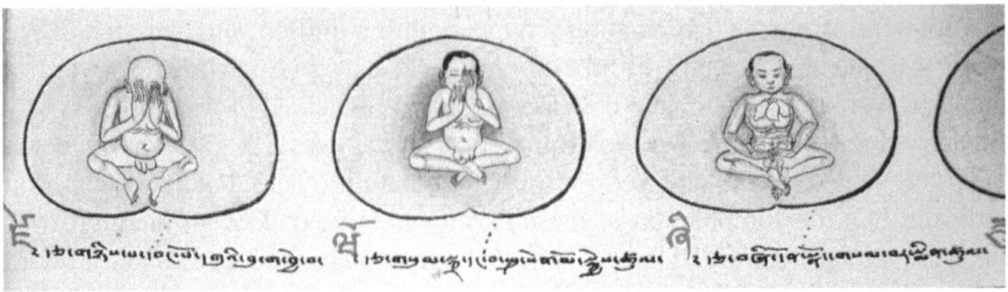

Figure 5.1 In the twenty-second week of gestation, the nine orifices open; in the twenty-third week, hair and nails develop; in the twenty-fourth week, the solid and hollow organs mature.

Conception and debates over the sequence of fetal development

The moment of entering the womb is illustrated in a Tibetan painting (see Figure 1.1), the transmigrating being rather humorously given a tiny human form that walks along the path of his or her karmic inheritance into the bed of the embracing parents. In medical texts, however, the precise mechanics of the transmigrating being's mode of travel is typically not addressed in great detail, although the transmigrator's state of mind is described, as I will explain below. In the *Four Tantras*, the topic of conception, not surprisingly, starts off the section on the growth of the body:

> First of all, the non-defective reproductive substance (*khu*) and blood (*khrag*) of the father and mother,
> the consciousness (*rnam shes*) impelled by karma, the afflictiv emotions,
> and the five elements assembled from tha
> are the causes of formation in the womb;
> it happens like the arising of fire from the friction of wood [9]

The text does not explain how the consciousness chooses the womb or how it enters it. Of greater concern here is specifying the ways in which the reproductive substances or the balance of the five elements may be defective, and what they are like when they are healthy. In chapter four, we noted how systemic imbalances in the reproductive substances would result in their turning "coarse, dark and astringent" in the case of a wind disorder, "sour, yellow and malodorous" in the case of a bile disorder, and so forth. The importance of the elements is also stressed:

> Without the earth element there is no formation; without the water element there is no integration;

> without the fire element there is no maturation; without the wind element there is no growth;
> without the space element there is no room for growth.
> The [male] reproductive substance should be white, heavy, sweet and abundant,
> the menstrual blood (*zla mtshan*) should be like the color of rabbit's blood, and
> [clothes should easily] be washed clean of it: if these are non-defective,
> [an embryo] will form in the womb.[10]

These details are not presented in the *Heart of Medicine*'s account of conception. The *Entering the Womb*, however, does focus its early discussion of human development on these very topics: disorders of the womb (defective male reproductive substances are not addressed) and the importance of the elements are presented in that text at length, as recorded in chapter two. While much of the *Four Tantras* is clearly derived from the Indic medical treatise, therefore, here it is more closely aligned with the Buddhist sūtric tradition.

The questions of how a transmigrating consciousness enters the womb and how an embryonic form is initially generated were difficult ones, and, in general, these were issues of more interest to Buddhist tantric traditions than to medical writers. Does the consciousness enter directly into the woman's vagina? Is it transmitted through the man's emission? Does it enter the combination of the male and female reproductive substances independently? How does an embryonic form emerge then, as if out of nothing? The *Four Tantras'* commentarial tradition bases its answers to these questions mainly on statements from the *Heart of Medicine* and the *Entering the Womb* sūtra, to the effect that the consciousness simply enters the womb on the occasion of finding a suitably matched combination of male and female reproductive substances. Tibetan medical commentators comment, based on Indic sources, that it occurs "invisibly":

> If you ask how the consciousness enters the mother's womb beyond the reach of sense faculties, this example teaches clearly: By the power of sun rays striking a crystal, grass or wood can be burned, even though you do not see the wood touching the crystal or the crystal touching the wood; like this case of burning, the consciousness enters the womb: it enters invisibly.[11]

The *Entering the Womb* sūtra speaks extensively about the moment beyond the consciousness's entry into the womb, clarifying how the embryo can be created out of nonexistence. The text notes that the body is formed by a combination of the three factors, in addition to the elemental functions. This interactive process is described with several metaphors: it is like butter is produced from the interaction of yogurt, a vessel and implements for churning, and the efforts of stirring; it is like insects will spontaneously emerge from a rotting mixture of plant matter, or from a pile of cow dung, or from aging yogurt. In other words, the sūtra explains that although you can not actually see the embryo itself among its causes and conditions (i.e., the reproductive fluids, transmigrating consciousness, or elements), it will, nonetheless, appear as a result of their combination.[12] These metaphors are repeated in the *Four Tantras'* commentaries of Kyempa Tsewang and Lodrö Gyelpo.

But then the question emerges of how different forms may arise from similar conditions: how is it that individual beings all look different when they have been caused by the same combination of causal conditions? Here, too, Indic metaphors are used: it is like how "from the single cause of wax and copper and so forth, you can make various different forms however you like." Kyempa Tsewang adds to these examples the response that particular forms emerge also due to karma and the predispositions.[13]

Also of interest is the related question of why it is that humans produce human children and, indeed, children that resemble their parents. The problem of how children come to resemble their parents is of concern in many cultures. Aristotle and other Greek writers, for instance, promoted a theory in which a child was developed after certain impressions given to the mother, particularly during intercourse, such that, for example, if a woman thinks of a monkey during intercourse her child will resemble a monkey. Doniger and Spinner point out that the notion that a child's appearance may be determined by something that the mother sees, thinks of, or does at the time of copulation or pregnancy also occurs in Hindu mythology, and Kinney cites Chinese texts with the same view.[14] Caraka repeats the idea that the child may resemble whatever the mother is thinking of at the time of conception, such that, if she desires a pale-skinned child, she should furnish her bedroom in white. In some Tibetan Buddhist traditions, in a twist on the Indic view, the thoughts of the transmigrating being itself in the final moments of its previous life are particularly important to the form the being takes in rebirth. Other Tibetan traditions note that the transmigrating being's state of mind while watching its potential parents copulate is what determines its gender. Thus in this context as elsewhere, paradigms of explanation that may involve the mother are rejected in favor of those that focus entirely on the being to be reborn.

For Tibetans, the question of the relationship between an original and its replication is not only of concern in the context of reproduction, but it is one that fits into a wider context of Buddhist thought. In Buddhist philosophy this is known as the problem of homologous cause and effect (*rgyu 'bras bu dang rjes su mthun pa*). Kyempa Tsewang and Lodrö Gyelpo both question how it is that such an infinite variety of forms can result from a limited set of causes, and they explain that effects only follow causes of the same class; results cannot arise from causes of a completely unrelated type. Likewise, whereas for each human being the causes and mode of conception are the same, various forms may result, although all of those forms will be human. The question of whether causes and effects must be homologous is a fraught one for Buddhist philosophers who are concerned with whether an enlightened mind is created newly as a result of practice, or whether it arises from a cause that is homologous to itself. If gnosis, or the enlightened mind, is the ultimate nature of one's ordinary mind, as opposed to a newly created mind that results from effort in contemplative practice, then "activating" that enlightened mind requires no more than emptying one's ordinary mind of conceptuality; in this case, cause and effect are homologous, because the cause (non-conceptuality) is homologous to the effect (the non-conceptual mind of enlightenment).[15] Most Tibetan tantric writers agree that progress in advanced meditation practices requires a homology of cause and effect, but the degree of homology is debated, as is what it means, precisely, to be "homologous." While Tibetan medical commentators seem aware of the Buddhist philosophical contexts of these problems in general, for the most part it is the child's own karma that is referred to as more important than any input provided by the mother. Sophisticated philosophical solutions to these problems are not addressed in any depth by medical writers, although the articulation of these matters as problems suggests a familiarity with this body of Buddhist philosophical literature.

These were not the only troublesome issues surrounding conception in the Indian sources available to Tibetans. Buddhist tantras, in particular, offered a range of descriptions of the process of conception that had to be negotiated by later Tibetan commentators. In his *Great Stages of Mantra*, Tsong Khapa summarizes views of Indian scholars such as Śrī Phalavajra or Vitapāda, which assert that the transmigrating being enters either through the mother's "lotus" (a tantric term for the vagina), or through the father's mouth, traveling from there to his "vajra" (tantric terminology for penis) and from the vajra to the lotus, or, alternatively, through the "crown-aperture," an opening at the top of the head.[16] Tsong Khapa cites the *Sheaf of Instructions* (*Saṃpuṭa*) tantra to explain that the Buddha taught that "In some divine cases the *gandharva* sentient being enters through the golden door, and in some cases through the mouth, and in some cases other ways."[17] The "golden door," also sometimes called "Vairocana's door," refers to the crown-aperture, Tsong Khapa clarifies (but there is some debate about whether it is there, or at the anus[18]); he notes further that "other ways" in this citation indicate the abhidharmic tradition of entry through the woman's vagina. A third entry place, the mouth of the father, is indicated in tantras such as the *Vajra Rosary* (*Vajrāvali*), the *Drop of Mahāmudrā* (*Mahāmudrātilaka*) or the *Arisal of Saṃvara* (*Saṃvarodaya*). Tsong Khapa comments that beings who are attracted to the "honey of the lips" enter through the mouth, those attracted to the hair enter through the top of the head, and those attracted to the mother and father enter through the vagina.[19]

Thus, the moment of conception elicited different concerns for different traditions. The *Four Tantras* and the Buddhist sūtric exoteric traditions were concerned with the causes of conception and, in particular, the role of the elements in early conception, and with the more philosophical questions of how something could arise from nothing, and how an identical set of causes could produce a differentiated variety of results. Buddhist tantras, by contrast, were primarily interested in precisely how the transmigrating consciousness enters the womb. For Tibetan medical texts in the *Four Tantras'* commentarial tradition, Buddhist tantric views on conception were not an issue, perhaps because the medical tradition was concerned mainly with the mechanics of conception for ordinary beings who were not substantially involved in tantric practice.

When it came to the issue of how the body grows, even exoteric sources disagreed on occasion. According to the *Four Tantras'* tradition, the navel is the first discernable part of the embryo's body to form, and thus the navel is referred to as the "cause" (*rgyu*) of the body's development. This is controversial, however, as are also the conventions for naming the early body of the embryo. The *Explanatory Tantra* states that during the first month after conception, the embryo is transformed from a substance that resembles curdled milk in week one, to a lengthened and thickened substance (*nur nur po*) in week two, and by week three it resembles the semi-solid consistency of yogurt. Although the descriptor "oval shaped" (*mer mer po*) is used in the *Entering the Womb* sūtra for the embryo in the first week immediately after conception, this term is not used in the *Four Tantras* tradition until the fourth week, when it describes one of the possible forms of the embryo as it comes to be identified as male, female or indeterminate in sex. Whereas the *Four Tantras* had followed a sūtric convention of detailing the possible defects leading to an inability to conceive and the importance of the elements, here, by contrast, it aligns itself more closely with Indian medicine in the use of this embryonic terminology.

After week three, the *Four Tantras* and its commentaries recommend, on the basis of the *Heart of Medicine,* that rituals be performed to transform the still undetermined sex of the embryo into that of a male. The text continues after a lengthy description of these rituals, stating that in the fourth week the embryo will take on a rounded (*gor gor po*), oval (*mer mer po*), or elongated (*nar nar po*) shape according to whether it will become a boy, girl or person of indeterminate sex (*ma ning*), respectively.[20]

In the fifth week of gestation, the navel forms and a week later the life channel (*srog rtsa*) extends from the navel. A preliminary form of the eyes develops in the seventh week around which the head grows the following week. In the ninth week, the upper and lower torso form, followed by the shoulders and hips in the tenth week, the nine orifices of the body in the eleventh week, the five solid organs in the twelfth week, and the six vessel organs in the thirteenth week.[21] In subsequent verses, the *Four Tantras* specifies which aspect of the body is formed each week, up to the thirty-seventh, as recorded in Table 5.2. The sequence of fetal development specified in the *Four Tantras* is accepted by subsequent Tibetan commentaries on that text, not surprisingly. As we will see below, however, despite this text's prominence in Tibetan medical history, it was not considered authoritative by a host of other Tibetan writers on matters of embryology and physiology.

Table 5.1 The use of terminology in early gestation

Wk.	*Heart of Medicine*	*Four Tantras*	*Entering the Womb*	Longchenpa's *Treasury*
1	*nur nur po*		*mer mer po*	*mer mer po*
2		*nur nur po*	*nur nur po*	*nur nur po*
3			*ltar ltar po*	*ltar ltar po*
4		*gor gor, mer mer,* or *nar nar po*	*mkhrang pa*	*gor gor po*
5	*gor gor, mer mer,* or *nar nar po*		*gor gor po*	*mkhrang 'rgyur*

The question of which parts of the body developed first was a difficult one. *Four Tantras'* commentators Kyempa Tsewang, in the fifteenth century, and Lodrö Gyelpo, in the sixteenth century, both explicitly reject alternate theories that suggest the head, legs, heart or other organs are the first to develop in the embryo. Their pointed objections suggest that such alternate views were well known. The rationale for their assertion of the originary function of the navel is a physiological description of the importance of the navel to the embryo's connection with the mother's body. As the bodily constituents (*lus zungs*) are metabolized in the digestive processes taking place within the woman's internal organs, the clarified essence (*dwangs ma*)[22] is collected in the reproductive vesicles (*bsam se'u*), which are the reservoir of that clarified nutritive essence. The reproductive vesicles are connected by two channels to the left and right side of the uterus or womb (*bu snod*). Those channels are also connected to the navel of the embryo residing inside the womb. Through these channels, the nutrients produced from the woman's food intake and stored in the reproductive vesicles are passed to the developing embryo. In this way, it is said, the embryo is nourished as a field is supplied water through irrigation canals that lead from a reservoir. Lodrö Gyelpo repeats statements of the Indic medical text, the *Heart of Medicine*, that it is the power of karma that generates the two channels that connect the reproductive vesicles to the navel of the embryo. In the *Heart of Medicine*, however, it is the woman's "heart" (*snying*) that is connected to the navel, not a reproductive organ. Playing on the ambiguity of the Tibetan term *snying*, which can mean "heart" in either a biological or an abstract sense, Lodrö Gyelpo claims that the heart in that text actually refers to the reproductive vesicles because the reproductive vesicles are the organs that integrate the "great nutrient" (*bcud*), which is the quintessential nutritive essence ultimately distilled from the woman's food and drink. Thus the reproductive vesicles are symbolically the "heart" of the developing embryo's nutritional supply.[23]

Although many, if not most, Tibetan-authored texts that describe gestation in any detail agree that the navel is the first aspect of the body to develop, curiously this sequence is not, in fact, present in three of the primary Indian sources for

Table 5.2 Development of the gross body, indicating which aspects of the body develop during which month

Mo.	*Heart of Medicine*	*Four Tantras*	*Entering the Womb*	*Drakpa Gyeltsen*	*Kālacakra*	*Kyempa Tsewang's summary of an (unidentified) tantric view*
1					blood, flui	wind and blood
2		navel, eye sense base, head	arms, legs, hips, shoulders, fingers, toes	five limbs, bu	heart, navel	
3	torso, head, hips, shoulders, five limb	torso, shoulders, hips, five solid organs	nine orifices, intestines, spine	head	four limbs and head	upper body
4	limbs	six vessel organs, arms, legs, digits	food is transmitted through navel, winds circulate	limbs develop	limbs develop	limbs
5		flesh, fat, ligaments, tendons, bones, marrow	sense organs, tongue, bones		bones, joints, sense organs	organs, bones, joints
6	sinews, channels, hair, digits, skin	nine orifices open, organs mature, hair and nails develop	flesh, blood, skin	limbs are complete	blood, fles	strength, two eyes
7		fetus is complete	fetus grows larger	fetus is complete	hair, orifice	ears
8		fetus grows larger			joints, bones, marrow, tongue, urine, feces	nose
9						tongue

Table 5.3 Development of circulatory channels

Mo	*Heart of Medicine*	*Four Tantras*	*Entering the Womb*	*Drakpa Gyeltsen*	*Kālacakra*	*Kyempa Tsewang's summary of an (unidentified) tantric view*
1				central, flavor and solitary channels form	no channels now, only blood and flui	central channel
2		life channel (*srog rtsa*)			channels begin to develop, first from the heart, then from the navel; 200 channels develop per day	every day 200 channels form
3						
4			detailed discussion of many channels			
5		all channels connecting the inner and outer body				
6	circulatory channels					

Note
None of these sources mention the growth of circulatory channels past the sixth month of gestation.

embryology available to Tibetans, the *Entering the Womb* and the *Abiding in the Womb* sūtras and Vāgbhaṭa's *Heart of Medicine*. In those texts, the navel's development is not mentioned until the third month of gestation. In the sūtras, the structural form of the embryo is created during the fifth through eleventh weeks of development. During those seven weeks the arms and legs, the finger and toes, the eyes, ears, nose, mouth, excretory orifices, and the empty spaces of the body are formed. Only after that do the nutrient-providing navel, the internal organs, and the circulatory channels form and begin to function. In Vāgbhaṭa likewise not until the third month, after the head, legs and arms are formed, does the navel connect to the mother and begin to nourish the fetus. Curiously, neither Lodrö Gyelpo nor Kyempa Tsewang acknowledge the inconsistencies in sequence of development between that of the *Four Tantras* and the model of the Indian sources that they laud so prominently in other contexts. What may account for this indifference?

Fetal development in tantric sources

With Buddhist tantric sources, the sequence of fetal growth is depicted in terms that clearly link embryonic development with contemplative practices. Although in the Nyingma scholar Longchenpa's fourteenth-century embryological narrative the navel does develop prior to the rest of the coarse physical body, in other respects his account of development differs vastly from that of the *Four Tantras* and its commentators. Writing at a time when the *Four Tantras* had accumulated some commentarial literature, but before the two major commentators discussed above, Longchenpa cites the *Tantra of the Sun and the Moon's Union* (*nyi zla kha sbyor*) to explain that "The bodily elements develop from the embryo's navel, and for nine months continue like this."[24] Longchenpa does not justify the navel's primacy with an explanation of female reproductive anatomy, however, and while the navel's development occurs in the fifth week and precedes that of the torso and limbs, as in the *Four Tantras* tradition, Longchenpa's account of early embryogenesis is primarily a detailed presentation of the growth of the subtle body. In his account, circulatory channels develop as early as the firs week of gestation; subtle letters appear within those channels and the two tiny "eye-like" essences, called the "eye of the lamps" (*sgron ma'i spyan*) and the "eye of the elements" (*'byung ba'i spyan*), are formed. Although in the firs several weeks the embryo is repeatedly destroyed and regenerated (activity that does not occur in any of the embryological narratives mentioned thus far), these channels, letters and other subtle body features nonetheless somehow continue to expand. During the second week, four new geographically-labeled channels stretch out from the center of the embryo: an eastern channel, southern channel, western channel and northern channel. The four element channels and the two tiny eyes become more clearly developed.

In the third week, according to this tradition, the embryo is again sequentially destroyed and reconstituted. During this week, the force of karmic wind causes a very subtle "quintessence of heat" (*drod kyi dangs ma*) to originate inside the western channel. This causes the essence (*dwangs ma*) of the embryo's consciousness to become very clear; during the next several days of churning, the bases (*rten*) of the consciousness are gathered together. By the end of the week, the embryo attains the "elongated" (*ltar ltar po*) stage and is roughly the size of a thumb. In the fourth week, the embryo is again destroyed and reconstituted and a series of subtle drops are formed, one each day. A quintessential essence (*thig le*) first originates in the eastern channel and inside that substance a non-conceptual consciousness (*rtog med kyi shes pa*) develops. Next, a white-colored essence (*dwangs ma*) of flesh forms within the southern channel, and within that there is a very subtle substance that is the basis of the psyche (*yid*) and mind (*sems*). Then, inside the northern channel the blue- and red-colored quintessence of breath (*dbugs*) originates, and based on this are the potential aspects (*rtsal*) of gnosis and awareness, along with the embryo's own consciousness. After this, a series of "bases" (*rten*) develop inside the western, eastern, southern and northern channels: the base of cognition, intellect and memory; the base of ignorance (*ma rig pa*) and afflictive emotions; the base of movements and psyche (*yid*); and the base of mind and conceptuality, respectively. The privileging of the appearance of these mental qualities in the very early weeks of gestation is substantially different than presentations of gestation found in sources based on sūtric literature, where the emergence of mental faculties is not mentioned until quite near the end of the process of fetal development.

In the second month of Longchenpa's account, as the embryo continues to be dissolved and reconstituted by the natural elements, the eyes, four channel wheels (*'khor lo*), and three vertical channels of the embryo are generated. With the development of the four wheels, the channels that are the basis for the fiv sense organs grow. The "elements eye" and the "lamps eye" appear first in the navel wheel and then in each of the other three wheels, at the heart, throat and top of the head. Extending from each wheel are a large number of additional channels. With the development of the wheels, the three main vertical channel columns running up and down the center of the body are formed. After this "firming up" (*mkhrang 'gyur*) phase, the embryo is again destroyed and reconstituted by each of the four elements in the next week. After this point the embryo has arrived at the "fish stage" of gestation, referring to the Indic scheme of Viṣṇu's ten incarnations that is used by many tantric accounts of fetal development, as we will see below. In the seventh week, the elements cause the sense faculties and essential and hollow organs to form, and the embryo is in the "tortoise-like" stage of gestation. From this point onwards, the embryo is no longer completely destroyed and reconstituted regularly and the actions of the elements, while still important, are more subtle. In the eighth week, the limbs of the body are formed, and the winds enter the central channel, which matures the five elements' abilities further. Also during this week, Longchenpa states that the three humors are formed and the afflictive emotions are activated. The body's flesh and blood are produced, and the embryo is in the stage of the "frog incarnation" of Viṣṇu.

Longchenpa's narrative of development ends here, at the end of the eighth week, a total of fifty-six days. During this initial period the body's fundamental form is created and for the remainder of gestation the elements continue to mature the embryo while the mother's nutrients cause the growth of skin, hair and so on. Longchenpa, therefore, focuses almost exclusively on the early development of the subtle body and all but ignores the details of development of the coarse body.

The developmental sequence in this account is completely unlike that seen in the *Four Tantras*, the Buddhist sūtra, or the Indian medical traditions. It may have similarities, however, to early Nyingma accounts. The *Tantra of the Secret Union of the Sun and Moon*, mentioned above, is part of the *Seventeen Tantras* anthology at the core of the Nyingma Heart Essence (*snying thig*) tradition. In that text, the fish, turtle, and frog stages are also compressed into the first seven weeks of gestation:

> From the seed, the primary cause of the father, and the blood, the secondary cause of the mother, the viscous embryo is born. After seven days it becomes oval, then going from state to state, from week to week it becomes solid and similar to a fish; a week later it is like a turtle, after another week, a frog; and this after seven weeks, in forty nine days, the body takes form, beginning at the navel and in nine months for man, or ten days for other kinds of beings, the complete body comes out of the mother's womb.[25]

This account suggests a precursor to Longchenpa's account in the Heart Essence collections, a link about which more research should be done.

Another tantric model of fetal development, in a text earlier than any mentioned above, including possibly even the *Four Tantras*, is found in Drakpa Gyeltsen's *Great Jeweled Wishing Tree*, a text that describes the growth of both the subtle and the coarse body. Drakpa Gyeltsen explains that when the embryo reaches the oval-shaped (*mer mer po*) stage, the central channel (*dbu ma*) begins to develop. By the power of the wind entering the central channel, the solitary (*kyang ma*) channel is formed, and when the wind emerges from the central channel, the flavor (*ro ma*) channel is formed. All other channels are produced after this. Structuring his account like some Indian tantras, Drakpa Gyeltsen arranges fetal development not by counting weeks from conception, but rather by organizing gestation into ten month-long stages named for the ten incarnations of Viṣṇu, although he uses an unusual list of those incarnations. Drapa Gyeltsen comments that such a scheme, as taught in the *Guhyasamāja* and the *Kālacakra*, was originally incorporated into those tantras "to attract followers of Viṣṇu."[26] In this scheme, during the first month of gestation the embryo resembles a fish, and in the second month, the five limbs protrude slightly and the fetus resembles a tortoise. In the fourth and fifth months, the limbs are define more clearly and the fetus resembles two Ramas, and in the sixth month the limbs are almost completely finished and the fetus looks like Kṛṣṇa. The fetus's body is completed in the seventh month, and it resembles the man-lion. In the eighth month it resembles a dwarf, and in the ninth a swan. At that time it desires release from the womb. In the tenth month, Drakpa Gyeltsen writes, the fetus is a Buddha "because it has completely perfected the tenth ground."[27] As stated above, the connection of the ten incarnations of Viṣṇu with human gestation is derived from various Indian sources, although the precise manner of linking the two varies. The *Vajramālā* tantra, for instance, correlates only the first five incarnations with the first five months of gestation.[28] The *Kālacakra* tantra correlates the ten incarnations with ten phases of human life both within and without the womb: the fish, tortoise and boar or wild pig stages occur during gestation, the man-lion stage occurs at birth, the period of childhood before one's teeth grow in is the dwarf stage, the period until one's baby teeth fall out is the Rāma stage, adolescence is the Paraśurāma stage, from then until the appearance of gray hair is the Kṛṣṇa stage, old age is the Buddha stage, and the final Kalkī stage is death.[29] Although this correlation with the ten incarnations of Viṣṇu is extensively recited in Tibetan tantric sources on fetal development, in the fifteenth century Khedrub Norsang Gyatso condemns the convention, calling it "lies and fabrications." Nonetheless, he too goes on to describe the fish-turtle wild pig correspondence, commenting that during the first two months the embryo does look rather like a fish, and during the third and fourth months, with its limbs beginning to protrude, the embryo looks indeed somewhat like a turtle! The manner of resemblance to a frog or wild pig is not clear, although the stages after birth are said to be easily justified by their similarity to events in the life of Viṣṇu.[30]

Drakpa Gyeltsen maintains that the coarse body, consisting of the aggregates, elements (*khams*), and sense-spheres, is established from the subtle body, consisting of the winds and mind. Like other tantric traditions, his account of fetal development is, therefore, largely focused on the growth of the subtle body and (as is also the case in the *Four Tantras*) the topic of "anatomy" (*lus gnas*) follows directly after embryology. Anatomy, for Drakpa Gyeltsen, is concerned with two main topics: one, the three "maṇḍalas" of body, *bhaga*, and *bodhicitta*; and two, the winds that actualize those maṇḍalas. The body maṇḍala refers to the coarse body and the subtle body – the coarse body including the torso, limbs and senses, and the subtle body including the circulatory system of channels and winds. The *bhaga* maṇḍala has coarse and subtle aspects too – the coarse refers to the sexual organs of the male and female, and the subtle refers to the letter channels. The *bodhicitta* maṇḍala refers to the male and female reproductive substances and five nectars.[31] He explains that the winds are what "activate" the maṇḍalas of the body and support the consciousness.[32] Drakpa Gyeltsen insists in this text, however, that understanding the channels is the basis for understanding all other aspects of the body. The topic of embryology, therefore, in which the origins of the channel system are taught, is of great importance.

Another Sakya esoteric work, *Profound Summarizing Notes on the Path Presented as the Three Continua* by Jamyang Khyentsé Wangchuk (1524–1568), also emphasizes the growth of the subtle body in early gestation, focusing additionally on the role of the transmigrator's nonrecognition of emptiness as a key causal factor for development. He explains that when the transmigrating consciousness enters the male and female reproductive substances, or white and red constituents, it dissolves into clear light. Because it does not recognize that clear light for what it is, namely an enlightened state of awareness, the central channel is immediately formed, followed by the left and right channels, thus beginning the process of physical embodiment. Gradually, coarse states of mind develop and their emergence is correlated to aspects of the subtle body as they grow in the fetus.[33] For Jamyang Khyentsé Wangchuk as for Drakpa Gyeltsen, knowledge of gestation is thus directly linked to knowing the path to (or away from) enlightenment. In order to proceed on the esoteric path, Jamyang Khyentsé explains, one must possess a womb-born body, because only humans may ripen their karma in this lifetime. Moreover, one must possess both the father's white constituent, which produced one's bone, brains and fat, and the mother's red constituent, which produced one's flesh, blood and skin; each of these qualities continue to exist throughout one's life in the bodies of men and women alike, and are, ultimately, the basis for enlightenment as the form of the human body.[34]

It should be striking by now how varied these accounts of early human development are. Exoteric medical and sūtric traditions are similarly interested in the sequence of growth, but they disagree about the details of that sequence and about terminological conventions. Esoteric traditions are interested in similar topics – sequence and terminology – but, again, the details are controversial. Exoteric traditions examine the growth of the gross physical body, whereas esoteric traditions focus on the subtle body's development. Were we to look more widely at Buddhist texts across Asian traditions, we would find a diversity even more extensive. In discussing Japanese Buddhist Shingon texts on gestation, for example, James Sanford describes a sequence of development in which the embryo's form first takes the shape of a stūpa, then the form of Mount Sumeru.[35] Another Japanese text, he reports, tells of how the embryo begins development with the form of "a monk's staff with small ears" and ends in the shape of a five pronged *vajra*, with its hands forming a *mudra* and its mouth intoning a *mantra*.[36] Yet another text describes the new embryo as eight lumps of flesh that are likened to an eight-petalled lotus blossom and the eight consciousnesses; the four stages of gestation are linked to the eight petals and to eight divinities, all of this connecting the embryo to the Womb Maṇḍala of Shingon.[37] A fourteenth-century scriptural fragment by Gonkaku, the *Aisen Myōō Initiation*, "equates the taking on of human form in the womb … with the attainment of perfect Buddhahood,"[38] casting the act of sexual intercourse as a religious initiatory ritual. In this tradition, Sanford writes, "The womb is a Buddharealm (Dharmadhātu; Jpn,

Table 5.4 Comparison of tantric stages of gestation

Mo.	*Kyempa Tsewang's summary of an (unidentified) tantra*	*Kālacakra according to Lodrö Gyelpo*	*Drakpa Gyeltsen*	*Kālacakra*	*Longchenpa's Treasury*
1	fis		fis	fis	
2	turtle	fis	tortoise		fish (sixth week); tortoise (seventh week); frog (eighth week)
3		turtle	wild pig	turtle	
4		tortoise	two Ramas		
5	wild pig	pig		wild pig	
6			Krishna		
7			man-lion		
8			dwarf		
9	man-lion		goose/swan		
10		man-lion	Buddha		

hokkai) and the fetus is the Dharmakāya (lit. "Dharma-body"; Jpn. *hosshin*) within that self-contained universe wherein ontogeny recapitulates ontology."[39] I will turn to similar examples of such recapitulation in Tibetan literature later in this chapter.

The fetal experience of conception, gestation and birth

We have seen so far that Tibetan embryological narratives disagree with their Indian source texts on the importance of the navel, and that the sequence of fetal development in general is described variously, partly depending on whether or not writers address the growth of subtle body elements (although even this does not account for all variances). Another category of inconsistency may be seen in disagreements over whether and to what extent the fetus itself is said to be aware of the events of conception and gestation. The exemplar of fetal awareness is, of course, the fetus who was to become Gautama Buddha himself. The *Lalitavistara* reports that,

> When the Bodhisattva had entered his mother's womb, his body assumed a form which appeared like a grand fire on the top of a mountain – a mountain fire which is visible even in a densely dark night at a distance of a yojana – and visible from a distance of five yojanas. Thus did his effulgence spread from the womb of his mother. His complexion was luminous, pleasing, agreeable; and seated on the bedstead in the pavilion, he looked exceedingly beautiful, like the lapis-lazuli set on native silver; and remaining in her fixed position, his mother could always see him in her womb.[40]

Indian Buddhist biographies of the Buddha depict him giving religious teachings from his mother's womb, which is described as a wondrously aromatic and bejeweled palace of multiple dazzling pavilions. His body was fully formed from the moment of entering the womb, and he sat cross-legged on a bed sized for a six-month-old infant, entertaining students in his uterine palace throughout his fetal life.[41]

Most fetuses have a different experience. There are various notions about what the transmigrating consciousness understands at the moment of conception. Some texts, including the *Four Tantras*, recount a tradition in which the ordinary transmigrating being is rendered senseless at the moment of conception, entering the womb without any awareness of the experience.[42] Another tradition, represented by the *Entering the Womb* sūtra, maintains that the transmigrating being will be assaulted by two types of deluded mind – attachment to one parent and aversion to the other – which will, in that moment, determine the gender of the fetus, as described above.[43] A third tradition, to be addressed further in chapter six, suggests that transmigrating beings with a large accumulation of merit will enter the womb with a more pleasurable experience than those with a smaller store of merit; the latter will have fearful visions upon entering the womb, and the former will have pleasurable visions. Similar to this is a four-fold sūtric tradition in which the experience of conception and gestation is morally coded: ordinary people enter the womb completely unaware of the moment of conception and oblivious to the entire process of gestation; universal monarchs (*'khor los sgyur ba*, Skt. *cakravartin*) and stream-enterers (*rgyun du zhugs pa*, Skt. *shrotāpanna*) are aware of their entering the womb, but then lose awareness for the duration of gestation. First-level bodhisattvas and solitary realizers (*rang sangs rgyas*, Skt. *pratyekabuddha*) also are "unconscious" during gestation, but they are aware of entering the womb and leaving the womb at birth. Higher level bodhisattvas are aware of the entire process.[44]

In addition to discussing the various levels of fetal awareness of the process of conception, Buddhist texts also provide vivid descriptions of what that process is like for the transmigrator. Just before entering the womb, the early Nyingma *Secret Union of the Sun and Moon* tantra says that "One feels the desire to move but feels held back by a net because one is blocked, like straw that has taken fire, or like being stuck in the mud. One is like a bird in a trap that has been dug in the earth: in the trap of desire without control, that is transmigration."[45] Teachings on "blocking the womb's door" to prevent rebirth, an esoteric practice about which more is said below, also offer a colorful picture of the transmigrator's experience just prior to conception. The transmigrator is told that:

> At this time you will have visions of couples making love. When you see them, don't enter between them, but stay mindful. Visualize the males and females as the Teacher, Father and Mother, prostrate to them, and make them visualized offerings! Feel intense reverence and devotion! Aim a strong will to request them to teach the Dharma, and the womb door will definitely be blocked[46]

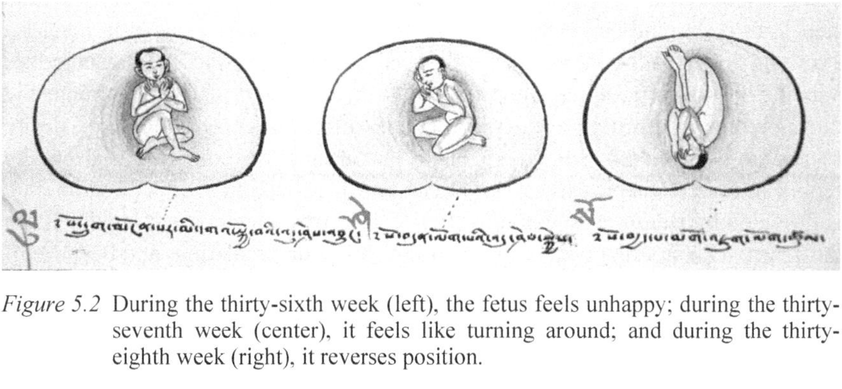

Figure 5.2 During the thirty-sixth week (left), the fetus feels unhappy; during the thirty-seventh week (center), it feels like turning around; and during the thirty-eighth week (right), it reverses position.

If that is ineffective, the text goes on to say, other sorts of visualizations may be tried. When the transmigrating consciousness feels attachment to one parent and aversion to the other, it should meditate intensely on the following thought:

> "Such a creature of negative evolution as myself will wander in the life cycle under the influence of lust and hate. If I still persist in lust and hate, I will know no end to my wanderings. I am in danger of being sunk forever in the ocean of miseries. Now I must give up lust and hate entirely. Alas! I must hold intensely the one-pointed will never to entertain lust and hate!" The tantras state that this meditation itself will close the door of the womb.[47]

If this still does not work, the transmigrator should contemplate the idea that all phenomena are like magical illusions, and if that is ineffective, a meditation on the mind's ultimate state of clear light is recommended: "Like water being poured in water, let the mind flow into its own reality condition; release it into its own nature. Letting it relax easily and openly will decisively and definitel block the womb door for all forms of rebirth."[48]

Beyond the moment of conception, there are also variations on how the fetus' own experience of gestation is described. In Vāgbhaṭa's *Heart of Medicine*, the fetus experiences pleasure and pain as soon as the head is formed in the third month, and its mind (*sems*) "becomes clear" in the fifth month. In the *Entering the Womb* sūtra, in the twenty-eighth week of gestation the fetus experiences "eight distorted conceptions" (*phyin ci log gi 'du shes*),[49] and in the thirty-sixth week it feels unhappy about being in the womb and wishes to escape. In the thirty-seventh week, five unhappy notions manifest: sensations of uncleanness, foul odor, a sense of confinement, darkness, and a premonition of the misery of birth.[50] These traditions are taken up by Tibetan writers as well, with a similar range of disparity. In Gampopa's twelfth-century *Jewel Ornament of Liberation*, the embryo experiences pain continually throughout gestation: in the first week it suffers unbearably as it if it is being boiled and fried, and when the nine orifices are opened in the eleventh week it feels as if it is being stabbed with a finger. By the thirty-seventh week, overwhelmed by the stench, dirtiness and darkness of the womb, the fetus craves escape. In Kyempa Tsewang's fifteenth-century *Four Tantras* commentary, the fetus recognizes happiness and suffering in the twenty-fourth week and, as in Gampopa, the thirty-sixth week brings an experience of suffering great enough to desire escape from the womb. Some texts claim that around this point of gestation, the fetus can remember past lives. An interesting justification of this phenomenon is provided by Butön, who explains that "during pregnancy, wind dwells within the central channel like a stick, without inhalation or exhalation, and because of this, a quasi-clairvoyance arises that remembers the past."[51] Reacting to this claim, Khedrub Norsang Gyatso adds that while for some traditions such clairvoyance is natural, other traditions argue that uterine experiences such as these

Table 5.5 Development of the mind/mental sensations over the course of gestation

Mo.	*Heart of Medicine*	*Four Tantras*	*Entering the Womb*	*Drakpa Gyeltsen*	*Kālacakra*
1					
2					
3	pleasure and pain recognized				
4					
5	mind (*sems*) becomes clear		mental sense power is completed		
6		pleasure and pain recognized			pleasure and pain recognized
7		memory is clear	eight distorted conceptions		fetus remembers past life
8					
9		desire to escape womb	desire to escape womb; five distorted conceptions	desire to escape womb	
10		boy feels attachment to mother and animosity to father; girl feels the reverse			

are only dreamlike (and therefore do not generate karma).[52] Kyempa Tsewang summarizes yet another model of gestation, which he attributes to the twelfth-century *Profound Inner Meaning* and which can also be found in the *Kālacakra*: in this version the fetus experiences suffering beginning only in the ninth month, because only then is its tongue developed and able to taste the foulness of its uterine environment.[53]

Certainly, the details of conception and development vary widely across Tibetan literary traditions. Stories of gestation provide descriptive accounts of embryogenesis that we may think of as "third person" accounts, but, interestingly, they also provide "first person" accounts of the fetus' own experiences of conception and growth. In one way, we may consider these to be literal reports of the process of gestation intended merely to satisfy a listener's interest in how this process works; in this sense, the central character of these narratives really is, simply, the developing embryo. But the phenomenological nature of these accounts in particular – their emphasis on the fetal experience of gestation and not simply a description of physical growth – underscores a sense that the story's discourse portrays an event that the listener him or herself may aspire to experience. In this way, these narratives are not simply a premodern approach to biological or scientific embryology, but are, instead or in addition, a prescriptive path of practice. This is not a hidden meaning of embryology; on the contrary, in many cases it is overt. As we will see in the following pages, Buddhist texts are explicit that the meaning and intention of embryological narratives lies in their direct relevance to religious practice, although that meaning varies by tradition.

Practicing the exoteric path

In the normative literature of exoteric Buddhism, the period of gestation and the event of birth are characterized, like ordinary existence, as hopelessly, insufferably wretched. The first of the Four Noble Truths posits the experience of suffering as the most basic feature of existence, and Buddhist traditions lavishly narrate the many ways that human existence is essentially an experience of suffering. Early Indian Buddhists saw the events of birth, aging and death as evidence of the inevitable misery of human existence. Labeling these life events the "enemies" of human existence, the author of the early Indian *Aṭṭhasālinī* likens birth to an enemy who carries a person off to the jungle, aging to an enemy who strikes someone to the ground, and death to an enemy who beheads a man.[54] In the *Entering the Womb* sūtra, the Buddha declares that conception essentially results in suffering: "The five aggregates of name and form, the moment they have taken on a body, are experiences of suffering."[55] This attitude toward fetal existence and birth is pervasive in Tibetan exoteric writings. Composed in twelfth-century Tibet, Gampopa's treatment of human development occurs within a tripartite presentation of suffering derived from the Buddhism of the Pāli Canon, a division that describes the suffering of conditioned existence, the suffering of change, and the suffering of suffering. A teaching on the vicious state of saṃsāra for the student of Buddhist meditation who needs an antidote to attachment to sensual pleasures, the topic of the "suffering of suffering," includes, first, a description of the "suffering of evil existences" and details the suffering of beings in the various lower realms, such as animal and hell realms, then next, a description of "the suffering of happy existences," which describes the forms of suffering of those born into the higher realms of existence, namely humans, demigods and gods. This fundamental Buddhist teaching claims that once one understands through meditation the transitory and miserable state of saṃsāric existence, one feels compelled to strive energetically toward a more enlightened manner of existence.

The embryological narrative in this tradition occurs within teachings on the suffering of ordinary existence. Gampopa's account states that if one becomes convinced of the suffering of entering the womb, one will want never to do it again. He cites the *Entering the Womb* sūtra, saying,

> Alas! Since this ocean of transmigratory existence is aflame, burns and blazes, not a single individual is unaffected by it. This blazing fire is that of attachment, antipathy and bewilderment, of birth, old age and death, of mourning, lamentation, distress and affliction. It is always burning and ablaze, not a single individual escapes from it.[56]

Gampopa's narrative summarizes the myriad ways a fetus suffers in the womb over the course of thirty-eight weeks. In the first week, the oval-shaped, runny substance feels as if it is being boiled and fried in a pan, and the consciousness and sense organs experience intense pain. In the second week, the embryo is transformed into an oblong, gelatinous substance and the four elements are manifested: earth, water, fire and wind, enabling solidity, cohesion, temperature and mobility. In the third week, wind strengthens the power of the four elements and the embryo becomes a ladle-shaped lump. In the seventh week, the hands and feet are produced, and the embryo experiences a pain as if it is being pulled by a strong wind and spread out with a stick. The nine orifices of the body are produced in the eleventh week, and the embryo suffers as if it were an open wound being jabbed by a finger. In the thirty-seventh week, the fetus experiences the need to escape the dirty, malodorous, imprisoning darkness of the womb, and in the thirty-eighth week wind pushes the fetus toward the mouth of the womb, an event which the fetus experiences as being crushed by machinery. Feeling as if it is being squeezed through iron netting, the infant is born.

Gampopa goes on to explain that the fetus is further victimized by the actions of its environmental host. If the mother eats cold food, the fetus feels like a nude person thrown onto ice. When she eats too much, it feels as if it is being crushed by rocks. When the mother has sexual intercourse, the fetus feels like it is being pummeled by thorns.[57] The reader is reminded that some children are stillborn, and others die during childbirth. Suffering only continues after release from the womb:

> ...when in the process of birth the child is put on the ground it feels the pain of being laid on a rough coat. At a later stage it suffers the agony of being scraped on the edge of a wall and of its skin being peeled (when it is washed the first time, as the skin is so sensitive). For a long time the newly-born stays in misery and suffers much pain, heat, darkness and unpleasantness. If you were offered three gold coins to remain two days and nights in an unclean closed pit, you would not accept, however much you might want the money, and yet the misery of being in a womb is worse than that.[58]

For the Buddhist narrator of Gampopa's story, the presentation of gestation and birth is an opportunity to demonstrate the intensity of suffering experienced in the human life. "If we are convinced of such misery," he argues, "we should be haunted by the fear of entering the womb."[59] His graphic description is a classic exoteric Buddhist account, mirroring that of the fifth-century Indian Buddhist commentator Buddhaghosa, who described life in the womb in his *Visuddhimagga* as follows:

> Here the suffering classed as "rooted in the descent into the womb" and so on, is this: when this being is born in the mother's womb, he is not born inside a blue or red or white lotus, etc., but on the contrary, like a worm in rotting fish, rotting dough, cesspools, etc., he is born in the belly in a position that is below the receptacle for undigested food (stomach), above the receptacle for digested food (rectum), between the belly-lining ... and the backbone, which is very cramped, quite dark, pervaded by very fetid draughts redolent of various smells of ordure, and exceptionally loathsome. And on being reborn there, for ten months he undergoes excessive suffering, being cooked like a pudding in a bag by the heat produced by the mother's womb, and steamed like a dumpling of dough, with no bending, stretching, and so on. So this, firstly, is the suffering rooted in the descent into the womb [60]

Like Gampopa, Buddhaghosa contextualizes early human development in a discussion of suffering. In this model of embryology, we witness the story of an individual who experiences little but the continuance of deprivation from lifetime to lifetime. The embryo perceives its uterine environment to be an abode of horror, and the reader or listener is urged to perceive his or her existence in the same way. This miserable character is offered the support of Buddhist practice as a means for escaping the thoroughly wretched cycle of ordinary existence.

The particulars of the misery of gestation and birth derived from the Indian sūtric traditions are fundamental in many Tibetan Buddhist presentations of suffering, both exoteric and esoteric, since, of course, the teaching of suffering is shared by all Buddhists. The sixteenth-century Sakya path text by Ngorchen Könchok Lhündrub (1497–1557), for example, explains that,

> Since birth is the root of all other sufferings as well as the result of the origination of suffering, its own nature does not go beyond suffering. Furthermore, as far as the womb is concerned, there is suffering of suffocation by bad odors when residing in the womb; the suffering like being pressed down upon when the mother eats food; the suffering like falling into a ravine when she moves about and stirs; and the suffering of being affected by heat and cold when she eats and drinks hot and cold food. During birth, there is the suffering like being drawn through a hole, and on being born there is the suffering like falling into a pit of thorns.[61]

In like fashion, the *Kālacakra* notes that "There is suffering for the fetus in the womb. There is suffering at the time of birth and in childhood as well."[62] The *Stainless Light* (*Vimalaprabhā*) expands on this sentiment: "The pain of fetuses, of transmigrating beings abiding in the womb, is similar to the baking of a potter's vessel. At the time of birth, it is like being crushed by the anvil and hammer. In childhood, it is like a hog feeding upon feces."[63] This model may, indeed, be one of the oldest paradigms of the process of birth in the Buddhist tradition, and is possibly inherited from much earlier Indian Upaniṣadic and Purāṇic sources: descriptions of human fetal development even in those traditions "want to induce in the reader repulsion for the return to the matrix, and thereby stimulate the desire to obtain *mokṣa*," or liberation.[64] The following pages will demonstrate, however, that quite unlike this paradigm, for esoteric tantric traditions the ordinary processes of birth and death are often not used as threats, but rather as *models* of spiritual progress.

Esoteric practices for closing the womb's door

Today for many people, knowing the details of human development is knowing something about medicine or science. In the examples here, however, knowing embryology is knowing religious practice. Let us look at another religious context for embryological detail, the practice known as closing or blocking the womb's door, mentioned briefly above, found within teachings on death and the intermediate state. In these teachings, which are common to all schools of Tibetan Buddhist practice and which derive from Indian *siddha* traditions, practitioners aim to end cyclic existence through yogic and meditative exercises played out in a re-enactment of the stages of dying, intermediate state existence, and rebirth. The Tibetan articulation of such teachings, originally conceived in India, involves a proliferation of intermediate state phases and a conflation of the notion of the intermediate state with the idea of the three bodies of the

Buddha. In a study of these developments, Bryan Cuevas explains that Tibetans created unique tantric conceptions of the intermediate state (*bar do*), articulating not only three, but as many as six separate intermediate states, many practices of which came collectively to be known as the six doctrines of Nāropa. He observes the growth of different practices of the intermediate state doctrine among Nyingma and Bön traditions, and then the eventual systematization of both Nyingma and Sarma versions of these practices between the fourteenth and fifteenth centuries. This systematization formed the basis for the funeral liturgies of the *Great Liberation upon Hearing in the Bardo*, one of the texts that is known commonly, if inaccurately, as the *Tibetan Book of the Dead*.[65]

The practice of closing the womb's door is aimed at the transmigrating consciousness about to enter a womb and be reborn. Derived from texts attributed to Indian *mahāsiddhas* such as Nāropa, this practice was expounded in Tibet by religious scholars around the time of the second diffusion, such as Gampopa for instance, as well as many others, and then transmitted in various forms through teaching lineages in each of the schools of Tibetan Buddhism. The tradition of Nāropa's six doctrines (*na ro chos drug*) thus exists in a diversity of forms across the spectrum of Buddhist schools.[66] The tremendously influentia Tibetan polymath Tsong Khapa (1357–1419), for example, synthesizing a comprehensive path of training based on Nāropa's six doctrines, integrates intermediate state teachings with instructions for the purification of the three life stages, practices to be addressed below. His discussion of this synthesis can be found in his *Treatise on the Stages of Training in the Profound Path of Naro's Six Dharmas*, now translated into English by Glen Mullin.[67] These practices involve training in contemplative subtle body yogas during one's lifetime that are then performed at the moment of death with the aim of experiencing one's death and transition into the intermediate state consciously, or, ideally, enabling an escape from that transition into a state of enlightenment. While the most advanced practitioners may achieve liberation through these practices directly, less advanced contemplatives may, instead, be able to control, to greater or lesser degrees, the experience and manner of intermediate state existence and rebirth.

If practitioners are unable to "close the womb's door" in this way, these teachings explain how one may encourage a transmigrating consciousness to choose a good womb. The *Tibetan Book of the Dead* tradition explains how, as a transmigrating consciousness, one can recognize the best place to be reborn – in our own world – and what sorts of places to avoid. The experience of choosing a rebirth destination are graphic and at times frightening. The transmigrator is advised,

> At that time when you are helplessly chased by butchers and are overwhelmed by terror, instantaneously visualize all at once the Lord Chemchok Heruka, or Hayagriva, or Vajrapani, and so forth, whoever is your Archetype Deity; gigantic in size, with bulging limbs, terrifying,

> furious, able to crush all demons to dust. By his blessing and compassion, you will free yourself from those butchers, and you will gain the power to choose a good womb.[68]

The text continues to explain two techniques: how to be reborn into a lotus bud in a Pure Land, and how to be reborn into an ordinary human womb. For those unwilling or unable to direct themselves into the Pure Land, the instructions for choosing a good human womb are as follows:

> Using your clairvoyance, enter a womb in a place where the Dharma has spread. Caution is required, for even if you were to be reborn magically in a heap of dung, you would get the notion that the impure mass smelled delicious and you would be reborn in it by the force of your attraction. Therefore you should not adhere to whatever appearance occurs, and you must discount any signs that trigger attachment or aversion. Then choose a good womb. And here the willed intention is important; so you must create it as follows: "Hey! For the sake of all beings, I will be reborn as a world-ruling emperor, or of the priestly class, sheltering all beings like a great shade tree, or as the child of a holy man, an adept, or of a clan with an impeccable Dharma lineage, or in a family where the parents have great faith. I must succeed in this coming life, by adopting a body that has great merit, to enable me to accomplish the aims of all beings!" Aiming your will in this way you should enter the womb. At that time, the womb you have entered should appear to you as if magically transformed into a divine palace. You should pray to the Buddhas and the Bodhisattvas of the ten directions, the Archetype Deities, and especially to the Lord of Great Compassion. And you should visualize that they are all anointing you in consecration as you enter the womb.[69]

Practices such as closing the womb cross sectarian lines and are directed at contemplatives aiming to choose particular rebirth states. In these accounts, more attention is focused on the experience of the intermediate state and the moment of conception; once conception has occurred, the objective of the practice has been met, and therefore the details of embryogenesis itself are of little concern.

Nowhere is the correlation between birth and liberation more overtly tied to Buddhist practice than in the tantras. Detailed contemplative practices modeled after the processes of human conception, development and birth are present in a wide range of Indian Buddhist tantras, such as the *Kālacakra*, *Vajrabhairava*, *Guhyasamāja*, *Cakrasaṃvara*, *Saṃvarodaya*, *Vajramālā* and *Hevajra* tantras, as well as in numerous exegetical works and *siddha* traditions. Knowledge of the mechanics of conception, gestation and birth were used for the conceptualization of spiritual enlightenment in general and for the articulation of specifi modes of practice. The requirements of a given author's preferred system of practice in turn affected how embryology was narrativized. For many Tibetan authors, therefore, the correspondence between fetal development and spiritual growth was overt. In the advanced tantric practice known as purification of the three life stages or "bringing the three bodies to the path" (*sku gsum lam 'khyer*), for instance, while the focus is still primarily the moment of conception, the details of gestation are also addressed in some detail. Let us turn to this practice now, considering it as articulated by the tradition of Tsong Khapa and his followers.

Purifying death, the intermediate state and rebirth

The founder of the Tibetan Buddhist Geluk tradition, Tsong Khapa's writings on religious practice and development spawned more than five hundred years of commentarial exposition and elaboration, and his treatment of human development and its religious symbolism is thus a prominent part of Tibetan Buddhist intellectual culture. Like the practice of closing the womb, this tradition describes activities in which religious contemplatives aim for liberation, at which point they stop the cycle of death and rebirth, through a series of meditations modeled after the actual processes of death, intermediate state existence and rebirth. The meditator is advised to gain control over these life stages by studying the tantric physiology of channels, winds and quintessential essences, and by performing practices that manipulate those aspects of the inner body, thereby mirroring the processes of death, intermediate state existence and rebirth.

The teachings in which these advanced practices occur appear at the pinnacle of the Buddhist fourfold classification of tantric texts and their practices into action (*bya*, Skt. *kriyā*), performance (*spyod*, Skt. *charyā*), yoga (*rnal 'byor*, Skt. *yoga*) and highest yoga (*bla med*, Skt. *anuttarayoga*) tantras. Each form of tantra prescribes a complex of different practices, which are said by some scholars to be aimed at practitioners of different contemplative capabilities.[70] The highest yoga tantra is generally distinguished by Geluk scholars from the other tantra classes by its claim to facilitate enlightenment within a single lifetime, and it thus involves the most esoteric of the esoteric, the most complex of tantric contemplative and ritual practices. The highest yoga tantra path itself is divided into a generation stage (*bskyed rim*) and completion stage (*rdzogs rim*). Generation stage practices are preliminary procedures, preparing the mind for later completion stage practices. Engaging in practices modeled after the ordinary life processes of death, intermediate state existence and rebirth, the practitioner is told to overcome ordinary conceptuality and the ordinary appearance of phenomena by visualizing him- or herself as a purified deity. The practice of generating an image of oneself as a deity is known as deity yoga (*lha'i rnal 'byor*), and the type of deity yoga that involves a mirroring of the three life stages is particular to highest yoga tantra forms of deity yoga.

A synthesis of a variety of Buddhist tantric sources on the subject, Tsong Khapa's *Great Stages of Mantra* (*Sngag rim chen mo*), describes generation stage deity yoga practices in which one begins to learn how to convert the three ordinary life stages into the three purified bodies of the Buddha: the purifie experience of death can transform one into a Buddha's Reality Body, the purified experience of the intermediate state can transform one into a Buddha's Enjoyment Body, and the purified experience of birth can transform one into a Buddha's Emanation Body. Success in this type of meditation is said to result in the winds of one's subtle body entering, remaining, and then dissolving inside the central channel, whereupon one may begin completion stage practices.

These advanced practices begin by combining a meditation on emptiness with one's knowledge of subtle physiology and the mechanics of dying. In an ordinary individual, the winds enter the central channel only at death – as an individual is dying, however, the winds of all seventy-two thousand channels throughout the body first gather in the right and left channels, then move into the central channel, until finally they dissolve into the channel-wheel at the heart. Losang Gyeltsen Senggé (b. 1757) explains that the special "indestructible" quintessential essence that is considered the basis of the wind and the mind, and therefore the basis of all phenomena, is located at the heart and survives until death. Death thus takes place at the moment when all other winds of the body dissolve into the indestructible quintessential essence and the very subtle wind at the heart.[71] Death occurs in this way, states the eighteenth-century Geluk scholar Yangchen Gawé Lodrö (1740–1827) in a *Guhyasamāja*-oriented treatise based on Tsong Khapa's work, "because, except for this very subtle wind, if the slightest wind that acts as a basis of consciousness dwells in any part of the body, death is not possible."[72]

The process of reaching this moment of death is explained as occurring in a series of stages during which the body's natural elements "dissolve" sequentially into each other. Internal and external signs are described that identify which stage of dying a person has reached. The functions of the body are gradually weakened: the body becomes thin and the limbs loose, one's vision and hearing diminish, food cannot be digested and one gradually loses consciousness.[73] The coarse types of mind then dissolve, and increasingly subtle forms of mind dissolve sequentially until only the mind of non-dualistic clear light (*'od gsal*) remains, at which point the individual has died. The clear light stage occurs when the white and red quintessential essences dissolve into the white and red indestructible quintessential essences at the heart, and the winds gathered in the central channel dissolve into the very subtle wind. "Through this," Yangchen Gawé Lodrö explains, "the very subtle wind and mind that have existed in the ordinary state from the beginning are made manifest." In other words, one manifests the components of conception itself, the white and red indestructible quintessential essences at the heart having been inherited from one's parents at conception. This experience is also referred to as an attainment of the "basic"

Reality Body, which may then be transformed into a Buddha's Reality Body (*chos sku*, Skt. *dharmakāya*).[74] It is this process of death that advanced contemplatives attempt to recreate in meditation.

An ordinary body generally remains in the state of clear light for three days. When pus or blood is seen at the nose and sexual organs, this indicates that the consciousness has departed the body, and the body may be discarded.[75] Once the consciousness has left the body, it experiences a reversal from its state of clear light back through the seven stages of dissolution and, once this has been completed, the intermediate state begins and the being will begin its search for a new body into which to be reborn. Yangchen Gawé Lodrö states that the actual moment of rebirth – that is, the moment that the intermediate state consciousness connects to the mixture of reproductive substances in the mother's womb – is the moment when the consciousness reaches the process of reverse dissolution upon entering the womb.[76]

When a practitioner has completed the stages of contemplative practice where death and the intermediate state are "purified," the practitioner begins the stage of purifying birth, imagining him- or herself undergoing the process of conception and gestation as a deity. The copulating parents-to-be are imagined as a deity couple in union, the deity couple understood to represent compassion and wisdom. The practitioner then imagines entering the parents' reproductive substances and traveling with them into the womb.[77] Tsong Khapa's account describes the meditative visualization of a "seed syllable," the form of a syllable visualized three-dimensionally, that signifies the consciousness that enters the male and female reproductive substances. In the language of tantric ritual, that seed syllable is transformed into a ritual implement called the five-pronge vajra, which is then likened to the fetus:

> from the seed (syllable) a hand implement is produced which is a five pronged vajra, and in the *Sheaf of Instructions* it is explained – gathering into sets of five – that the five prongs of one end (of the vajra) are the (embryo's) four limbs (legs and arms) and the head above the neck, and that the five prongs of the other end (of the vajra) are the five digits on the feet and hands and the five senses on the head [78]

In a contemporary account of this process, the Geluk scholar Kelsang Gyatso describes the practice as follows. After being told to visualize a maṇḍala in which is centered a union of male and female reproductive substances, the meditator is instructed to imagine entering these substances: "With the motivation to benefit all living beings, we … develop a strong wish to be reborn inside this union of Father Heruka's sperm and Mother Vajravarahi's ovum."[79] Conception occurs, and Kelsang Gyatso equates the subsequently visualized development of the syllable *Hum* with the growth of the fetus. He explains that this practice transforms the ordinary experience of rebirth in a way that facilitates the later achievement of a Buddha's Emanation Body.[80] These practices are not limited to

Gelukpas; a contemporary Nyingma scholar, Gyatrul Rinpoche, describes a similar meditation practice. While meditating on the deity, he explains, one visualizes a red lotus seat on which a red sun and a white moon lie flat – these three form the throne of the deity. During the practice of purifying birth, the lotus represents the channels and channel-wheels, the sun represents the practitioner's heat (*me drod*), lying below the navel, and the moon represents the father's seed, imagined as a white upside-down *Ham* syllable at the crown of the head. By yogic practice of manipulating the winds, heat travels up the central channel and melts the seed syllable in the crown. In a subsequent stage of the practice, the sun represents the mother's reproductive substance and the moon represents the father's reproductive substance, and when the seed syllable falls onto these disks, this corresponds to the moment when the consciousness enters the union of male and female reproductive substances. At that moment, the seed syllable transforms into an implement held by the imagined deity. Light radiates out from and is absorbed back into the implement, this action purifying the moment of conception, when the consciousness enters the womb. A repeating cycle of light radiating out from and being absorbed back into the deity then corresponds to the growth of the fetus. Gyatrul Rinpoche explains that "the particulars of the phases of growth during the nine months of human gestation are given detailed attention in the more extensive generation stage teachings."[81]

For the Gelukpa, this type of deity yoga, involving a meditative generation of oneself as a deity and the performance of certain activities in that form, is posited as the practice that distinguishes tantric from sūtric practice, and it is presented as a direct way of generating a Buddha's Form Body (*gzugs sku*). When a practitioner is exhorted to purify ordinary death, intermediate state and rebirth through the method known as "bringing the three bodies to the path" (*sku gsum lam 'khyer*), these practices are thus ultimately aimed at actualizing the Buddha's three bodies.[82] When the practitioner reaches the point of taking birth from the imagined womb, he or she perceives that experience as birth into a purified m ṇḍala with the body of a Buddha.

Tsong Khapa's presentation of actualizing the Buddha's bodies through practices modeled after the three life stages is not without controversy, even within the Geluk system itself. Yael Bentor has studied debates recorded in the writings of Tsong Khapa and his student, Khedrub Jé (1385–1438), over topics such as whether the transformation of birth is the only practice performed during the generation stage or whether all three transformations occur there, and whether it is only womb-born humans that may engage in these practices, as opposed to those born by one of the other three modes of birth. She cites interesting deliberations by authors in Tsong Khapa's tradition, before and after his lifetime, on the issue of purifying each of the four modes of birth. As mentioned in chapter two, Buddhist sūtras offer four possibilities for birth: beings may be born from eggs, from wombs, from warmth or moisture, or miraculously, from "space." Bentor explains that Butön Rinchen Drub, in Tsong Khapa's own *Guhyasamāja* lineage, claims that for purifying birth from an egg, one should practice the "generation of deities from a seed enclosed in the midst of embracing sun and moon"; for purifying a womb birth, one should practice "generation in a manner of invoking with a song a seed that has entered into the womb of the Father-Mother and has dissolved there"; for purifying a birth from warmth or moisture, one should practice "generation from just a seed, signifying the consciousness of the intermediate being, on top of an open lotus, with a sun ray signifying warmth, and a moon signifying moisture"; and for purifying a miraculous birth, there is "the instantaneous generation of enlightened beings."[83] Tsong Khapa and Khedrub Jé disagree with this view, however, claiming that these purifica tion practices are only for the womb-born, and yet the purification of the four modes of birth was, nonetheless, a widespread teaching. Bentor cites a number of other examples: a fourteenth-century figure Barawa, for instance, offers a *Hevajra* version of the purification of the four modes of birth [84]

Beyond speaking of conception itself and directing oneself to an appropriate womb, tantric traditions across sectarian lines explicitly link the subsequent stages of fetal growth with spiritual progress. Tsong Khapa cites Indian tantric sources that correlate the stages of gestation with the paths of spiritual attainment: he assigns the path of seeing (*mthong lam*) and the path of meditation (*sgom lam*) to the ten months of gestation, the moment of birth to the path of no more learning (*mi slob lam*), and the period from birth up to the next occasion of entering a womb to the path of preparation (*sbyor lam*).[85] The fourteenth-century Nyingma scholar Longchenpa cites a similar correspondence as found in the *Seventeen Tantras of the Great Perfection* collection, which also states that the spiritual stages are experienced in the ten months of gestation.[86] A contemporary Nyingma account of the generation stage practice of purifying the act of rebirth mirrors this tradition: Gyatrul Rinpoche links the time in the intermediate state to the path of accumulation (*tshogs lam*), the moment just prior to conception to the path of preparation, the moment of conception to the path of seeing, the period of fetal development to the path of meditation, and birth to the path of no more learning.[87] In one *Kālacakra* tradition, the four types of the Buddha's perfect awakening are similarly expressed through a connection to fetal stages of growth[88] and in another, the four bodies of the Buddha are linked to those gestational stages.[89] The general association between stages of gestation and stages of attainment has a long history and is not originally a tantric tradition, as it occurs in a commentary by Vasubandhu and elsewhere in exoteric Buddhism.[90] It is the esoteric Buddhist traditions that bring this linkage between embryogenesis and the spiritual path to its fullest expression, however, such that the entirety of the religious path is explicitly tied to conception and the stages of fetal development.

The ultimate reason for performing these purification practices is to assist sentient beings and oneself in the movement toward Buddhahood. Khedrub Norsang Gyatso explains that fetal development is taught so that one may "know and understand the bases of purification for the generation and completion stages."[91] Gyatrul Rinpoche notes that these practices "result in birth as an enlightened being,"[92] and that the purification of birth practice eliminates "the habitual tendency to take rebirth and helps one directly understand the non-dual nature of appearance and emptiness."[93] Ngawang Dargyé notes that knowledge of conception and fetal growth is essential because it is the basis for knowing how to return from an illusory body into a gross body in order to teach ordinary beings.[94] Drakpa Gyeltsen argues that contemplative practices can only be performed with a clear understanding of the body, including how it is conceived and its early development.[95] Scholars of tantra across the centuries emphasize the importance of special attention to the nature of, and usage of, one's own ordinary physical body and one's subtle body physiology. With detailed knowledge of the physiological processes that occur during ordinary death, intermediate state and rebirth, the tantric practitioner uses these processes as objects of purifi cation during generation and completion stage meditation. The practitioner's embodied condition is thus central to these practices. This provides a rationale for the detailed study of physiological processes: human physiology is itself the guide to the most advanced forms of soteriological practices. The main character of these embryologically-articulated stories is one who has systematically mastered the technicalities of ordinary gross and subtle physiology, and who can effect one's own transformation by proceeding methodically through a sequence of physiologically presented practices while visualizing oneself as an enlightened being. One brings sentient beings and oneself toward Buddhahood through detailed knowledge of, and manipulations of, one's own body.

The embryologic vision of reality

During the same fifty year period as the scholastic synthesis and expansion of Indian Buddhist sources in which Tsong Khapa entwined models of human development with contemplative practice, a tremendously influential scholar of the Nyingma school was also at work on a similar task. In his *Treasury of Precious Words and Meanings*, the fourteenth-century Nyingma scholar Longchenpa records a reworking of tantric paradigms of enlightenment that relies on poetic uses of traditional Buddhist symbols. Central to Longchenpa's work is an account of the human body – including a very long narrative of embryogenesis – in which the body itself hosts a playful dance of delusion and enlightenment. According to Longchenpa's cosmologically-oriented presentation of the esoteric Great Perfection doctrine, existence itself spontaneously arises from "the Ground" (*gzhi*), which, prior to its manifestation, is illustrated with a uterine metaphor as a "youthful body in a vase" (*gzhon nu bum pa sku*). The drama that ensues upon the Ground's manifestation is scripted by the ordinary human's perception and interpretation of experience: as long as karmically-determined, distorted perceptions dominate human experience, cyclic existence continues. Releasing oneself from this distorted mode of perception, thereby allowing progress toward enlightened experience, is the project of the Great Perfection contemplative, and, as in other tantric traditions, the worksite for this project is the body itself.

Hierarchically correlating to the esoteric Geluk highest yoga tantra tradition described above, the Great Perfection is considered the supreme vehicle in the Nyingma system of nine traditions, or "vehicles," of thought and practice. While the eight lower vehicles emphasize practices such as merit accumulation and purification of obstacles, Great Perfection practices are aimed at accomplishing a direct understanding of innate wisdom (*ye shes*, Skt. *jñāna*). Like their Geluk counterparts, Great Perfection contemplatives begin with practices from the lower vehicles, advancing only after completion of the standard set of "preliminary practices" (*sngon 'gro*), which involve taking refuge, prostration, generating *bodhicitta*, making offerings and performing purifications. Highest yoga tantra practices of the generation and completion stages, common to other schools of Tibetan Buddhism, are also performed by Great Perfection contemplatives. Only after mastering these complex systems do practitioners engage in specific Great Perfection practices known as "breakthrough" (*khregs chod*) and "direct transcendence" (*thod rgal*). Here, I will consider one aspect of the dialogic relationship between these contemplative practices and the articulation of embryology in Great Perfection literature.

In the early chapters of the *Treasury*, Longchenpa locates within each sentient being's body an enlightened essence, which is identified with the Ground. In chapters two and three of the *Treasury*, this pure energy of the Ground is identified as the very source of our physical and psychic being. As such, it is said to be located in literal and symbolic ways throughout the psycho-physical body. Enlightenment depends on a recognition of this essence that will allow its energies to surface from the obscuring depths of perceptual error. This, of course, is the traditional Buddhist teaching that all beings possess within themselves a "Buddha-nature," which is explicitly the subject of the *Treasury*'s third chapter. Longchenpa's presentation of the discovery of enlightenment within the ordinary body ties that process to gestation and birth, arguing in his *Seven Treasuries* that "birth and death are the optimal measures of familiarization with reality itself."[96] He cites a poetic passage from the *Garland of Precious Pearls* (*Mu tig phreng ba*), a tantra from the *Seventeen Tantras of the Great Perfection* collection, that explains how the changes of embodied human existence are events in the storyline of spiritual progress:

> Entering the womb
> Is the manifestation of self-awareness from the Ground;
> With the initial seven weeks of the embryo's development,
> The measures of contemplative realization are attained;
> With the total ten months, the spiritual stages are traversed;
> Birth is arising in the Spiritual Bodies;
> Your body's development is the objective sphere of the Ground-presenting,
> While remaining in your body is the Ground;
> Through aging, distortion is cleansed away;

Sickness is the assurance of realization,
And through death you are freed into reality's emptiness.
Manifesting thus, all sentient beings
Are effortlessly and primordially free...[97]

The normal life cycle events of one's own birth, illness, aging and death are used here as symbolic correlates to spiritual progress, which are articulated as a sequence of embodied events. As with other tantric traditions, spiritual attainments are thus presented as events that are understood not primarily through intellectual speculation, but rather through the experience of the body itself.

Emphasizing the ultimate purity of cyclic existence, Longchenpa associates ordinary, impure physical objects with the pure dimension of existence from which they originate. "Since all the appearances of cyclic existence's three realms are initially apprehended and abstracted out from the dimension of the [Ground's] expanse," Longchenpa explains, "each exists in intimate correlation with that dimension."[98] Explaining that enlightened reality is present within the body at all times, Longchenpa links the stages of human existence to the three spiritual bodies, although differently than in other tantric traditions: birth (*btsas pa*) is correlated with the Emanation Body, taking form in a physical existence (*lus gnas*) with the Enjoyment Body, and death (*shi ba*) with the Reality Body.[99] In the Great Perfection model as in other Buddha-nature traditions, enlightened reality is not a distant goal to be manufactured, but rather an inherent aspect of the existence humans inhabit right now. The purity that is symbolically represented by the five Buddha families appears during embryogenesis as fiv tiny letters, or syllables, that manifest inside the channels of the embryo. These letters are also linked to pure seed syllables that are said to yield the Buddha Bodies during contemplative visualization practices. As in the Geluk example above, this physiology justifies religious practices that require an intimate knowledge of the body. Longchenpa explains that "by understanding the characteristics of the body's origination, you attain certainty as to the Reality Body."[100] Although the three Buddha Bodies are located within the ordinary human body, during the process of ordinary embryonic development this pure dimension was generated in a distorted way. This doctrine thus justifies the importance of embryology as a topic of study for the religious practitioner: it is essential to understand the process of embryogenesis in order to fully comprehend the causes of saṃsāric existence and the true nature of our essential enlightenment. Understanding the distortions that result in ordinary saṃsāric existence is the key to purifying or reversing the process, clearing up the distortions and revealing one's pure enlightened existence.

The general notion that for a soteriological end one can meditatively re-enact one's birth and the physiological processes of fetal development that result in birth, is similar in the Geluk and Nyingma esoteric traditions described in this chapter. But Great Perfection literature goes a step beyond correlating the stages of human existence to spiritual rebirth. For Longchenpa, the very details of embryonic growth are explicitly scripted to express the relationship between the generation of an ordinary being and the generation of an enlightened being. The esoteric Nyingma account of the uterine growth of the subtle body is unique. As described above, in Longchenpa's embryological narrative, circulatory channels emerge in the embryo's body during the first two weeks of gestation, and two tiny "eyes" are formed within them. These embryonic eyes are associated with subtle innate wisdom (*ye shes*), a discursive turn that is essential to the presentation of Longchenpa's contemplative system, which appears later in the *Treasury*. The eyes are especially important to Great Perfection practice because they act as the conduit for the transmission of enlightened energy from internal to external areas of the body. It is the eyes that give birth to enlightenment.

Longchenpa's embryology describes a series of very subtle light channels (*'od rtsa*) throughout the body, two of which travel from the eyes to the heart, the heart being the primary location of the individual's enlightened essence.[101] A network of pathways running throughout the entire body and originating in the heart, these light channels are a distinctive feature of the Great Perfection tradition. David Germano points out that unlike the network of channels typically described in other systems of tantric physiology, which are said to operate in both impure and pure modes, carrying the ordinary bodily fluids of saṃsāric existence as well as the purified substances and energies of enlightened existence, the light channels are conduits of pure energies alone. The tradition explains that during the contemplative practice known as direct transcendence (*thod rgal*), when a portion of this enlightened essence has left the heart through the light channels and exited the body at the eyes, it manifests as visions. Contemplatives see maṇḍalas of rainbow-colored light that are to be understood, therefore, as an outflowing of their own enlightened essence. As such, they are, in fact, visions of the true nature of reality seen without the distortions of ordinary saṃsāric conceptuality. Ultimately, in the course of these practices, the contemplative's material body may dissolve completely, leaving only the rainbow-colored light of the enlightened essence, a form of spiritual liberation known as achieving a "rainbow body" (*'ja' lus*).

In direct transcendence meditation, the enlightened essence concentrated at the heart is aroused by focusing on an external light source, such as the sun or a lamp, and it flows outward through the light channels via the eyes, which are known as the "door" or "gateway" (*sgo*) of innate wisdom. Explaining the origins of these light channels in the embryonic body, Longchenpa cites the *Blazing Lamp* (*Sgron ma 'bar ba*), another tantra of the *Seventeen Tantras of the Great Perfection* collection:

> At the time of residing in the mother's womb
> When one's own body is first developing,
> Within the vibrant energies of the entire body
> The great channel knot of the navel wheel originates,
> And in its triangle at the embryo's center

> Via the vibrant energies of the paternal cause and maternal condition
> The eyes' orbs develop.
> Furthermore, the eyes' combination of white and black
> Derives from the paternal and maternal elements respectively;
> The gateways of innate wisdom's shining forth are these two eyes.[102]

The two eyes mentioned here are those that develop in the embryonic form during the first week of gestation, the "eye of the elements" and the "eye of the lamps." The father's reproductive substance, said to be white in color, and the mother's, said to be black or red, are here given direct responsibility for the development of these eyes, the most important part of the developing embryo's body. Germano notes that elsewhere in his corpus, Longchenpa refers to *The Totally Radiant* (*Thig le kun gsal*) as another early source that supports the view of the embryological primacy of the eyes; that text explains that

> The initial origination of the body takes hold from the eyes,
> Via being connected to the two eyes at the navel;
> They come into being within the channel-knot.[103]

What is fascinating about this tradition is the uniqueness of its embryology, which has few ties to any known Indian medical or religious accounts, and which is so tightly intertwined with the particulars of Nyingma practice. The subject of Longchenpa's story is encouraged to see him- or herself as essentially enlightened. The process of religious transformation for this figure involves relaxing the rigidity of distorted, ordinary perceptual habits and releasing a radiant, internal enlightenment through practices that require intimate knowledge of physiology. By placing the development of the eyes in the earliest stages of embryogenesis, the embryological narrative itself is manipulated to provide a roadmap for a particular type of spiritual practice in the very origins of the body. Thus, in this instance, it is especially clear that not only do narratives on meditation draw on embryological symbolism, but the reverse is also true: embryological narratives rely on religious or philosophical discourse.

Inconsistency, ignorance, or innovation?

In Tibet, there is not one single tradition of embryology – there are many. If we think of embryology within a scientific paradigm, where it would be a single body of knowledge, developing and changing throughout history but nonetheless driven by a model of correspondence to *how embryos actually grow*, the history of embryology we have seen in this book is puzzling, even incomprehensible. But was embryology incomprehensible to pre-modern Tibetan thinkers? What was it that made their embryological narratives true? Human development was a topic that captivated scholars and practitioners from all schools of intellectual life, and it took on importance in various and shifting ways throughout history.

Although well-known Indian medical and Buddhist texts had much to say about the growth of the embryo, for some reason this grew as a topic only loosely guided by Indian scriptural authority, and Tibetan authors allowed themselves here to exercise their own discretion. Although the sequence of psycho-physical development was carefully detailed in the *Entering the Womb* sūtra, a text considered authoritative on other matters of embryology, no subsequent Tibetan text adopted these details. Likewise, no subsequent Tibetan text repeats the sequence described in the *Heart of Medicine*, the early Indian medical text that served as the basis of much of Tibetan medicine. While those texts that are explicitly commentaries on the *Four Tantras* did agree with the sequence of development noted in the *Four Tantras*, other contemporaneous and subsequent embryologies presented a completely different model. Gampopa's presentation of fetal development, for example, focuses primarily on growth as an experience of recurring pain and suffering. Longchenpa's very detailed description, by contrast, stressed the volatile actions of the four elements and the emotions. Strangely, as we saw earlier, given the importance of the "humoral" and digestive systems in medical etiology and pathology, embryological narratives themselves are generally silent on the role of the systemic processes, or humors, and that of digestive heat. Indeed, very few Tibetan descriptions of fetal development – in religious *or* medical texts – even mention the development of the three systemic processes in the body, despite this being one of the most important aspects of Tibetan medical physiology.

Although the topic had been canonized in scriptures, the matter of precisely how the fetus grew was often addressed without requiring much, if any, external legitimatization. If an author's presentation diverged from known authorities, no justification was required. Drakpa Gyeltsen in the twelfth century summarized the varying accounts of embryogenesis known to him, but without denouncing those diverse views – rather, he says, in effect, that such details are only part of what is to be understood from embryology.[104] The medical commentator Lodrö Gyelpo insists that agreeing with the sūtra's account of the function of the winds in gestation, as he does, does not require approving of everything else set forth in the sūtras.[105] Pointing out that such discrepancies occurred even in early Indian texts, the eighteenth-century religious scholar Yangchen Gawé Lodrö likewise explains away embryological variances by pronouncing that, really, it all means the same thing.[106]

If the details of sequence of fetal development are not what embryology is really about, however, why then did Tibetans consistently make note of these events? The fact is, such details, however idiosyncratically represented, were regularly included in any significant embryological narrative. Observing this lack of attention to tradition, we may wonder whether the choices Tibetans made when writing about the body's development were somehow simply arbitrary. Even in such matters, however, where issues are apparently resolved through independent authorial discretion, this chapter argues that Tibetan writers were making deliberate choices – choices about whether the head develops first, the feet or the eyes – according to some principle. What, therefore, might the operative principles have been in these authorial decisions? If not empirical or scriptural, perhaps they were aesthetic principles. The authorial need to fill out certain details in the literary presentation of an issue can certainly be a question of literary aesthetics. Or, prioritizing parts of the body at the embryonic level may have harmonized with a given writer's philosophical or contemplative system, a matter of philosophical or logical aesthetics. Some embryological statements may, therefore, be assertions of aesthetically justified fact. In other words, descriptions of human development were firstly aesthetic or philosophical issues, not questions of empirically verifiable fact

While the details are quarreled over – Which limbs develop first? What degree of awareness does the fetus experience? – there is one important commonality in most of these accounts of growth. One of the very few consistencies across Tibetan texts with respect to the sequence of fetal development occurs in their classification of development into *stages*. As I mentioned in chapter two, most Tibetan texts describe the appearance of the early embryo using a vocabulary – *nar nar po, mer mer po, gor gor po* and sometimes *ltar ltar po*, which are variously correlated to the Sanskrit terms for the stages of embryonic development, *kalala*, *arbuda*, *budbuda*, *peśī*, and *ghana* – that goes back as far as the *Mahābhārata* and the Pāli Canon.[107] Some texts, such as Drakpa Gyeltsen's mid-twelfth-century *Great Jeweled Wishing Tree*, continue past these initial weeks by organizing development into abstract stages utilizing tantric vocabulary. In that text, we saw that the ten incarnations of Viṣṇu designate ten stages of fetal development spread over ten months. Longchenpa uses some of this vocabulary, although not consistently. Kyempa Tsewang and Lodrö Gyelpo, the two famous medical commentators, acknowledge these tantric models in their discussions of embryology as alternatives to the *Four Tantras*' view. Each of these scholars, however, presents the model differently. Kyempa Tsewang spreads the ten incarnations over ten months, as does Drakpa Gyeltsen, although the two disagree on the sequence of these stages.[108] While Longchenpa places the fish, tortoise and frog stages all within the first two months, Lodrö Gyelpo reports on a tradition in which three stages – fish, tortoise and pig – encompass the entire period of gestation.

The fact that these writers share an impulse to describe abstracted *stages* of development, rather than agree upon the actual details of what develops, suggests a structural correlation between embryology and stages of religious path that are prevalent across Buddhist literature, and this association is made explicit in tantric traditions. The prolific publication in Tibetan literature after the twelfth century of texts describing spiritual "grounds and paths" point to this as a significant conceptual methodology in thinking about spiritual development. Grounds and paths literature provides contemplatives with a detailed map of the Buddhist path. It is a map not of physical geography but of spiritual development; the grounds and paths are not physical locations but rather states of consciousness. Where grounds and paths literature describes a development of consciousness, embryology describes a development of physicality, and yet both are accounts of development or growth. If the compelling nature of the embryological narrative as a literary device in Tibet during these centuries can be explained in part by its structural affiliation with the popular grounds and paths genre of literature, what might this add to our understanding of how to read the plot of embryology? Firstly, it might indicate, as I have said, that embryology is often not so much about the growth of the literal embryo as it is about suggesting models of growth or change in general. If this is true, the author of an embryological narrative is governed by imperatives other than correspondence to the physical reality of an embryo. If we read embryology as the presentation of an abstract, idealized notion of growth or as the description of an acceptable model for change, then we can see the natural links between narratives of human development and tales of the Buddhist path of spiritual progress.

The question of whether an ordinary human's body is host to an enlightened essence has been of great importance in the intellectual history of Buddhism. The Great Perfection, with its poetically narrated Buddha-nature teachings and positive descriptions of enlightenment, is often contrasted to the more scholastically narrated, logically rigorous Geluk tradition. The latter is sometimes accused of describing enlightenment negatively, as an absence of defilements rather than positively, as the presence of enlightenment. While we must be cautious about exaggerating this bifurcation, the significance of narrative discourse must be noticed. Buddhist literature of the Nyingma school is known in general for its heavy reliance on allegories and metaphorical, poetic language, a stylistic choice that implies a rejection of the logical analytical rhetoric favored by much of Buddhist scholasticism. Thus the Ground is poetically rendered as the "youthful body in a vase," where the young body, symbolic of fresh, unsullied potential, is concealed within a vase, the former representing the Ground's spontaneous presence and the latter the Ground's emptiness or original purity. The uterine image of the youthful body in a vase also refers to the Buddha-nature, the enlightened nucleus that lies within the body of each sentient being and yet is obscured by the perceptual errors of sentience. Such a poetic use of language is sometimes said to value the emotional experience of the audience or the reader in reaction to the sound, appearance or syntagmatic connotations of the language used. Contrasted to a use of language that depends on the existence of a correspondence between the "correct" interpretation of words and the confirming presence of a structure that is described by them, the key to poetic language and its function steps beyond such necessary correlation. Poetic metaphors, in which odd terms are placed together to create an act of "semantic impertinence" (referencing Ricoeur), work to create new meanings that step beyond the literal, and this type of language places a special importance on the reader's imagination and the ability to see something as something else, despite differences. This understanding of metaphorical language also puts emphasis on an aesthetic appreciation of the world, which may be experienced in ritual, symbolic or artistic activity, and which serves to help re-create one's life-world, a central goal of much religious activity. Uterine metaphors of containers and their contents are frequently used in Great Perfection descriptions of the possibility of enlightenment: containers may be vases, bodies, hearts, eyes, wombs or eggs, and they hold within them a concentrated, essentialized form of the Ground, pregnant with potential. Such images also emphasize the experience of the human body – surely the most intimately direct experience of a container, and the most prominently used container metaphor in Buddhist tantra in general. The metaphor of birth is used to reflect experiences of being propelled forth toward a new existence, just as the direct transcendence contemplative experiences of projected vision release that which was held within toward an experience of boundary-less integration with one's environment. Such poetic and dramatically rendered embryological metaphors – containers pregnant with potential, the bursting forth of interior energies that realize themselves in exterior manifestation – are characteristic of many Nyingma narratives.

By contrast, in the highest yoga tantra teachings synthesized by Tsong Khapa not long after the writings of Longchenpa, embryology, while still important symbolically, is portrayed in a more procedural manner. The subject of the Geluk story is led along a sequential path shaped by the technicalities of physiological processes and is encouraged to perform, in the guise of another, a series of methodically hierarchical practices that are literally modeled after ordinary life-stage events. The subjects of both of these tantric narratives, however, share more similarities than differences when compared to the miserable subject of Gampopa's narrative. The lurid discourse of the misery of the womb is used in that exoteric model as a threat to instill religious values in the figure burdened by the suffering of existence itself.

In this chapter, I have recounted stories of transformation that situate the seeds of change in the very origins of the human body. In the literal realm, these narratives start with conception and end with birth; in the symbolic realm, they start with saṃsāra and end with Buddhahood. In these examples we have also seen the workings of the narrative's plot – Ricoeur's "intelligible whole that governs a succession of events in any story"[109] – in the soteriological priorities articulated by each tradition. These stories have been enacted by characters of different types. Some looked to the model of birth as liberating, as an opportunity to re-create or re-envision one's body, and therefore one's existence, in a deified form. Others looked at birth as evidence of the unarguable wretchedness of saṃsāra. Significantly, metaphors in each of these embryologies are crafted from the perspective of the embryo and not the perspective of the pregnant woman; it is the embryo, or the practitioner who imagines him- or herself embryologically, who will ultimately be released, liberated into a more integrated, less confined form of existence

This chapter has considered the fictional, "intended" audience (the meditator as reader) of religious embryological narratives, who is also simultaneously cast as a character (the embryologically envisioned meditator). But there is more to say about how a story progresses and about what moves it along. A feature of narrative that I have not yet addressed involves an explication of the necessary connections between events. The next chapter, therefore, will be about what makes the story move. What causal elements drive the events of the story? This will also tells us more about how the discourse of embryology is used to market acceptable models of change, and in so doing, we will consider the ethics of storytelling, for when we tell a story we inevitably value certain courses of action over another.

6

GROWTH, CHANGE AND CONTINUITY

Describing the most dramatic transformation we can experience, embryology is about becoming as much as being. There has always been a tension in Buddhism regarding the discourse of being, and this is a topic that has long been closely tied to thinking about human development. The Buddhist aversion to a language of the self required early Buddhists to modify known Hindu accounts of human development. Indian Buddhist scriptures grounded refutations of the self in the complex task of defining "self," although, in fact, early Buddhist definitions of self were often difficult to distinguish from those of the non-Buddhists.[1] In many texts the existence of a self was not denied outright; Indian Buddhists simply rejected the existence of a *permanent* self. In other writings, an aggressive rhetoric outlawed the possibility of an existent self of any kind. Variations in this issue led to hermeneutic maneuvers in which later commentators labeled certain teachings as definitively the word of the Buddha, and others as only interpretively so.

But the issue of "becoming" was arguably of greater importance. If it can be said that many European philosophical systems are based primarily on a study of being, by contrast many of the most influential Buddhist doctrines reflect on the notion of becoming. Buddhists throughout history have concerned themselves with describing how change and development occur in the various realms of human experience. Defining such metaphysical concepts and integrating them into systems of thought and practice is central to Buddhism from its earliest origins in India, and embryological narratives turned out to be a compelling means of expressing these difficult concepts

The effort to explain the nature of phenomena without positing their permanent existence led to highly developed theories of causality in Buddhist literature. Specific theories about how events are caused – how things become – abound in early Indian thought; prominent scholars have gone so far as to claim that the very foundation of Buddhism is a theory of causality.[2] In *Causality: The Central Philosophy of Buddhism*, Kalupahana cites early Buddhist texts that situate the central role of causality in every realm of existence: in the inorganic and organic physical worlds, in the sphere of thought or mental life, in the social and moral realm, and in the realm of higher spiritual life.[3] In the last chapter, I considered the symbolic subjects of embryological narratives and the discursive strategies used in those narratives to describe the religious path. That chapter showed that for Tibetan writers the composition of such narratives was far from formulaic, and that some authors carefully crafted the details of human development to support their doctrinal systems. Embryology allows these writers to temporalize doctrinal issues: doctrines are embedded into narratives of human growth that allow readers or listeners to imagine themselves as characters in those plots. The "emplotment" of embryological narratives transforms the sequence of events in human development into stories with specific rhetorical functions, thereby imbuing doctrine with a sense of time. As narrative theorist D. Ezzy writes, "Emplotment endows the experience of time with meaning;"[4] Ricoeur explains further that "The plot, therefore, places us at the crossing point of temporality and narrativity: to be historical, an event must be more than a singular occurrence, a unique happening. It receives its definition from its contribution to the development of a plot."[5] In this chapter, I will continue the discussion of embryological stories and their plots by considering the mechanics of causation in rebirth and growth. At the same time, I will consider the "emplotment" of the narration of Tibetan embryology itself. How did embryological narratives interact with each other and with their literary environments during this period of Tibetan history? What might embryology tell us about the historical transformation of medical and religious forms of literature?

Karma and the Buddhist problem of causality

In the doctrines of the Pāli Buddhist canon, humans are said to be composed of five aggregates (Pāli, *khandhas*): the material body, feelings, perception, predispositions, and consciousness. The proportions of these aggregates are continually shifting and an individual, therefore, is not continuous from moment to moment as a stable, unchanging entity. Misperception of the basic fact of substantial instability, or impermanence, and the imposition of a stable, constant "self" upon this shifting configuration of aggregates is, in Buddhism, considered the central downfall of humankind. Belief in a self that underlies or unites the aggregates into one, the Buddha taught, is the root of all human suffering.

The problem with this theory is how to deal with the continuity asserted by the process of rebirth. The fifth-century abhidharma writings by Vasubhandu explain that both individuals and worlds are created by the acts of sentient beings. An act, in Sanskrit *karman*, involves an intention, a physical or verbal action, and the results of the action, and actions leave upon the actor an imprint that travels with the individual across lifetimes. The question of how the karmic imprints are transferred across lifetimes is especially thorny given the Buddhist doctrines of impermanence and no-self, and untangling this quandary has been a contentious issue for Buddhist philosophers throughout history.[6]

The notion of karmic causality is thus a historically and systematically complex phenomenon. Although it is but one aspect of Buddhist causality theory overall, karmic causality is at the root of much of Buddhist thought and practice. In discussions of the body at the level of fetal development, concerns with the workings of karma and the effects of behavior are at the heart of various debates in both medical and religious systems. Many of these systems award karma a significant, motivationally shaping role in the creation of the human body. In this chapter, I will discuss how embryology is used to express a range of Buddhist notions of causation, change and growth by focusing on four models of growth found in that context: a model where the primary causal force is karma, another where the primary forces of growth are the natural elements, yet another where the principal forces are the body's energetic winds, and, finally, a model where the chief force of growth is the wisdom of a Buddha. Over the course of this chapter, by examining the presence in embryological discourse of competing models for causation and human growth, we will see that while karma was vital to some models, others emphasized the power of different psychosomatic features of the individual to effect change. In this discussion, we will observe once again that embryology is at the center of a fundamentally *Buddhist* concern.

How growth occurs is critical to a study of gestation for obvious reasons. What is interesting here is how an embryological narrative's view on growth and causality is part of a broader intellectual perspective on change and causation. As I trace these four models in a variety of embryological writings, a relationship between these notions of causality and the complexities of Buddhist practice will become evident as well. Theories of causality are the framework for a particularly divisive problem central to the definition of Buddhism as it spread throughout Asia, that is, a problem often known simplistically as the dichotomy of "sudden" versus "gradual" enlightenment. This is an idealized polarity between those who conceptualize enlightenment as an effortless leap into an ineffable, fundamentally innate state of experience, on the one hand, and those who present enlightenment as a gradual process of growth in which there are identifiable stages of development to be learned and mastered, on the other. Around this basic polarity, which flavored the various stories of transformation in chapter five, hovered a number of related concerns pivotal for Buddhist thinkers. Is suffering a mere perceptual delusion, or is it predetermined by karmic conditioning? How does the enlightened essence exist in the unenlightened individual, and how can it be encouraged to present itself? Do innate enlightenment or Buddha-nature teachings contradict the Buddhist no-self teaching? Is the subitist's positive language simply an expedient rhetorical strategy aimed at those intolerant of the apparently nihilistic edge to emptiness teachings? What different does any of this make?

Although the number of Indian Buddhists devoted to the Buddha-nature doctrine was relatively small, these teachings took on great importance in Central and East Asian Buddhism. Although representing an opposition between spiritual cultivation as either intuitive or effortful, the sudden-gradual dichotomy is not black and white; as Luis Gomez explains, it is rather "a very general, sometimes vague, intuition of a tension or polarity between two approaches to knowledge and action."[7] Still, the sudden-gradual conflict covered a network of epistemological, ethical and ontological issues that were integral to the workings of Buddhist thought, practice and teaching. In this chapter, by examining how causation is expressed in the context of human growth, I will continue to address the role of embryology in this and other subjects of concern to Buddhist thinkers.

Causality, the individual, and the cosmos

How it is that karma works, and how exactly karmic causality could be effective from one lifetime to the next, is an issue that has been debated since the beginning of Buddhism. The earliest of Buddhist texts feature dialogues between the Buddha and his students on the topics of causality in the context of rebirth; this topic has been analyzed by Dasgupta, McDermott and others.[8] Karmic causality is an integral part of both Āyurvedic and Buddhist Indian sources on rebirth, and all Tibetan authors who write on embryology – whether affiliated with medical *or* religious traditions – acknowledge the role of karma in human conception and development. For some writers, the role of karma is quite significant, but for others, the role of karma is played down in favor of different factors influencing conception and embryonic development. Karma's role in embryology manifests on two levels, both in the larger context of the Buddhist law of interdependent origination, and in the context of specifi causes of conception and fetal growth.

One of the most fundamental teachings of Buddhism, the law of interdependent origination is an important aspect of abhidharma teachings. It is a doctrine that explains the ultimately interdependent nature of all phenomena, a notion that is the basis of the Buddhist thesis that all phenomena are impermanent, arising through causes and conditions, and therefore creators of suffering. It is interpreted variously by all schools of Buddhism and is arguably the philosophical helm of Buddhist thought. The Vaibhāśika, for example, using the theory to refute early Indian philosophies that posited a permanent original creator, explained that according to interdependent origination, there could be no genesis without cause. Later formulations, such as that of the Mādhyamika, used the "twelve links" of interdependent origination to go beyond a theory of causality to justify their position that because all phenomena are interdependent, they must therefore be intrinsically selfless or empty.[9] From this perspective, there are no things causally connected – there is only causal connection.

The specific expression of the doctrine of interdependent origination in the form of twelve linked stages is designed to explain causality in the case of living phenomena. Very briefly, the first of the twelve links, "ignorance" (*ma rig pa*), refers to a misconception of the true metaphysical status of all phenomena, including that of the human individual. The second link, "action" (*'du byed kyi las*), refers primarily to meritorious or non-meritorious acts committed in a previous lifetime. The nature of these actions are imprinted on the "consciousness" (*rnam shes*), the third link, and their ethical quality determines one's type of rebirth. As a new being is conceived in a womb, the fourth link, the physical aggregates of "name and form" (*ming gzugs*), are created as the body of the embryo. The fifth link, "sources" (*skye mched*), are the developing individual's six sense powers (the eye, ear, nose, tongue, body and mental powers). "Contact" (*reg pa*), the sixth link, arises when the sense powers, the objects of the sense powers and the consciousness join together in the effort to classify external objects as pleasant, unpleasant or neutral, and "feeling" (*tshor ba*), the seventh link, is consequently defined as the feelings of pleasantness, unpleasantness or neutrality toward that contact. These feelings serve as the basis of "attachment" (*sred pa*) to objects deemed pleasurable, the eighth link; the ninth link, "grasping" (*len pa*), is a more intense experience of attachment. Due to attachment and grasping, "existence" (*srid pa*) – that is, existence as a newly conceived individual – occurs, followed by "birth" (*skye ba*) and inevitably "aging and death" (*rga shi*). A single cycle of twelve links thus follows an individual through three lifetimes.[10]

The doctrine of interdependent origination serves as a mediating concept, a "middle way," between the two extremes of eternalism, on the one hand, a belief that the individual, or an essential portion of the individual, continues unchangingly throughout a series of lifetimes, and nihilism, on the other, a belief that the individual is completely annihilated at death. The doctrine of interdependent origination allows Buddhists to speak of a causal chain connecting deeds and their effects without asserting a permanent transmigrating entity. It allows a connection to be drawn between rebirth and the morally loaded Buddhist notion of ignorance. Significantly, it also means that the cause of ultimate liberation is the cessation of rebirth and the mechanics of karma. This places embryology – where the mechanics of rebirth is taught – squarely at the center of Buddhist soteriology.

While all religious and medical Tibetan embryological narratives are naturally complicit in the doctrine of interdependent origination, some Tibetan authors contextualize their discussion of early human development more explicitly within a discussion of the doctrine. Fetal development is situated by Longchenpa, for example, within a cosmogonic process that is sparked into operation by metaphysical ignorance at a cosmic level, an act referred to as the Ground's "straying" (*'khrul ba*). The consciousness that manifests in cyclic existence through that process then begins the cycle of rebirth into various forms of existence as determined by individual beings' karmic actions. The cycle of rebirth is inextricably linked to the ethical quality of action, whether actions are virtuous, non-virtuous or neutral determining how the process develops. Longchenpa uses the twelve links to narrate the process of individual human conception and development. After death, he explains, the intermediate state being is drawn toward the next life due to a misunderstanding of the self-originating nature of intermediate state visions. A particular being's karmic conditions lead it toward rebirth and as the embryo develops, the fourth link, "name and form," is manifested. The sense organs develop and sensations are experienced through that contact. The individual begins to grasp at and become attached to objects and consequently is reborn, giving rise to old age and inevitable death.[11] The story of early human development is told here as the story of interdependent origination, and this serves as a preface to a more detailed discussion of embryogenesis. We will see in the pages to come that while Longchenpa does in this way acknowledge the general influence of karma in the perpetuation of cyclic existence, however, other factors play a crucial role in human development as well.

Kālacakra traditions of generation stage contemplative practices use the twelve links of interdependent origination as markers for meditative development, which is described embryologically. As the practitioner begins the phase of meditation in which he or she imagines taking on the body of a deity, the twelve links are sublimated in a process that is also marked by the stages of fetal development. The firs act in this practice represents the moment of conception, imagining oneself as the Buddha Kālacakra standing on the sun, moon and Rāhu, embodying the mother's blood, father's reproductive substance and the consciousness, respectively. Subsequent phases of the practice involve imagining various actions performed by the Buddha Kālacakra that aim to sublimate the mental obscurations, and each phase is correlated to one of the twelve links of interdependent origination and to a particular month of fetal development. Later stages of practice involve purifying life stages after birth, and thus "the tantric adept imaginatively transmutes his entire life, from the time of conception until death, into the state of Buddhahood."[12] Knowledge of the particulars of the stages of ordinary life, including the period from conception to birth, and of how these are expressed in the Buddhist doctrine of interdependent origination, is thus essential to the performance of complex meditative rituals such as those described in the last chapter.

At the root of the association of human embryogenesis with the more abstract notion of phenomenal causality that is the doctrine of interdependent origination is the parallel association of the human individual with the entire cosmos. This latter correlation is the basis of Buddhist notions of being and becoming. Unlike many Euro-American cosmological traditions, which focus on the cosmos as an entity distinct from the individual, Buddhist cosmology is explicitly concerned with defining the interactive relationship between the human individual, his or her environment, and the cosmos. Much has been written about the explicit correlation made in many Asian traditions between the generation of the universe and the generation of the individual, where the notion that the microcosmic individual is linked to the greater macrocosmic environment and is the basis of understanding the body. The Indian medical tradition's embryological presentations are explicitly linked to cosmogony in this way, and many Indian tantric traditions, such as that of the *Kālacakra*, similarly embrace this connection. Tibetan astrology is accordingly intertwined intricately with practical Tibetan medical concerns as well. Because the five natural elements give rise to the three systemic processes (*nyes pa*) and dictate their balance in the body, a physician's diagnosis requires understanding the movements of the planets, the changing of the seasons, and the effects of these on the condition of the human body.

The alliance between cosmogony and embryogenesis can be addressed from two perspectives. The discursive structure of some Tibetan religious texts that narrate embryology (though seemingly not that of medical texts) explicitly links individual with cosmos; but beyond this, within the narratives themselves, thematic and rhetorical elements also demonstrate the commitment of many writers to communicate the inseparable nature of the individual and the cosmos through embryology. Making the direct correlation between cosmogony and embryogenesis explicit, many Tibetan religious texts are structured as are both the classical Indian Āyurvedic treatises and many religious tantras, introducing the subject of embryology (the creation of a human) directly following a discussion of cosmogony (the creation of the universe). The *Kālacakra*, a text particularly influential in early Tibetan writings on embryology, is organized by such a structure: the first two chapters of the *Kālacakra* are devoted to the cosmos and the individual, respectively, and comment directly on the relationship of the cosmos as macrocosm and the individual as microcosm. The first chapter, the "outer Kālacakra," which presents a complex description of the cosmos and its origins, is followed directly by the "inner Kālacakra" chapter, which begins as the sage Sucandra asks the Buddha, "How can the entire three worlds be within the body?"[13] The chapter explains the stages of life, beginning inside the womb, as provisional experiences of the bodies of the Buddha and asserts that both the ultimate and conventional nature of the individual, as well as its manner of creation and destruction, are identical to that of the cosmos.

Similarly organized is Longchenpa's *Treasury of Words and Meanings*, which begins with an explanation of why beings stray away from their primordial state of enlightened existence, known as the "Ground" (*gzhi*), into the materiality that characterizes ordinary human existence. The chapter describes this process of birth into ordinary human existence on a grand, cosmological scale: in the beginning was the Ground's "presencing" (*gzhi snang*) or manifestation, which is poetically described as an event during which the (personified Ground fails to recognize its own nature in a manifested display of lights and self-reflective consciousness. If these manifestations are seen as something other than itself, the Ground strays into a saṃsāric world of reified materiality; Longchenpa cites the *Adamantine Hero's Heart-Mirror* tantra to report that at this critical moment, "this darkened cognition reflects, 'Have I emerged from that over there, or has that over there emerged from me?' In this way, the protoconsciousness goes astray merely by force of thought."[14] With rebirth ultimately initiated by ignorance (*ma rig pa*), a being is thus embodied as a result of not recognizing the true nature of things. Above, we considered Longchenpa's analysis of this evolutionary process in terms of the twelve links of interdependent origination, which is sparked into operation by the Ground's straying. Here, we notice the explicit organizational ties in Longchenpa's text between cosmogony and embryogenesis.

While dramatically different in content, the discursive structure of Gampopa's *Jewel Ornament* is similar. In this text an account of human conception and development follows a graphic description of the unfortunate condition of saṃsāra into which beings are born. In Buddhist cosmology, beings are said to be reborn into one of either five or six realms: abhidharma texts delineate fiv (hell realms, the realm of hungry spirits, the animal realm, the human realm and the realm of the gods) and later Buddhist schools added a sixth (the demigods). The hell, hungry spirit and animal realms are considered the worst rebirths, but the inhabitants of all realms are subject to suffering, entrenched in the misery of endless desire. Gampopa's depiction of saṃsāra begins with the Buddhist cosmological classification of eighteen hot, cold or otherwise unpleasant hell realms, their precise locations in the universe, the suffering one experiences as a resident in each of these hells, and the typical life expectancy for those residents. His explanation of birth into the human realm of saṃsāra is thus seated in the context of these frightening cosmological pictures, emphasizing here too the integral relationship between individual and cosmos.

The connection between the conception of the individual and that of the cosmos reaches around the Buddhist world. James Sanford, in an article on conception and embryonic development in Japanese Shingon texts, points to the presence of a theme in which conception and development are described as a secretly transmitted initiation and an "inner proof of the body" that accords to the cosmogonic stage when Heaven and Earth were still united and chaos had not yet manifested differentiated forms.[15] Thus, Sanford continues, "procreation is made one with Creation." Sanford sees narratives of embryonic growth to be directly derived from Buddhist cosmologies. "The first substantial trace of this cosmogonic process in the womb," he writes, "is the emergence of an inner sun and inner moon that parallels the emergence at Creation of the worldly sun and moon."[16] Elsewhere in East Asia, this connection has been documented as well. Charlotte Furth's work has identified the deep cosmological roots of Chinese medicine and their particular ties to notions of gestation and birth. She notes that philosophical and religious traditions, which considered birth to be "a replication of cosmogenesis," had a significant impact on the role of knowledge of gestation and birth in Chinese medicine.[17] Significantly, while the connection between cosmogenesis and embryogenesis is explicit in the discourse of Buddhist texts, and while the connection is also clear in some Indian Āyurvedic works (but not in the *Heart of Medicine*), this explicit connection is not a feature of Tibetan medical works in the tradition of the *Four Tantras*. The connection between cosmogenesis and embryogenesis is thus primarily made in the context of religious writings on human development, not medical writings, at least in the early centuries of Tibetan medical scholarship.

The deep and pervasive interrelationship between Buddhist cosmic and individual creation is also exemplified within stories of embryogenesis themselves, a link that becomes clear when we consider the importance of the natural elements, which organize and direct the universe and everything that exists within it, to human growth. This correlation is not unique to Buddhism, nor is it unique to Asia.[18] From the time of the earliest Buddhist theories about the universe, nature was understood as a causal system guided by discernable laws. Early Indian Buddhism posited foundational particulate and energetic elements in its explanation of the make-up of the universe. Abhidharma writings explain these particulate elements (Skt. *paramānus*) as, "the smallest part of matter, uncuttable, unable to be destroyed, taken up, or grasped. They are neither long nor short, neither square not round. They cannot be analyzed, seen, heard, or touched."[19] These particles do not exist independently but occupy space only when combined together into larger conglomerations. All matter is further composed of energetic forces called the "four great elements" (Skt. *catvāri mahā bhūtāni*): earth, water, fire, and wind. These qualities allow the conglomerated matter elements, the *paramānus*, to be perceived, and the particular combination of energetic elements acting on a given *paramānus* is what gives the *paramānus* its distinguishing characteristics. Other Buddhist traditions added a fift element, space. Although later schools of Buddhist thought embrace the notion of phenomenal and personal "identitylessness" or emptiness, many still accept the heuristic use of the early Buddhist natural physics founded on conventionally established atomic particles and energetic elements.

In Tibetan accounts of conception and fetal development, as is also the case in classical Āyurveda, these natural elements – the building blocks of the universe itself – play an essential role. Successful conception is said to result from the mixture of male reproductive substance, female blood and the transmigrating being's consciousness, interacting with the energetic processes of the five elements inherent in those three substances. The body is defined from the moment of conception as a particular equilibrium – characterized by the balance of elements – of bodily constituents and systemic processes. As we will note below, medical commentator Lodrö Gyelpo is highly critical of those who question the need for all the elements in the growth of a new human body (despite the

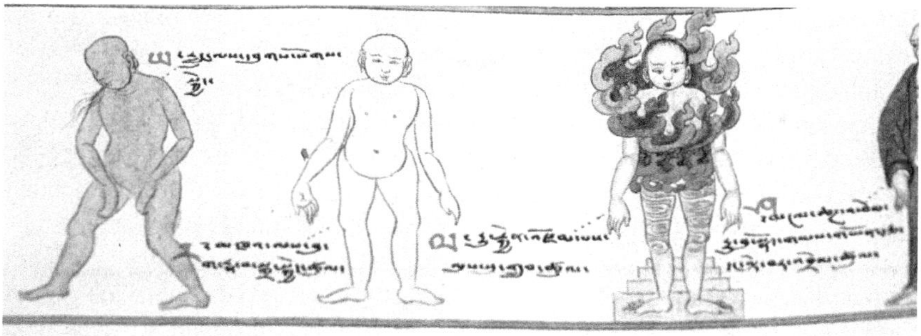

Figure 6.1 The painting shows the influence of the natural elements on the growth of the fetus: the wind element (left) contributes movement and the space element (center) contributes the openings of the body and the sense of hearing. The accumulation of all the elements (right) thus creates the body.

absence of the elements as causal factors for fetal growth in Vāgbhaṭa's *Heart of Medicine*, one of his primary medical sources).[20] Both the reproductive fluids of the parents and the transmigrating consciousness, Lodrö Gyelpo argues, are necessarily possessed of subtle forms of the five elements and, therefore, it is impossible for conception to occur without the presence of all elements. While Lodrö Gyelpo speaks adamantly on the causal necessity of the natural elements on conception and fetal growth, the relative importance of their contribution is, in fact, contested, as we will see in the following pages.

The fact that analysis of individual human embryogenesis often sequentially follows presentations of cosmogony explicitly links the individual with the cosmic process, lending issues of human conception and development a tenor of profound significance. Interestingly, however, the structural correlation that joins cosmological and embryological narratives in a particular work exists primarily in religious texts. This discursive format is absent in the *Four Tantras* and in the earliest commentaries on the *Explanatory Tantra*'s embryology. By the fifteenth century, most Tibetan authors – religious and medical writers alike – agree that the natural elements must be discussed in embryology as essential conditions for human conception and growth, clearly tying the make-up of the individual to that of the universe. But the earliest of Tibetan medical writers were relatively unconcerned with the role of the elements during fetal development. We will see that the increasing interest in the material nature of the human body, and in connecting the human individual with the cosmos at the material level, may be an idea that comes to medical thinkers as a result of the increasing influence of Buddhism on Tibetan scholarly communities. In other words, in the context of human development, Buddhism offers to medicine a basis for explaining the material world and material embodiment.

The power of karma in the context of conception and development

But let us first return to the issue of karma's role in human development. Narratives of embryogenesis address the problem of karma directly in the context of explaining the causes of conception and fetal development. All sources agree that conception is caused by three main factors: the joining of the two healthy reproductive substances of a man and a woman in intercourse and the consciousness of the transmigrating sentient being, which is generally said to be propelled toward the copulating man and woman by its own karma and afflictive emotions. Most (but not all) sources comment that this combination is then nurtured by the presence of the natural elements. This basic model of conception is featured in Vāgbhaṭa's medical text, the *Heart of Medicine*, which was widely influential in the subsequent development of Tibetan medical literature. This is also the model present in the Buddhist sūtra, *Entering the Womb*, the most widely cited source for Tibetan embryology, and it can be seen in the earliest of Buddhist texts, such as the *Majjhima Nikāya* and in abhidharma texts as well.[21]

There is little disagreement among Tibetan Buddhist religious or medical writers on this key process of conception, and although we will see that in other aspects of human development the issue of causality is more problematic, to this degree and in this context, karma is important to all. Over the next few pages it will become clear, however, that while the larger metaphysical connections between rebirth and karma that are described by the law of interdependent origination, for example, are traditionally Buddhist, when we take note of the details of embryological narratives, the role played by karma in the processes of conception and growth may be more closely linked to Indian medical traditions, at least for the earliest of medical writers in Tibet.

In the earliest extant medical examples of Tibetan embryology, such as the *Four Tantras* and its twelfth-century commentaries, the discussion of the causes of conception introduces the main factors required for conception (the healthy reproductive fluids, the consciousness driven by karma, and the natural elements), in a model that is followed by commentators in later centuries. In Kyempa Tsewang's fifteenth-century commentary on the *Four Tantras*, the topic of embryology is divided into three main themes: the causes of the body's formation, the conditions of its growth, and the signs of birth. In this and other *Four Tantras* commentaries, the cause of embryonic formation – that is, conception – is a significant, heavily commented-upon topic. All the factors necessary for conception are described in the context of this topic: the non-defective male reproductive substance (*khu ba*), the non-defective female reproductive "blood" (*khrag*), a transmigrating consciousness (*rnam shes*) that is drawn toward the man and woman in sexual union, and the five elements (*'byung ba*). Menstruation is also addressed in this context, explaining when a woman can conceive. Following the *Four Tantras* primarily, of course, Kyempa Tsewang also cites the *Entering the Womb* sūtra as authoritative in this section, and other works such as the *Heart of Medicine* and the *Kālacakra*.

As discussed earlier, according to these traditions if these necessary factors are defective or not present, conception will not take place. Systemic imbalances – that is, an inappropriate placement or function of the systemic processes (*nyes pa*) – in either the female reproductive blood or male reproductive substance will make them unsuitable to cause normal development, resulting either in unsuccessful conception or in development of a fetus that is severely physically deformed, as described in chapter four. Furthermore, if the reproductive substances are not defective but there is no karmic connection between the transmigrating consciousness and the potential parents, there will be nothing to draw the consciousness to those parents, and thus in this case also, conception will not occur. Early Buddhist scriptures – sūtra and jātaka – are cited as evidence for this view. Kyempa Tsewang explains that, additionally, the presence of each of the five natural elements is required for successful conception, a fact that is noted in the *Four Tantras*, although he backs this up by citing the *Entering the Womb* sūtra.[22] The elements provide the material and energetic opportunity for development: the substance of the embryo is composed by the earth element, its fluidity and flexibility by the water element, its maturation by the fire element, its growth by the wind element, and the space in which it grows is provided by the space element. Each of these conditions must be in place for fetal development to occur. The developing fetus is thus bound by the same laws of natural physics, as it were, as every other impermanent phenomenon in the natural world. Other requirements for successful conception include the woman's being of an age to menstruate and her being at the proper stage in her menstrual cycle. As the *Four Tantras* states, when the womb is open (*mngal kha bye*), conception can occur. The womb is open for up to twelve days per month – during the firs three of these days, menstrual blood is collected in the womb and conception can occur there up to the eleventh day. After this time the "old blood" is eliminated, Kyempa Tsewang explains, and the womb closes.[23]

In the sixteenth century, nearly a hundred years later, Lodrö Gyelpo's *Transmission of the Elders* again addresses the causes of conception and how the embryo is formed. Lodrö Gyelpo condemns scholars who only make passing note of how conception occurs, contending that simple explanations cannot adequately describe how the consciousness enters the womb or precisely how the body is established.[24] He argues that one should explain conception fully as the simultaneous occurrence of the following factors: one, the healthy wind, bile and phlegm processes that are present in the father's and mother's reproductive substances; two, the transmigrating consciousness that is impelled toward this particular human rebirth by karma and the afflictions; and three, the very subtle forms of the five elements that exist within the blood, male reproductive substance and consciousness. Only with these causes in place, if the healthy man and woman copulate, will a transmigrating consciousness be able to enter the womb.

Buddhist writers also considered the details of conception, as discussed in some depth earlier. Drakpa Gyeltsen, for instance, contrasts that which he calls "birth from substance and non-substance" (*dngos po dang dngos med las skyes ba*) with a variety of opposing views ("substance" here refers to the male and female reproductive substances, and "non-substance" to the transmigrator's consciousness). To take a body into a womb, he explains, many causes and conditions must occur: during intercourse of a man and woman, when the white and red quintessential essences are poised at the tips of their respective sexual organs, a transmigrating consciousness who is of a compatible karmic disposition with the potential parents may enter the area, riding on a stream of wind, whereupon the three become indistinguishably mixed. Gender identificatio occurs instantaneously, he claims, as the emotions of the bardo consciousness ally themselves with either the man's or the woman's substance. While this is the theory he proposes, however, Drakpa Gyeltsen comments that there are alternative views. He remarks that,

> Some speak of birth from the three minds, some conceive of birth from karma, some conceive of birth from the three [which are] body, speech

> and mind, some conceive of birth from reproductive substance (*khu ba*), blood and wind, and some conceive of birth from particles, darkness and courage.[25]

Interestingly, Drakpa Gyeltsen does not reject these alternate views outright as incorrect, stating obliquely that one should accept aspects of various views rather than hold dogmatically to a single view.

Whereas medical commentaries on the *Four Tantras'* verses on conception draw primarily upon Vāgbhaṭa's medical text and Buddhist sūtra, when we move to the next main commentarial topic, that of how conception is experienced by the transmigrator, the religious tantras begin to play an important role, as discussed in the last chapter. While Indic medical texts and exoteric scriptures are used to support an emphasis on karma's role in conception, the tantras bring forward the causal significance of the winds to the event. (Paradoxically, however, we will see later in this chapter that, in fact, it is sūtric narratives that champion the role of the winds in fetal development.) Lodrö Gyelpo begins the discussion by explaining that the transmigrating consciousness, driven by karmic predispositions and afflictions, is caused by the winds to observe a man and woman in copulation, whereupon karma impels the consciousness into the womb. (Curiously, he attributes this tradition to the *Guhyasamāja.*) At the time the consciousness melts into the mixture of reproductive substances, it experiences a moment of senselessness, as if intoxicated.[26] Lodrö Gyelpo cites a corroborating tantric account by Rangjung Dorjé, emphasizing the role of the winds as well as the karmic predispositions in bringing the transmigrating mind into the womb, noting likewise that the mind enters the womb in an "unconscious" state. In this tradition, the mind is said to feel as if it is being blown by wind and rainstorms and, therefore, needs to take shelter in the womb.[27] As we discussed in the last chapter, such pre-conception visions are common in religious texts; the seventeenth-century Kagyü and Nyingma teacher Tselé Natsok Rangdröl's *Mirror of Mindfulness* explains similarly that just prior to conception the visions one has are indicative of one's direction of rebirth: those to be reborn in Pure Lands will see lovely figures such as swans or running horses. "On this continent of Jambudvipa," however, "one will either be born as an ordinary human in one of the unfree states if one feels that one is entering into a mist, or one will attain a precious human body if one has the experience of arriving in a mansion or city or among many people."[28] Lodrö Gyelpo cites an alternative interpretation as well, one we have seen from sūtras, in which the transmigrating being enters the mixture of reproductive substances and immediately reacts to one or the other substance in a way that instantaneously determines its gender: attracted to the mother's substance, it becomes male, or attracted to the father's substance, it becomes female. As noted earlier, this abhidharma account makes gender identification central to conception itself

In the context of conception, karma is given responsibility for more than pushing the transmigrating consciousness toward the copulating man and woman. Citing the *Entering the Womb* sūtra, Lodrö Gyelpo explains that the transmigrating being must possess virtuous karma of an adequate level to be born as a human, and also that the karma of the transmigrating being and that of the parents must be equivalent in "type" or "class" (*rigs*) and level of meritorious distinction. In many texts, karma also plays an important role in what *type* of rebirth one obtains. Lodrö Gyelpo summarizes another tradition present in the *Entering the Womb* sūtra, one also repeated by Gampopa, that transmigrating beings entering the womb are of two types, possessing some degree of merit or possessing less merit. Gampopa's narrative explains that all intermediate state beings possess miraculous abilities, such as walking on air and seeing with divine eyes, but eventually the strength of their karma causes them to experience frightening visions, such as that of a storm, heavy rain, a darkening sky, or the roar of a crowd of people. Then they envision entering a place, such as the second story of a house, a throne, a thatched hut, a leaf house, a shelter of grass, a jungle or a rocky crevasse. Those with exceptional merit will see palaces or mansions, while those with low merit will be directed toward the rocky crevasse. Arriving at their envisioned destination, they are immediately attracted to either the father's or the mother's reproductive substance. Colored by this emotional reaction, the consciousness enters into the mixture of the reproductive substances, whereupon conception occurs.[29] Tselé Natsok Rangdröl explains likewise that, according to one's karma, one will be reborn into one of the six classes of beings with one of six experiences of entering the womb: those destined to be animals will experience conception as if entering a cave or earthen pit, those destined to be hungry ghosts will feel as if entering a deep forest, those being reborn in hells feels as if being led into a black pit.[30] Lodrö Gyelpo explains that, according to sūtra, while ordinary beings experience a loss of awareness upon entering the womb, the classes of beings with higher levels of spiritual realization have different experiences.[31] As mentioned earlier, universal monarchs and stream-enterers are aware of the moment of entering the womb, but then are "unconscious" during gestation; first-level bodhisattvas and solitary realizers are aware of the processes of conception and birth, but not that of gestation; and bodhisattvas never lose awareness.[32] In chapter four, I addressed how embryological narratives are used to express Buddhist taxonomies of embodiment; here, we see them also used to teach about the organization of individuals by their moral status.

The shaky foundations of karma's role in becoming human

Following models inherited from Indian texts, for Tibetan authors karma played a critical role in causing rebirth and in directing the type of rebirth one takes. Despite the ubiquitous presence of karma as a force of conception in these accounts of creation, however, we have also seen that some medical commentators use tantric texts as authorities for attributing a causal role to the winds in conception. Some of these same accounts admit, furthermore, that the effects of karma can be overwritten by ritual intervention or medicinal application. In some contexts, therefore, one's own karmic destiny could be overcome by an external human intermediary. Medicinal or ritual intervention was said to be able to affect the health of one's reproductive substances, for example. For conception to occur successfully, male and female reproductive substances must be healthy, and Lodrö Gyelpo notes that reproductive defects can be caused by karma. Rejecting the suggestion of other scholars that it is impossible to evaluate the health of the reproductive substances because they are hidden within the body, he counters that with clinical experience one can observe many signs of texture, color and taste elsewhere in the body that are adequate indications of the health of these substances. When the reproductive substances are defective, conception will not be possible, and yet some types of defects can be treated medicinally. For the details, however, Lodrö Gyelpo simply refers the reader to texts by Vāgbhaṭa and his commentators in which appropriate treatments are described. He notes that these sources also provide rituals that men and women can do themselves to promote healthy qualities in their own reproductive substances.[33]

More dramatically, these texts claim that the very sex identification of the fetus could be changed medico-ritually. As explained in chapter three, the issue of how to guarantee the birth of a male child is of great importance in medical embryologies, although this is a matter ignored by religious texts. The rituals described in the *Four Tantras* and its commentaries, as derived from Vāgbhaṭa's *Heart of Medicine*, are alchemically and astrologically oriented and do not involve direct propitiation of deities; it is thus not divine but human intervention, by largely ritual means, that is being advocated here.[34] The *Four Tantras* and its commentaries claim that these procedures should be performed during the third week of gestation. Expanding on the *Four Tantras'* verse that outlines this and other practices, Kyempa Tsewang explains, for example, that according to the *Heart of Medicine* tradition, rituals such as those noted on the

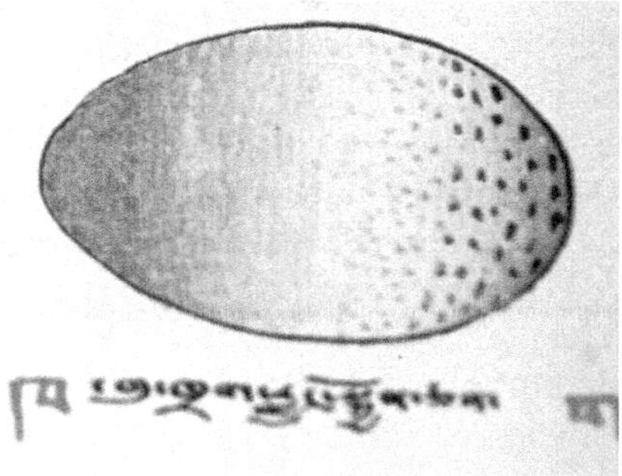

Figure 6.2 A series of images depict male and female reproductive substances with various sorts of defects: here, a wind defect is illustrated.

first page of this book can ensure development of a male child. He argues that although generally the sex of the fetus depends on its karmic inheritance, because additional factors do play a role in development, rituals may still be effective. He offers medicinal preparations that he claims to be a more powerful method for sex transformation, and he narrates an additional procedure in which a statue is entwined in a protection cord made from the wool of a sheep with male offspring, and then wrapped around the pregnant woman's waist.[35] Interestingly, such rituals are not described in the *Entering the Womb* sūtra, where the issue of sex transformation is not mentioned at all, nor is it a subject of interest for Buddhist tantric texts. This point may simply remind us that medical practice is linked to the concerns of lay people, many of whom want boy children, whereas the concerns of the lay and religious audience of Buddhist texts are of a different sort.

Clearly, although karma is accepted as a primary cause of rebirth and cited by many as the determinant of body type, there is nonetheless a conflict between the apparent predeterminism of the karmic model of causality, on the one hand, and the need for medical systems to assert that human intervention can be effica cious, on the other. Medical interventions are regularly given the power to override the effects of karma, even in the matter of forming the human body. While medical commentators do recommend such ritual procedures, however, for further detail they refer readers to the Indic medical sources in the Tibetan canon or to Tibetan astrological sources.[36] Although medical scholars are comfortable with the presence of these rituals in this context, therefore, they are not prepared to go into significant detail about them there, acknowledging that the proper place for such matters is somewhere other than the medical corpus.

The role of the elements in causing growth

The firm foundations of karma's predeterministic role in rebirth are shaken by more than this, however. Beyond the moment of conception, there are varying positions on the relative importance of karma and other factors during the process of gestation. While most embryological narratives state that the natural elements are essential factors at the moment of conception itself, Tibetan descriptions of the precise role of the elements in subsequent fetal development, by contrast, are far from consistent. Some authors emphasize the essential role of all the elements, others ignore three or four elements in favor of the wind element alone, and yet others neglect to mention the elements at all. Neither the *Heart of Medicine* nor the three earliest extant commentaries on the *Four Tantras* mention the role of any of the natural elements in fetal growth. Some authors, such as Gampopa, provide details on the activities of the wind element, but overlook the activities of other elements. The *Entering the Womb* and *Abiding in the Womb* sūtras do discuss the importance of the elements for conception, as noted earlier, but as will see in the coming pages, they downplay the role of four out of five elements in the subsequent process of fetal growth

In his *Transmission of the Elders*, Lodrö Gyelpo is highly critical of those who question the need for all the elements in gestation. Both the reproductive fluids of the parents and the transmigrating consciousness, he argues, are necessarily possessed of subtle forms of the five elements, and therefore it is logically impossible for growth to occur without the presence of all elements. The natural elements, he explains, refer not to static material substances but rather to qualitative, dynamic functions. For instance, the earth element refers to the quality or function of hardness, and the water element refers to the quality or function of cohesiveness, flexibility or coolness. The elements are thus the very functional interactivity that make change and growth possible.[37] Acknowledging the *Heart of Medicine*'s neglect of this matter, Lodrö Gyelpo looks to another Indian source and notes that the *Entering the Womb* sūtra does clearly state that each element is essential for growth. He explains,

> When the body itself is generated, the parents' reproductive substance and blood, the four great elements and the consciousness (*ngo bo*) become undifferentiated, because by the earth element solidity is made; by the water element liquidity is made; by the fire element heat is made; and by the wind element movement is made.[38]

Lodrö Gyelpo defends the presence of the elements in the transmigrating consciousness especially, maintaining that consciousness and the five elements necessarily exist interdependently. As tantric sources say, he argues, "These great elements should be known as the support of life. Likewise, life is that which is supported [by] them."[39] How is it that we can confirm the existence of these very subtle elements if they cannot be seen? Lodrö Gyelpo notes that imperceptibly subtle forms of the elements must be present to make growth possible, and he cites a number of tantric sources as evidence for this claim. One source, for example, links the emergence of the elements to components of the sexual act that results in conception:

> By connecting the penis with the fruit [of the mother's vagina],
> the latent trace of tangible hardness,
> the earth [element], is brought forth.
> From the nature of the *bodhicitta* substance (*byang sems khu ba*),
> the water element emerges.
> From the exertion [of the parents], the heat [of the fire element] is generated;
> [their] movement establishes the wind [element], and
> [their] bliss is the space element.
> By these five, the consciousness is encircled[40]

There is here a clear causal link between the elements and the manifestation of the fetal form. In his own words, Lodrö Gyelpo asserts that taking hold in the womb is the role of the earth element, generating the fetal form is the role of the water element, ripening the form is the role of the fire element, growing the form larger is the role of the wind element, and providing the opportunity for all of this is the role of the space element. The elements are held responsible for the development of the sense powers and other aspects of the body, and the six tastes are correlated to the elements as well. Khedrub Norsang Gyatso, similarly, in his fifteenth-century *Kālacakra* commentary, describes the responsibilities of the elements in fetal growth: the fire element enables fetal growth, and the space element allows room for growth.[41] While the majority of Tibetan writers on early human development discuss the functions of the elements only at the time of conception, it is esoteric traditions that typically consider their importance to human growth beyond conception. Lodrö Gyelpo's focus on this tradition signifies the strong influence of tantric traditions on his presentation of embryology. He insists that the five elements are responsible for generating various aspects of the body throughout the course of its development. Intrinsically part of the reproductive substances and consciousness that join in the womb at conception, the initially subtle elements grow stronger during gestation as a result of the nutrients consumed by the mother.[42] As the fetus grows, supported by the mother's supply of nutrition, the strength of the elements increases.

Roughly a century earlier, Longchenpa's description of fetal growth is dominated by the activities of all of the elements. During the first two weeks of development, he organizes development into seven-day cycles according to the functions of the elements: during days one through four, each of the four elements is sequentially predominant; on days five and six they operate in pairs; and on the seventh day they function together as a group. This organizational principal is said to pertain to the entire period of gestation, although Longchenpa's account only provides details for the first two weeks. His explanation of the first week of development describes the four elements' activation of four very subtle channels in the embryo's body: Named for the elements themselves, these are a water channel, an earth channel, a fire channel, and a wind channel. The space element operates on the seventh day to provide a place for the four elements to gather together. In the second week, the work of the elements continues as the embryo is dissolved, compacted, baked and scattered about, dispersing "like fluffy clouds in the sky." On the eighth evening, by the power of karma and predispositions, these fragments are gathered by the water element. In the third and fourth weeks, the embryo is again sequentially destroyed and reconstituted as new structures and energies of the subtle body are formed within the embryo.

In this unusual presentation of the role of the elements in human development, Longchenpa also distinguishes between "conventional" (*kun rdzob*) and "ultimate" (*don dam*) elements. Through what he designates as the male cause and female condition, the conventional elements become functional; these conventional elements are responsible for the development of physical features during gestation. The activity of the conventional elements thus generates the

Table 6.1 The names of the winds responsible for fetal development during each week of gestation

Mo.	*Week*	*Entering the Womb*	*Kyempa Tsewang's summary of an (unidentified) tantra*
1	1		life-sustaining wind
	2	*kun sdud*	
	3	*mdzod kha*	
	4	*nang rab tu 'byed pa*	
2	5	*yang dag par sdud pa*	downward expelling wind
	6	*zas*	
	7	*'khyil bar byed pa*	
	8	*zlog cing sgyur bar byed pa*	
3	9	*rnam bar 'byed pa*	upward-moving wind
	10	*sra bar byed pa*, and then also *kun nas sgo* (*Mngal na gnas pa* has *kun nas skye ba)*	
	11	*rdo rje* (*Mngal na gnas pa* has *bug snang ba*)	
	12	*yon po'i sgo*, and then also *spu brgyus pa*	
4	13	*bkres shing skom par byed pa* (*Mngal na gnas pa* has *snga ma*)	pervasive wind
	14	*skud pa'i sgo*	
	15	*pad ma*	
	16	*bdud rtsi 'gro ba*	
5	17	*'bri gdong*	fire-accompanying win
	18	*brtan par 'gyur ba* (*Mngal na gnas pa* has *dri med pa*)	
	19	none mentioned	
	20	*shin tu sra ba* (*Mngal na gnas pa* says *shin tu brtan ba*)	
6	21	*yang dag skyed ba*	nāga wind
	22	*kun tu rgyal ba*	
	23	*yongs su dag par 'dzin pa*	
	24	*sprin 'dzin* (*Mngal na gnas pa* has *kun tu 'phyo ba*)	
7	25	*grong khyer 'dzin*	tortoise wind
	26	*skye ba mngon par grub ba*	
	27	*sman yon chen po*	
	28	none mentioned	
8	29	*me tog phreng ba*	chameleon wind
	30	*lcags kyi sgo*	
	31	none mentioned	
	32	none mentioned	
9	33	none mentioned	Devadatta wind; bringing-forth wind
	34	none mentioned	
	35	none mentioned	
	36	none mentioned	
10	37	none mentioned	dhananjaya wind
	38	*thogs pa'i rgyen*, and *kha thur du lta ba* (*Mngal na gnas pa* has *yan lag sdud ba*, and also *kha thur du lta ba*)	

body's blood, flesh and breath, as well as many of the mental abilities of cognition, perception and awareness. Through the mind and wind, which are contributions of the transmigrating being, the ultimate elements become functional: they allow the intermediate state consciousness to take hold of the new body, and they initiate the maturing energies of differentiation and assimilation, mentioned above, that enable fetal growth. The ultimate elements generate the eyes, four wheels and three channels of the embryo. With the parents' reproductive substances causing physical development and the consciousness' contribution causing the organizational impulse for development, the role of the natural elements is discussed in a much more subtle and detailed way in this Great Perfection account than by any other tradition.[43] And here again, we see how a central Great Perfection doctrine is made prominent in the narrative of embryology. David Germano explains the central importance of the elements to this tradition, and their relationship to the Great Perfection articulation of soteriology. "In the Great Perfection tradition," he writes, "these five elements are understood as the congealed solidification of the pure light intensities referred to as the five lights, a materialization which takes place by virtue of our failure to recognize the lights as self-presencing, and our consequent straying into the alienation of cyclic existence."[44] The significance of the natural elements here, then, goes far beyond their role as the building blocks of material reality. In the case of the Great Perfection, the emphasis on the activities of the natural elements during gestation is justified by the tradition's overall philosophical and soteriological system.

Attributing causality to winds

While karma plays a leading role in some aspects of conception and development, according to some traditions, its power is questioned by the authority of ritual interventions and its influence is countered by the responsibilities of the elements in human growth. In some cases, however, the significance of the elements as a group is overshadowed by a strong argument for the importance of just one of these, the wind element. By the time of the second diffusion, Tibetans had available to them two Indian textual models for the causal function of the winds in embryology. The Indian medical model, as we have seen, ignores the role of the winds in favor of karma, even during the process of gestation. The Buddhist canonical model, as revealed in sūtras and tantras, by contrast, emphasizes the causal function of the winds over that of karma. These canonical narratives offer intricate schemes for attributing growth during gestation to a host of variously named winds. Indeed, the emphasis on winds as a causal force in religious accounts of creation may be quite old, predating Buddhism itself. Zysk notes that the *Atharvaveda* contains a verse attributing the winds with the force that causes birth; the verse submits that, "A human being breathes out (*àpānati*) and breathes in (*prāṇati*) when inside the womb (*gàrbhe*). When you, O *Prāṇa*, urge him on he is born again."[45] As we will see, while we might expect karmic causality to be fundamentally religious and a causality based on the natural elements to be fundamentally medical, it appears rather to be the reverse.

In Tibetan medical and religious embryological narratives alike, we have seen again and again that Buddhist sūtras are referred to as authorities on the process of transmigration, the nature of the transmigrating entity, the workings of karma and the four elements, the relationship between the mind and the body, and other topics relevant to human growth. The primary source for sūtric embryology, the *Entering the Womb*, makes note of independently named winds (shown in Table 6.1) that are responsible for fetal growth during each week of gestation. These details are extensively cited by many Tibetan authors who write about human development in both medical and religious traditions. In the early twelfth century, Gampopa named gestational winds from this sūtra in his *Jewel Ornament of Liberation*, crediting the sūtra specifically. The *Entering the Womb* is arguably the main source on embryology, aside from the *Four Tantras*, for three major Tibetan medical commentaries on the *Four Tantras* – the commentaries by Kyempa Tsewang, in the late fifteenth century, Zurkhar Lodrö Gyelpo, in the mid-sixteenth century, and Sanggyé Gyatso, in the mid-seventeenth century. Citing the *Entering the Womb* repeatedly, Lodrö Gyelpo notes that it is very important in embryology to get the names of the weekly winds correct, and that this is an issue about which other scholars are often mistaken. The names and functions of the winds, as taken from the Buddhist sūtra, are the most prominent and consistent details these medical commentators add to their accounts of the body's weekly development.

Another context for embryogenesis in which specific causal forces for fetal growth occur – that is, forces other than karma – is that of the tantras. Here, there are various traditions. Some narratives link each of the five primary winds (the life-sustaining, downward-clearing, fire-accompanying, upward-upholding and all-pervasive winds) and five branch winds (the serpent, tortoise, chameleon, Devadatta, and bow-victor winds) of Tantric physiology, mentioned in chapter three, to each of the ten months in the womb. Others simply note the general role of the five primary winds throughout the growth process. Still others, as described above, generally attribute gestational causality to each of the four elements, one being wind. Surprisingly, given the overall importance of winds in tantric contemplative practices, even in the earliest Tibetan embryologies oriented toward tantric, rather than sūtric, teachings, the winds in general play a less important role than they do in exoteric traditions. Neither the *Great Jeweled Wishing Tree* by Drakpa Gyeltsen nor the early Nyingma Heart Essence text, *Union of the Sun and the Moon*, mention the role of the winds in their accounts of gestation.[46] Drakpa Gyeltsen does mention the wind's role in forming the three channels in the embryo, explaining that "through the power of the wind entering [the central channel], the solitary channel [is formed], and by its gradually emerging [from the central channel], the flavor channel [is formed]."[47] Beyond this statement, however, he does not attribute growth during stages of development to the winds specifically, as in the sūtric model. While some tantric narratives do discuss the causal relationship between the winds and the general stages of fetal growth, it therefore seems to be primarily a sūtric tradition in which individual winds are enumerated for each week of development.

As is the case in the Buddhist sūtras, and to a lesser extent in the tantras, many important Tibetan religious and medical scholars felt that intermediary causal forces – that is, forces other than karma – are essential to the growth of the body. Some early scholars in Tibet who wrote about early human development do not mention such intermediary forces at all, as we have noted, leaving karma as the sole causal force. In the *Heart of Medicine*'s model of embryology, it is karma alone that provides the impetus, at the time of conception, for the growth of the body, and over the course of fetal growth no other force, not even that of the winds, has any causal function. The *Four Tantras* is also largely silent on the role of the winds in the body's development. Its chapter on human development does not describe the names and effects of individual weekly winds, although it does state ambiguously that the wind element is active during thirty-eight weeks of gestation. It is unclear whether this verse refers to the activity of thirty-eight winds, or whether it simply refers to the general effect of wind on the thirty-eight weeks of gestation. The commentators who wrote most immediately after the *Four Tantras* do not clarify the question of whether thirty-eight winds are indicated when they address this particular verse. It appears to have taken more than a hundred years for the sūtric explanation of thirty-eight winds with individual names to be used to expand on this *Four Tantras* position, despite the fact that Buddhist writers in Tibet at the time of the *Four Tantras* or before, such as Gampopa, certainly knew about the sūtra.

It is clear that Buddhist canonical materials are the source for the importance of the winds in gestation, and that Indian medical models, by contrast, emphasize the role of karma. Earlier narratives of embryology in the medical tradition – for example, those from the eleventh or twelfth centuries – are significantl less likely to attribute causality to the winds, or indeed any of the natural elements, than are later embryological accounts, where doing so becomes almost ubiquitous. What is interesting here is the absorption of the Buddhist canonical model into the Tibetan medical commentaries. By the fifteenth century, medical texts focus heavily on the intermediary causal role of the winds during gestation. The *Entering the Womb* sūtra is the central source for embryology for these medical commentators. In the matter of identifying causal forces responsible for the growth of the body, it seems that over time the Buddhist canonical model, emphasizing the causal influence of the winds, won out in Tibet over the early medical model, which left developmental causality up to karma.

Growth caused by the power of gnosis

Up to this point we have seen that, as in the Buddhist sūtras and tantras, many Tibetan religious and medical scholars felt, or came to feel, that causal forces other than karma are essential to the growth of the human body. Those other forces, the winds alone or all of the natural elements, are themselves integral components of the newly developing, ordinary body of the fetus. In these models, the various features of the growing body themselves thus serve to cause further gradual development. Notably, however, these forces are impure, part of the world of saṃsāra. Now, we will turn briefly to a uniquely Buddhist model of causation in human growth, one that differs substantially from other presentations, and one in which change is motivated by an eminently pure phenomenon, the wisdom of a Buddha.

First let us recall that Vajrayāna Buddhism in general is characterized by an emphasis on the inherent purity of all phenomena and a focus on harnessing one's physical and mental purity as a tool along the path to enlightenment. A rarified experience of the mind, bringing forth an innate and pure wisdom that is normally clouded by mental afflictions is, for tantric adepts, at once the aim of all tantric practice and also the means toward that aim. That wisdom is, moreover, for many Vajrayāna traditions the ultimate ontological reality of all phenomena, often articulated as the Reality Body of the Buddha, an expression of Buddhahood as pure knowing. This idiom places the origin, basis, path and result of enlightened experience rhetorically in *knowing*, more than in *being* (although the two are then equated). Not exclusive to Vajrayāna Buddhism, of course, the notion of an innate and pure wisdom that is the basis of all phenomena, including one's own mind and body, and that is an instance of the Buddha's very existence, is the core of the Mahāyāna Buddha-nature doctrine, and also the hub of the so-called sudden-gradual debate, both of which became especially pivotal in the formation and articulation of Buddhist traditions outside India. Much has been written about these topics, in Buddhist and non-Buddhist secondary literature alike. Ruegg, for instance, examines the fundamental problem of discerning the relationship between the fruit (*'bras bu*) that is enlightenment, the basis (*gzhi*) of all phenomena, and the path (*lam*) of practice through a series of etic categories, bringing themes of contrast to Buddhist doctrine: enstatic concentration versus intellectual analysis, "spontaneism" and "simultaneism" versus "graded acquisition and reinforcement through progressive cultivation," ethical quietism versus effort, or cataphatism versus apophatism.[48] We have examined some of these relationships already, considering in the last chapter different models of the religious path, and emphasizing, for example, a contemplative expression of innate purity, on the one hand, and the energetic effort of external practices and ritual interventions, on the other. In addition to touching upon these dualities, we see two further Buddhist themes illustrated in stories of human growth, the pairings of impure/pure and lay/monastic.

In the models of development examined so far, growth is caused by impure forces. Longchenpa's Great Perfection embryological narrative, by contrast, exemplifies a tantric model of propelling growth by purity. Longchenpa's model is unusual not only for its particular attention to the causal role of the natural elements, as discussed above. Also remarkable is his discussion of the formation of the eyes in the embryo. In chapter four, I outlined the Great Perfection theory of fetal development which describes the formation of two tiny "eye-like" features, called the "eye of the lamps" (*sgron ma'i spyan*) and the "eye of the elements" (*'byung ba'i spyan*). In Longchenpa's account, these eyes appear within the circulatory channels during the first week of gestation. Germano's research points out that for this Great Perfection tradition, the tiny "eye of the elements" directs the development of the physical body, and the "eye of the lamps" is given ultimate responsibility for the subtle body and, therefore, also for the visionary experiences felt during specific contemplative practices. The designation of these forces as "eyes" and their placement in the very earliest stages of human development is dictated by the importance of vision in Lonchenpa's contemplative system, as discussed in chapter four. In this context it is notable that, by attributing causal force in embryonic growth to these "eyes," which are explicitly correlated to innate wisdom (*ye shes*), Longchenpa has effectively given the Buddha's wisdom the power to cause human growth. In this model, therefore, a purified form of knowing is explicitly the causal agent of human existence. Contrasting this model with the earlier model valuing the role of karma, here we see a primacy of epistemology over ethics, or a valorization of cognitive over moral transformation.

Pointing to the systematic Buddhist contrast between karma (*las*) and innate wisdom or "gnosis" (*ye shes*), Germano characterizes the Great Perfection as a "gnostic reinterpretation of Indian Buddhism."[49] Gnostic traditions are those in which the Buddha's wisdom, or gnosis, is the central, pre-existing agent in the creation of cosmic and individual existence. These are contrasted to karmic traditions, for which the Buddha is an end point arrived at through substantial effort. Germano argues that in Longchenpa's work all phenomena – at both the universal, cosmogonic level and the individual, embryonic level – originate with the movement of innate wisdom or gnosis, and that karmic processes are thus relegated to a position of secondary importance. Thus, the wisdom of a Buddha – not karma – is the primary causal operative in Great Perfection notions of generation. Here, again, we see how embryology is portrayed in ways that are aligned with a tradition's broader agenda, as the emplotment of fetal growth is scripted to the service of larger Buddhist themes. Stories of fetal development are stories of the religious path, of the innate purity of phenomena, or of the inherent suffering of existence.

The forces of creation

In Chapter 4, I presented embryological narratives as a means for Tibetan authors to define human bodies, and to say something about what it is (or what it should be) to be human. In addition to deciding what counts as a body, embryology divides bodies into a range of body types. The typology of bodies is done according to some underlying organizational principle; in many societies, for example, bodies are sorted by explicitly racist or sexist schemata. Indeed, the problem of how bodies are differentiated is one that all religions try to solve. Why are some born healthy, some beautiful, some ugly, some into poverty and distress? Why does illness and misfortune strike some and not others, why does it strike when it does?

An answer is provided in Buddhism by the concept of karma, which rationalizes and moralizes that which otherwise would seem random, instructing humans to cherish their human embodiment as a precious opportunity to generate good karma and obtain a better rebirth. It is also karmic merit or demerit, however, that ultimately keeps one locked in the perpetual cycle of rebirths until final salvation. In early Indian Buddhism, one's karmic destiny was largely only a matter of one's own concern – that is to say, one's karmic effects were carried solely within one's own lineage of rebirths and did not affect to a significan extent the rebirth paths of others. With the Mahāyāna bodhisattva ideal, the notion of karmic destiny was expanded beyond one's own line of lifetimes: the bodhisattva was to generate a karmic force powerful enough to liberate all beings from their own karmic destinies. In Vajrayāna Buddhism, the emphasis on ritual action came to be seen as an essential intervention, as many traditions relied on the power of the divine – whether embodied within oneself or called upon as an external force – on the path to enlightenment.

In this chapter, we have seen that for Tibetan authors karmic causality was far from the only pattern of thinking about the causation of the human individual. We began by understanding that karma as articulated in embryological narratives – both in its involvement with the Buddhist law of interdependent origination, and in its specific role as a causal agent in conception and human growth – was held by some early Tibetan embryologists to be the sole causal agent in human rebirth and development. Karma is an integral part of the law of interdependent origination, propelling the transmigrating being along the path toward physical embodiment and defining the nature of that embodiment. Karma is also responsible for the type of body a transmigrating being can obtain: transmigrators carrying superior moral achievements can obtain psycho-physiologically and soteriologically superior bodies.

We also saw, however, that a karmic theory of causality was not enough for all embryologists, and that sometimes other characters, such as winds, the four elements or one's Buddha-nature, are the dominant causal contributors to the formation of the new human being. Indeed, as I suggested in chapter five Tibetans often seemed little constrained by the authorities of scripture or empiricism, apparently free to write the details of embryonic growth as they liked. Tibetan embryology germinated the individual human body with a scholar's own specialized narrative about causation and growth. Embryological narratives defined certain acceptable paradigms for change and growth. Change and growth happen in stages, as with Drakpa Gyeltsen and other texts, that outline the religious path structure. They are characterized by suffering, as for Gampopa. They are completely integrated with both the emotions and the workings of the natural elements, as with Longchenpa, and in that tradition, moreover, they are ultimately driven by an enlightened form of knowing. In some narratives, change and growth are innately present as potentials within the fetus; in other narratives, they require the successful workings of an intricately coordinated complex of sequentially generated causal forces. These narratives thus imbue religious doctrines with specific, personified models of causality and temporality.

Disputes about the significance of karma and rebirth are nothing new in Buddhism, and several good volumes of secondary scholarship have addressed the varied ways karma has been interpreted throughout the history of Indian and Tibetan thought.[50] In this chapter, my claim is not that these embryological debates add much of sophistication to Buddhist arguments over doctrines such as causality or the sudden-gradual problem. Rather, a more interesting conclusion at this point is that the *existence* of these controversies, and the ways in which they are played out, in medieval Tibetan embryology – a subject of significance that spans the disciplinary boundaries of religion and medicine – has additional historical and methodological implications.

Despite the availability of Indian Buddhist models, such as that of the *Entering the Womb* sūtra, that marginalized the role of karma in human growth in favor of other causal factors, we have seen that many early Tibetan narratives, such as that of the *Four Tantras* and its earliest commentaries, attributed dominant causal responsibility for embodiment to the force of karma. On this matter, early Tibetan medical texts are more closely aligned with the Indic *Heart of Medicine*. Thus, initially, karmic causality is more important for medical traditions, and an elemental or material causality is more closely associated with religious traditions. If these associations are a surprise to some readers, consider José Cabezón's reminder to examine our own preconceptions about science and religion, which may reify Buddhism as a discipline of the mind and science as a discipline of the material world. To the contrary, in fact, medicine has much to say about ethics, for instance. According to Tibetan medicine, ethical behavior is a key shaping element throughout an individual's lifetime – according to medical theory, the body's constitution in health or illness is literally created by ethical action. The vital role of karma is ubiquitous in all Tibetan medical notions of embodiment, seen at the level of embryogenesis and also at the level of an adult's maintenance of health. Because health is defined as a particular balance of the individual's humoral constitution, and human action is a central feature in defining this balance, the human body is quite literally defined, or created, by one's moral agency. Likewise, we have seen that at the very core of Buddhism is a complex theory of the material world. Thus, the early association of medicine with karma and Buddhism with theories of the natural elements is less astonishing than it may seem.

Tracing the dialogue between religious and medical writers on these topics for the next several centuries, however, we begin to see that by the fifteent century, the influence of Buddhist theories that downplayed the role of karma won out in Tibetan medical literature. By that time, medical texts focused heavily on the causal role of the winds during gestation, and Buddhist sūtras were the central source for embryology, even for medical commentators. As Tibetan intellectual sectarianism became more prominently pronounced in the thirteenth-fourteenth centuries, the Indian medical model of causality in which karma is the dominant force (a model adopted by the *Four Tantras* as well) was thus slowly overshadowed by a collection of alternative views. Tibetans increasingly emphasized the possibility of intervening in the dictates of karma, and relied on Buddhist sources that featured the causal role of other forces for growth, such as the winds and the natural elements. In medical traditions, this shift may thus indicate an increasing acceptance of the authority of the Buddhist metaphysics of the abhidharma, the sūtras and the tantras, as the theoretical basis of the topic of embryology, and perhaps also physiology as a whole. Paradoxically, however, this occurs even as medicine is increasingly defined as a "secular" tradition in the developing spirit of sectarianism and disciplinarity in Tibet.

How can we make sense of this situation? One possibility is to recognize that the nature of this problem has to do with where we are defining the boundaries of religion and medicine. Although it is sometimes vaguely stated that medical theories are fully integrated with religious doctrines in Tibet, the two are still defined as distinct disciplines. What has been missing in these discussions is the question of what counts as "medicine." It appears that while Tibetan historiography typically marks medicine as a "secular science," by the fifteenth century certain topics within medical literature, most notably embryology, anatomy and physiology, had been largely absorbed into Buddhist conceptual frameworks. As it turns out, what has become increasingly evident in the last two chapters is that it is less the case that religious traditions borrowed embryology from medical traditions, as is generally assumed by Western scholars,[51] than the reverse – that is, embryology is most fruitfully a *religious* topic. For religious writers, embryological narratives were a means of embedding doctrinal messages into human identities: such embryologies are religious doctrines that are narrativized into human lives. For medical writers by the fifteenth century, embryological narratives became a forum for religious theorizing. The topic allowed medical scholars, most of whom by that time were Buddhist monks or otherwise seriously educated in Buddhist literature, the opportunity to theorize about issues of vital importance in Buddhist literature. By this point in history even medical writers considered the topic of human development fundamentally a religious topic – that is, a topic for which the central concepts, sources and arguments were part of Buddhist literary history and discourse.

As contemporary Euro-American scholars interpreting Tibetan intellectual culture, then, we must be careful. The modern positivist or scientistic perspective, in which we might evaluate the truth of Tibetan embryology as primarily a part of Tibetan medicine, would lead us to think that the tradition is simply *wrong* about the details of conception and gestation. Indeed, still today, most

Euro-American writings on Indian and Tibetan embryology do just that: "how quaint," they imply, are these extraordinary, sophisticated writings. When we read embryology in another way, for example, as philosophical or religious narrative, we see that it effectively communicates religious or social taxonomies, moral or political reflections, and a variety of other cultural aims and positions

Narrative theorist D. Ezzy, like Ricoeur, promotes the narrative form as particularly effective in the effort to integrate notions of identity and temporality. He writes that "the unity of the self, however transient and changing, is a temporal unity that locates past and future in the present, through the act of role-taking."[52] Buddhist embryological narratives impose upon the otherwise discordant present of the human identity a temporal unity of the past and future. These narratives "emplot" identity, suggesting an organizing theme for one's identity and its path of growth. At the same time, the heterological narratives of embryology record the narrative of the history of Buddhism in Tibet. As medieval Tibetan scholars sifted through inherited texts and theories, embryology fell clearly to the side of religion, eventually becoming a place for religious and medical theorists alike to contemplate metaphysical questions of being and becoming, while topics such as pharmacology and nosology were left to shape the domain of "secular" medicine. Correspondences made between aspects of embryology and religious thought are deeply imagined by many Tibetan writers. This is not simply a superficial schematic repetition of structures or paradigms from earlier traditions, but rather, highly creative interpretative work, using embryology to discuss Buddhist philosophy. Tibetan embryology is linked to issues of fundamental importance in Buddhist thought and culture: to cosmology and astrology, to causality, salvation, ethics and the complexities of Buddhist practice.

EPILOGUE

Historiography recapitulates embryology

I began this book by suggesting that although we may think we know where the boundaries of religion and medicine lie, a look at the history of these disciplines makes it clear that our current views are historically and culturally particular. Our understanding of Buddhism even today is shaped by the ideological concerns of Europeans who first encountered the tradition, and the history of the interaction between religion and science in eighteenth- and nineteenth-century Europe has a special role in our perception of Buddhism. This not only limits our understanding of what Buddhism is, but it hampers our learning about a range of intellectual concerns that were critical to the history of ideas in Tibet. Science historians delineate several models for the interaction between religion and medicine or science. The traditional "conflict thesis" is largely rejected now as too simplistic, as it ignores the close alliance often found between the religion and science and their proponents. Instead, many now advocate a "complexity" thesis, which emphasizes the changing and multifaceted relationship between religion and science throughout history. In this book, I have found it necessary to see the relationship between religion and medicine in Tibet as a complex one, as a living interaction that changes over time and that must be addressed on a granular basis rather than with broad disciplinary strokes. I proposed, moreover, that rather than use scientific paradigms to examine Tibetan accounts of early human development, where the standard of truth would ultimately lie with empirical observation and objectivity, a more fruitful way to examine embryology could be to see writings on the topic as narratives, with particular characters, narrators, plots and story lines that we could examine individually.

Because instances of these narratives of human development are products of particular times and places and existed within a larger literary context derived from India, primarily, but also from elsewhere, it was necessary first to become aware of this textual inheritance. Chapter 2, thus surveyed the Indian and Chinese precedents to Tibetan medical and religious thinking on embryology in particular, and human physiology more generally, which served as the basis for the development of indigenous Tibetan writings on the topic. Embryology is clearly a contentious topic in non-Buddhist writings in India, and philosophical concerns are at the heart of much of that literature. In the case of Indian medical accounts of embryology, caring for the pregnant woman, as well as the developing fetus, is a prominent concern. Embryology is also a topic of interest from the earliest period of Buddhist writings. Buddhists texts, however, are unconcerned with the woman's experience of gestation, and these writings are primarily crafted as a moralistic lesson in impermanence or suffering. With the rise of Buddhist tantric literature in India and its positive valuation of the human body as a tool for movement toward enlightenment, embryology is linked to a range of broader concerns, such as contemplative and ritual practice and cosmology. A brief look at Chinese texts on human gestation indicates that in that context too, embryology is, as in Buddhist tantra, intricately related to broader concerns of religion, philosophy, ethics and cosmology. As Tibetan scholars began to work with these inherited ideas, how did they adapt them to meet their own concerns? As Tibetan literary and intellectual life became increasingly complex in the renaissance period of the thirteenth-sixteenth centuries, during which time scholarship was classified along sectarian and disciplinary lines, how was the relationship between religion and medicine articulated? Where were the lines drawn between these bodies of thought and writing?

These are not easy questions, and Tibetan historians themselves were troubled by the relationship of medicine to Buddhism. In some cases, they portrayed medicine, particularly in the early period, as internationally cosmopolitan and not especially influenced by Buddhism. In other contexts, though often within the same historical presentation, medicine is portrayed as entirely integrated within the history of Buddhism. For these conflicted historians, Tibetan medical knowledge was derived from the contributions of South, East and Central Asian scholars, and it was also inherited in its entirety from an Indic lineage traced back to the Buddha himself. Taking this historiographical conflict as evidence of increasing pressure to make medicine Buddhist, we saw human physiology fall prey to this demand. A traditional Buddhist discourse of physiology can increasingly be observed within medical literature. Because the discourse of physiology is not itself a part of Tibetan medicine historically, the organized exposition of physiology and embryology in medical literature is therefore, for the most part, derived from Buddhism. Texts on nosology, pharmacy and *materia medica*, forming the bulk of medical literature, do not typically include independent discussions of the structure or functions of the human body, adult or fetal. With the exception of the *Four Tantras* and its commentarial tradition, it appears that only a fairly small percentage of circulated work on Tibetan medicine is likely to have contained material on organized presentations of embryology, or even of topics we might call physiology or anatomy, especially in the earlier periods of medical history. According to a rough quantitative evaluation of the range of pre-fourteenth-century texts classified by Tibetan historians as being on Tibetan medicine, the explicit explication of the human body simply was not a very important topic for medical writers. While religious thinkers from the beginning were fascinated by the origins and workings of the human body, this was not so in the early medical tradition. We see a change by the fifteenth century, however, when the influence of religious texts and religious education increasingly defined medical scholarship in new ways

The organized exposition of physiology and the taxonomy of embodiment are essential parts of all forms of Buddhism. Medicine is also concerned with understanding human bodies, of course, but not in the systematic way of Buddhist literature. And the focus is different: medical physiology is most centrally based on an understanding of systemic (humoral) processes and the metabolic heat of the digestive process, and this physiological paradigm is, for the most part, not shared with Buddhism. Interestingly, we see little evidence of this paradigm in presentations of human embryology. The physiology of the circulatory system, by contrast, is a key part of tantric Buddhism, and it is also shared with medicine, particularly in later medical literature of the renaissance period; the physiology of the circulatory system is also a key part of medical embryologies of that period. Thus, we saw that as Tibetan intellectual life was increasingly pervaded by Buddhist ideologies, the presentation of human development in medicine drew closer to Buddhism. One result of this shift is that the woman's experience of pregnancy was neglected in favor of a presentation of female reproductive physiology in isolation. Because the topic of embryology was firmly a part of Buddhist doctrine, not medical or clinical attention, the woman had little role to play.

What is it about gestation that so intrigued Tibetan scholars? A study of medical commentaries during the renaissance period shows that even for medical writers, the problems of gestation are fundamentally Buddhist problems. Knowing about embryology is knowing about religion. Medical commentators seem little troubled by the many traditions of gestation, perhaps because it is not the (empirical) "facts" of gestation that are critical to the writing of embryology. The emphasis in many embryological accounts on the fetus' own experience of gestation suggests that narratives of gestation are about something that the reader may actually experience. How is it that embryological knowing is religious knowing? In renaissance Tibet, one of the most widespread topics of writing was the religious path, and gestation turned out to serve theorizers of the path perfectly. When the exoteric path teaches suffering, gestation is about suffering. When the esoteric path teaches liberation through bodily practices, gestation is about rebirth into an enlightened body. Practices such as that of "closing the womb's door" require knowledge of conception and gestation; in the practice of "bringing the three bodies to the path" too, knowing embryogenesis is knowing religion. Gestation is thus scripted to serve religious ideology. As an exemplar of the religious path, gestation is ultimately about growth and change. It is about the contemplative as developing fetus (and not at all about the pregnant woman developing that fetus).

If embryology is about change and how change occurs, then it is also about karma, both cosmic and individual in scope. Embryological narratives are linked explicitly to cosmology, both by their discourse or style and by their story, that is, the meaning indicated by the arrangement of events or themes in a given presentation. Medical commentators' increasing need to emphasize the role of the natural elements – and the winds in particular – in gestation is further evidence of the essentially Buddhist quality of this topic in their eyes. Here our expectations are surprised as we find that it is Buddhist canonical models of growth that highlight the role of the winds, and Indic medical models that rely primarily on karma as a motivator for growth.

In Tibetan accounts of early human development, we can see many attributes of the narrative – a central subject, a well-marked beginning, middle and end, a narrative voice, the suggestion of necessary connections between events – and reading embryologies as narratives reveals them to illuminate the richly colorful ways in which Tibetans constructed human identities by the creative act of authorship. Embryological narratives allowed Tibetan scholars to write about the body, about human identity, and about what it means to be human. The subject is a discursive tool for the articulation and promotion of acceptable models of identity, continuity and change. We have seen Tibetan authors wield this tool variously, and although the stories of gestation were controversial, all were stories of transformation that situated the seeds of change in the origins of the human body. In this book, we looked at Tibetan embryological narratives as aesthetic objects, rather than as statements of scientific or empirically observable fact. In the end, we saw that embryology is most richly a religious topic: scholars of human development embedded doctrinal messages into human identities using the discourse of embryology, narrativizing religious aspirations into human lives. Throughout this book, we have seen the thematic and structural comparison of embryological accounts point to both convergences and divergences between modes of discourse in Tibetan literature.

Reversing Buddhist historiographical style, which moves from the vastness of cosmic history to the discreteness of human lives, let us now move from small to large: from considering the transformation of the human individual to thinking about the formation of social institutions that produced those narratives. Investigating the embryonic "historiography" of individual identity leads me to think about the historiography of social identity too, for if embryology is a narrative that defines individual identity, history, surely, is the narrative that defines social or institutional identity. Might we expand the inquiry into narrative and identity by examining aspects of Tibetan historiography? Can we see parallels between models of expressing human identity and models of expressing social identity? What are the organizing themes of histories in Tibet, and how are their characters described?

Like embryological narratives, which claim to record the personal history of the individual, histories of traditions or institutions are often recorded as stories – stories with characters who enact or are affected by events that are organized temporally and driven by a plot. These stories are essentially tellable, and they arrange events in a rhetorically purposeful manner to express a point or teach a lesson.[1] In chapter one, I wondered whether we might find similarities in compositional form between embryological and historical narratives. Hayden White maintains that themes of authority are common in histories, as is the latent or manifest desire to moralize the events they address, and, indeed, we have seen these to be central issues in embryological narratives.[2] In this book, I have written about what embryology tells us about the relationship between medicine and religion in Tibet. This "cultural poetics" of embryology has contributed to our understanding of the interactions between religious and medical literary culture during a period of several centuries in Tibet. But how is the history of medicine presented by Tibetan medical historians themselves? How is the main character – the tradition of Tibetan medicine itself – portrayed in the historiography of medicine? What are the stories told in histories of medicine, and how are these stories narrated? What do these stories tell us about how medical traditions distinguished themselves from other systems of thought and scholasticism in Tibet?

Zeff Bjerken's writing on Tibetan historiography articulates key features of Tibetan historical narratives, which are typically highly stylized and which share "tropes, categories, and techniques of emplotment."[3] He illuminates rhetorical strategies used by Tibetan historians of Buddhism to express notions of moral authority and continuity; we have seen that Tibetan historians of medicine also adopted these strategies. Historical discourse emphasizes specific notions of causality and relationality; Tibetan histories are structured to emphasize logically predetermined chains of events, unbroken lineages, and neatly catalogued textual and geographic records. Bjerken argues that historical narratives thus accurately represent the "Buddhist desire for continuity in the face of change and impermanence, so that the events recorded manifest a coherence, integrity, and fullness that proves so elusive to realize in our partial perspectives and transitory experience."[4] This, indeed, is the aspect of the narrative form that Ricoeur calls central to the expression of narrative identity. Describing a remarkably Buddhist notion, D. Ezzy explains that the term "narrative identity" as Ricoeur uses it suggests that "what we call subjectivity is neither an incoherent series of events nor an immutable substantiality, impervious to evolution. This is precisely the sort of identity which narrative composition alone can create through its dynamism." He goes on to say that, "narrative identity is coherent but flui and changeable, historically grounded but 'fictively' reinterpreted, constructed by an individual but constructed in interaction and dialogue with other people."[5]

The narrative identity – fluid and changeable, constructed interactively – provided by embryology for the human individual is created similarly for social groups or institutions by histories. Earlier, I discussed the significance of semantically charging the spaces in which a narrative's events take place: for some embryologists the womb was described as a horrific site, while others emphasized the womb's function more hopefully as a container of potential for enlightenment. Such emphasis on physical space is a key feature of Tibetan historical narratives as well. Biographies of important Tibetan figures take great care to note where people traveled. Biographical and historical accounts are often so focused on travel that the geographic tracking of an individual across the soils of

Asia provides the structural basis for the biographical narrative itself. Important figures are generally identified by their region of provenance. Despite their great travels, therefore, individuals possess an inherent relationship with a certain region, even when they may end up spending much of their lives elsewhere. They did not simply live *in* a certain place; they were, in a fundamental way, *of* a certain place. Places are themselves often deeply historicized as well, and many important historical figures are famous precisely because of their connections with specific physical locations. In Tibetan histories, the recording of travels to India in particular was a means of emphasizing Tibet's essential connections with that culture. While Sanggyé Gyatso identifies many Tibetans who studied medical texts with Rinchen Zangpo, some still traveled to India for additional medical training, among them Zhang Zijibar from Yarlung, who went to study at Nalanda, and Könchok Kyab, student of Drapa Ngönshé.[6] The biographies of both Yuthok Yönten Gönpos are largely organized by their travels to India: each Yuthok is said to have trekked the arduous trail between Tibet and India six times.[7] The identity of a text was contrived similarly. Whether texts were products of the Tibetan landscape or imported by travelers to foreign lands, the exact geographical source of a text was of great importance to its claim to authority. Just as individuals were inherently identified by their place of origin, the geographical origin of an important text was a key identifying feature of the text; just as an individual's travels comprised central biographical details about his or her life, the travels of a text across continents, or across local regions as it passed hands, was duly noted as a key feature of the text's identity.

The eleventh and twelfth centuries represented a period in which Tibetans transformed their relationship to the environment. The land was built upon furiously throughout this period, dominated by monuments of human construction, and wide regions of land were mapped out as the exclusive possession of particular religious communities. This land also spoke back to its inhabitants, as it were, offering forth an increasing number of important treasure texts. We might speculate that newly developing attitudes toward geographical space during this period coincided with changing notions about the human body. If this period is characterized by the fervent creation of physical sites for religious activity, we might indeed count the human body as one of those sites, as tantric traditions located religious meaning in the body. Detailed organizational schemata in tantric traditions mapped the body in a manner not unlike the mapping of the landscape. Anatomical or physiological representations of the human body identified key centers of dominating function within the bodily structure, contrasting these with peripheral functions, in a layout that resembles how religious centers were surrounded by peripheral temples and communities. Metaphors of building were widespread: they are used to describe a teacher's important disciples, as in the *Blue Annals*, where students are known as pillars, beams, door bolts, rafts or planks.[8] The human body is described in the *Four Tantras* using architectural and imperial metaphors: inside the structure of the body-as-castle, the organs are imaged as courtly inhabitants, with the heart as the king and the other important organs his queens and attendants.[9] The concern with identity construction and self-validation that characterizes this period in Tibetan history thus made geographical space one of its key players. Geographic and geometric conceptualization, whether for individuals, texts or internal organs, was an important form of self-identification and validation, and, arguably, it was often the most significant factor enabling a Tibetan notion of history in which history itself serves as validation of the present.

Not only was the vastness of space called upon, but also the depths of time. In Buddhist historical thinking, individual persons are tied to the past, and to the identities of other individuals, in various ways. As embryology teaches us, each individual is continuative with his or her own endless succession of past lives. Many are part of a genealogy of personal reincarnations. They are linked to their teachers, and their teachers' teachers, and ultimately to the very beginnings of time, lists of succession thereby legitimizing the present through the past in the most forceful way possible. Tibetan communities articulated their identities in similar ways: while recognition of a geographic origin or of a distinctive philosophical or theoretical doctrine was part of this self-identification, also important was the naming of a select group of members organized genealogically. The various kinds of lineage seen in Tibetan literature – royal genealogies, monastic genealogies, divine genealogies and so forth – each have their own socio-historical origins and particular characteristics. Tibetan historical and biographical literature, as exemplified by the *rgyal rabs, chos 'byung*, or *deb ther* genres, assigns necessary characteristics to the members of these groups, such that qualified members must have studied with certain teachers, mastered certain texts and doctrines, or traveled to certain places. This association of a particular set of personal and professional characteristics with each member of a genealogy serves not only to identify a given individual, but also to define the entire group to which the individual belongs.

Tibetan medical historical and biographical literature clearly adheres to this genealogical model of narrative self-identification. There were other ways of distinguishing medical traditions during these centuries, such as the predominantly text-focused lineage system. On the upper cartouche of most of the Tibetan medical paintings commissioned by Sanggyé Gyatso in the seventeenth century, for example, there are depictions of lineage holders for several other important medical texts, such as the *Heart Essence of Yuthok*, the *Ten Million Relics* (*Bye ba ring bsrel*), and Padmasambhava's *Vase of Nectar* (*Bdud rtsi bum pa*).[10] Through transmission along a continuing lineage, the teachings are likened to endlessly reborn lives; like human beings themselves, the teachings are alive, and the qualities of continuity and eternity are valorized. Historiography meets embryology here, too.

One of the most conspicuous characteristics of Tibetan historical narrative is its vast temporal scope. Following an Indic cosmological model that views contemporary events from an ultimately cosmic perspective, Tibetan histories often begin with the origins of the universe. Bjerken suggests that the karma-driven, cyclic "moral-temporal structure" that is based on the evolutionary narratives of Buddhist cosmology – and, I will add, embryology – are the very foundation for the plot of every Tibetan historical narrative.[11] Here, again, we see a fascinating recapitulation of embryonic growth in the very manner of recording history (or, it could be, a recapitulation of history in the manner of embryonic growth). Recall the modeling of some embryologies, such as that of Longchenpa's *Treasury of Words and Meanings*, after the Buddhist cosmogonic paradigm in which the universe begins with alternating phases of destruction and creation. In Longchenpa's model, the embryo, just like the universe, is sequentially destroyed and reconstituted repeatedly during the first weeks of gestation. The patterns evident in various models of embryonic growth are intricately related to standards of religious order and causation.

Matthew Kapstein's research suggests that the correspondence of models of historical change with models of embryological change may have a polemic history in early Tibet. In *The Tibetan Assimilation of Buddhism,* he notes that Dunhuang documents provide evidence for the vigorous promotion of Buddhist teachings about karma and saṃsāra prior to the tenth century (implying that these teachings were somehow problematic to Tibetan audiences at the time).[12] Notions of time and causality promoted by the embryological paradigm, therefore, may have begun to rise to prominence in the context of this imperial push to emphasize Buddhist soteriology. "From the perspective of normative Buddhist doctrine," Kapstein explains, "cosmology is thought of above all in terms of moral causation, involving, in traditional terms, the crucial teaching of rebirth." He goes on to note that we see during the imperial period in Tibet a rise in the "production of an indigenous Tibetan didactic literature whose primary aim is the propagation of the doctrines of rebirth and moral causation."[13] Kapstein suggests further that there were political reasons for encouraging these Buddhist notions of change, noting that "the cosmology of karma and saṃsāra comported well with an imperial interest in legislation; that is to say, law and order may be reinforced by assenting to cosmic justice and order."[14] Subsequently, in the centuries to follow the royal period, the embryological paradigm remained a central means for expressing notions of change, time and identity, perhaps defining also the historiographical method

Like stories of human gestation, histories offer various sorts of information. Although many readers will mine a historical text only for the details it may offer about events that really happened and people that really existed, on another level, these texts can also provide a view of how authors and narrators choose to portray time, change and identity. Just as it would be of limited value to read embryological narratives only for information on how embryos grow, there is, in the same way, much more to be understood from a historical narrative than simply what events occurred. Reading histories as narratives illuminates a wealth of information about Tibetan culture, history and belief. Notions of ethics, causality and identity shape the creative construction of social history just as they do the creative construction of personal history, as the stories of embryogenesis have told us. Embryological and historical narratives alike are concerned with explaining discontinuity as continuity, and with making whole selves out of fragments. Asking how we can account for discontinuity, they are centrally about change: how it happens, why it happens, and how it should happen, were we able to gain control of the process. These narratives are also about the creation of bodies: a personal, material body in the case of a human individual, and a public, social body in the case of a tradition. Indeed, in two important contexts in which one might talk about identity – namely the contexts in which we describe the growth of the human being (embryology) and the growth of the social being (history) – Tibetan writers have felt an impulse toward the use of the narrative form. Looking at embryology or history as narrative allows us to see their shared characteristics in a way that we could never do were we to consider embryology as "science," arcane and "traditional" at that. Writings about embryology, cosmology, history and the religious path are united in structure and rhetoric in Tibetan literature, forming together a genre of thinking and writing focused on articulating how change occurs and what constitutes identity despite change.

NOTES

1 BECOMING HUMAN IN TIBETAN LITERATURE

1 Skyem pa tshe dbang, *Mkhas dbang skyem pa tshe dbang mchog gis mdzad pa'i rgyud bzhi'i 'grel pa bshugs so*, vol. 2, New Delhi: Bod gshung sman rtsis khang, no date, 133. Referred to hereafter as *Rgyud bzhi'i 'grel pa*. The first of these procedures is described briefly in Vāgbhaṭa's *Heart of Medicine* (Aṣṭāṇgahṛdayasaṃhitā, Tib. Yan lag brgyad pa'i snying po bsdus pa); see *Vāgbhaṭa's Aṣṭāṇga Hṛdayam (Text, English translation, Notes, Appendix and Indices)*, trans. K.R. Srikantha Murthy, vol. 1, *Krishnadas Ayurveda Series*, Varanasi: Krishnadas Academy, 1991, 367. In Tibetan, Pha khol, "Yan lag brgyad pa'i snying po bsdus pa," in *Bstan 'gyur nang gi gso ba rig pa'i skor gyi dpe tshogs: gso rig pa'i rtsa 'grel bdam bsgrigs*, ed. Rdo rje rgyal po, Mi rigs dpe skrun khang, 1989, 258. I do not know the origin of the other recommendations; Vāgbhaṭa includes several suggestions that are not included in Tibetan sources.

2 Klong chen pa, *Tshig don mdzod*, in *Mdzod chen bdun*, Gangtok, Sikkim: Sherab Gyaltsen and Khyentse Labrang, 1983, 200. The first five chapters of this work have been translated in David Germano, "Poetic thought, the intelligent universe, and the mystery of self: the tantric synthesis of Rdzogs Chen in fourteenth-century Tibet," Ph.D. Dissertation, University of Wisconsin, 1992. The remaining chapters are translated in David Germano, "Longchenpa's The Treasury of Precious Words and Meanings," 9/13/94 manuscript. Translations of Longchenpa's *Treasury of Precious Words and Meanings* in this book are based on Germano's translation, but with minor modifications made so that terminology will correspond to that used in the present work. His translation of this passage is at "Poetic thought," 193.

3 Edward Grant, *Science and Religion, 400 B.C. to A.D. 1550: From Aristotle to Copernicus*, Baltimore: Johns Hopkins University Press, 2004, 61–67.

4 Philip van der Eijk, "Introduction," in *Magic and Rationality in Ancient Near Eastern and Graeco-Roman Medicine*, ed. H. F. J. Horstmanshoff and M. Stol, *Studies in Ancient Medicine*, Leiden: Brill, 2004, 5.

5 Ibid., 4–6.

6 For an overview of the contemporary history of such debates, see Edward Grant, *Science and Religion*.

7 Ibid., 169–176.

8 Ibid., 176–190.

9 Wilhelm Halbfass, *India and Europe, An Essay in Understanding*, Albany: State University of New York Press, 1988, 158. On this topic also see Philip C. Almond, *The British Discovery of Buddhism*, Cambridge: Cambridge University Press, 1988; Tomoko Masuzawa, *The Invention of World Religions: Or, How European Univer-*

salism Was Preserved in the Language of Pluralism, Chicago: University of Chicago Press, 2005.

10 Three of these options are suggested by David B. Wilson, "The Historiography of Science and Religion," in *Science and Religion: A Historical Introduction*, ed. Gary Ferngren, Baltimore: Johns Hopkins University Press, 2002, 14.

11 Richard G. Olson, *Science and Religion, 1450–1900: From Copernicus to Darwin*, Baltimore: Johns Hopkins University Press, 2004, 2–7.

12 Colin A. Russell, "The Conflict of Science and Religion," in *Science and Religion: A Historical Introduction*, ed. Gary Ferngren, Baltimore: Johns Hopkins University Press, 2002, 7.

13 Ibid., 8–9.

14 James R. Moore, *The Post-Darwinian Controversies: A Study of the Protestant Struggle to Come to Terms with Darwin in Great Britain and America, 1870–1900*, Cambridge: Cambridge University Press, 1979; cited in David B. Wilson, "Historiography," 23.

15 David B. Wilson, "Historiography," 15. Also see John Hedley Brooke, *Science and Religion: Some Historical Perspectives*, Cambridge: Cambridge University Press, 1991.

16 B. Alan Wallace, "Introduction: Buddhism and Science – Breaking Down Barriers," in *Buddhism and Science: Breaking New Ground*, ed. B. Alan Wallace, *Columbia Series in Science and Religion*, New York: Columbia University Press, 2003, 7.

17 Ibid., 8.

18 José Ignacio Cabezón, "Buddhism and Science: On the Nature of the Dialogue," in *Buddhism and Science: Breaking New Ground*, ed. B. Alan Wallace, *Columbia Series in Science and Religion*, New York: Columbia University Press, 2003, 36.

19 Ibid., 42.

20 Ibid., 58.

21 Vincanne Adams, "The sacred in the scientific: Ambiguous practices of science in Tibetan medicine," *Cultural Anthropology* 16, no. 4, 2001, 543.

22 Ibid., 550.

23 Ibid., 555.

24 *Gso ba rig pa'i bstan bcos sman bla'i dgongs rgyan rgyud bzhi'i gsal byed baidur sngon po'i malli ka zhes bya ba bzhugs so*, Dharamsala: Tibetan Medical and Astro Institute, 1994. The medical paintings are reproduced in Gyurme Dorje and Fernand Meyer, eds., *Tibetan Medical Paintings: Illustrations to the "Blue Beryl" Treatise of Sangye Gyamtso (1653–1705)*, 2 vols., New York: Harry N. Abrams, Inc. Publishers, 1992.

25 This topic is skillfully covered in Clara Pinto-Correia, *The Ovary of Eve: Egg and Sperm and Preformation*, Chicago: University of Chicago Press, 1997. Also see Norman Ford, *When Did I Begin? Conception of the Human Individual in History, Philosophy and Science*, Cambridge University Press, 1988.

26 R. Dix, "Organic Theories of Art: The Importance of Embryology," *Notes and Queries*, 1985, 215. On the organic theory of art and its relation to European philosophical thought, also see John Zammito, *The Genesis of Kant's Critique of Judgement*, Chicago: Chicago University Press, 1992.

27 Joseph Ziegler, *Medicine and Religion c. 1300, The Case of Arnau de Vilanova*, Oxford: Clarendon Press, 1998, 171.

28 Richard Sorabji, "Foreword," in *The Human Embryo: Aristotle and the Arabic and European Traditions*, ed. G. R. Dunstan, Exeter: University of Exeter Press, 1990, ix.

29 I model my approach here on Leslie Kurke, *Coins, Bodies, Games, and Gold: The Politics of Meaning in Archaic Greece*, Princeton: Princeton University Press, 1999, 31.

30 Ibid., 23.
31 Ronald M. Davidson, *Indian Esoteric Buddhism: A Social History of the Tantric Movement*, New York: Columbia University Press, 2002, 6.
32 Because numismatic and epigraphic evidence are not utilized in this study, I will not address stretching the boundaries of "literature" beyond that of texts recorded on paper or woodblock, although in another context one might make a point of doing so. Similarly, although many of the texts I will consider quite possibly originated as "oral literature," because the forms we have access to now are written, I will refer to them as written literature.
33 José Ignacio Cabezón and Roger R. Jackson, "Editors' Introduction," in *Tibetan Literature: Studies in Genre*, ed. José Ignacio Cabezón and Roger R. Jackson, Ithaca: Snow Lion Publishers, 1996, 17. In the twentieth century, Tibetan writers began to use the term *rtsom rig* as an equivalent to the English term, "literature."
34 Jerome Bruner, *Actual Minds, Possible Worlds*, Cambridge: Harvard University Press, 1986.
35 Charles Leslie and Allen Young, eds., *Paths to Asian Medical Knowledge*, Berkeley: University of California Press, 1992, 3. Also see Don Bates, ed., *Knowledge and the Scholarly Medical Traditions*, Cambridge: Cambridge University Press, 1995; Karl Figlio, "The Historiography of Scientific Medicine: An Invitation to the Human Sciences," *Comparative Studies in Society and History* 19, no. 3, 1977; Karl Figlio, "The Metaphor of Organization: An Historiographical Perspective on the Bio-Medical Sciences of the Early Nineteenth Century," *History of Science* 14, 1976.
36 Wallace Martin, *Recent Theories of Narrative*, Ithaca: Cornell University Press, 1986, 7.
37 Donald Polkinghorne, *Narrative Knowing and the Human Sciences*, Albany: State University of New York Press, 1988, 36.
38 Hunter, "Narrative, Literature and the Clinical Exercise of Practical Reason," *Journal of Medicine and Philosophy* 21, 1996, 304.
39 Ibid., 307. See D. Burrell and S. Hauerwas, "From System to Story: An Alternative Pattern for Rationality in Ethics," in *Why Narrative? Readings in Narrative Theology*, ed. S. Hauerwas and L. G. Jones, Grand Rapids, MI: Eerdmans, 1977; A. MacIntyre, *After Virtue: A Study in Moral Theory*, Notre Dame: University of Notre Dame Press, 1981; M. C. Nussbaum, *Love's Knowledge: Essays on Philosophy and Literature*, New York: Oxford University Press, 1990.
40 Hayden White, "The Value of Narrativity in the Representation of Reality," in *On Narrative*, ed. W. J. T. Mitchell, Chicago: University of Chicago Press, 1980, 7.
41 Daniel Punday, "A Corporeal Narratology?" *Style* 34, no. 2, 2000, 227.
42 Ibid., 228.
43 Hayden White, "The Value of Narrativity," 4.
44 Ibid., 14.

2 THEORIES OF HUMAN DEVELOPMENT

1 From Gerald Larson, "The Concept of Body in Āyurveda and the Hindu Philosophical Systems," in *Self as Body in Asian Theory and Practice*, ed. Roger Ames, Thomas P. Kasulis, and Wimal Dissanayake, Albany: State University of New York Press, 1993, 110. Translation by Gerald Larson.
2 *Caraka saṃhitā*, trans. A. Chandra Kaviratna and P. Sharma, 2nd ed., vol. 2, *Indian Medical Science Series* No. 42, Delhi: Sri Satguru Publications, 1996, 461–469; hereafter referred to as *Caraka saṃhitā*. For surveys of conflicting views, also see *Caraka saṃhitā*, 496–497; Surendranath Dasgupta, *A History of Indian Philosophy*, 5 vols., New Delhi: Motilal Banarsidass, 1975, vol. 2, 302–319; Bhagwan Dash, *Embryology*

and Maternity in Ayurveda, New Delhi: Delhi Diary, 1975; P. Kutumbiah, *Ancient Indian Medicine*, Calcutta: Orient Longmans Ltd., 1962, 2–6; Jyotir Mitra, *A Critical Appraisal of Ayurvedic Material in Buddhist Literature*, Varanasi: The Jyotiralok Prakashan, 1985; Alex Wayman, "The Intermediate-State Dispute in Buddhism," in *Buddhist Studies in Honour of I. B. Horner*, Dordrecht: D. Reidel, 1974.

3 Surendranath Dasgupta, *A History of Indian Philosophy*, vol. 2, 316. Also see *Caraka saṃhitā*, 497.

4 Minoru Hara, "A Note on the Buddha's Birth Story," in *Indianisme et bouddisme: melanges offerts a Mgr Etienne Lamotte*, Louvain-la-Neuve: Universite catholique de Louvain, Institut orientaliste, 1980, 154, ff. 49; Lakshmi Kapani, "Upanisad of the Embryo and Notes on the Garbha-Upanisad," in *Fragments for a History of the Human Body*, ed. Michael Feher, Urzone, Inc., 1989. For references to secondary literature on this text, see Hara, "A Note on the Buddha's Birth Story," 151, ff. 37. For a discussion of embryology in the eleventh-century Agni Purāṇa, see Sarita Hamda and Jyotirmitra, "Agnipurana ka garbhakranti sarir," *Journal of Research in Indian Medicine* 13, no. 3, 1978. For additional Vedic references to the process of human fetal development, also see Gian Giuseppe Filippi, "The Secret of the Embryo According to the *Garbha Upaniṣad*," *Annali di Ca' Foscari* 31, 1992; K. Kaladhar, "Niruktopaniṣad and Garbhopaniṣad: The Vedic Sources of Studies on Human Embryology," *Bulletin of the Indian Institute of History of Medicine: Hyderabad* 24, no. 1, 1994; P. Rolland, "Un fragment medical vedique; Le premier khaṇḍa du Vārāhapariśiṣṭa bhūtotpatti," *Munchener Studien zur Sprachwissenschaft* 30, 1972. On Jain embryology, see C. Caillat, "Sur les doctrines medicales dans le Tandulaveyāliya," *Indologica Taurenesia* 2, 1975.

5 Surendranath Dasgupta, *History of Indian Philosophy*, 2: 305–312.

6 Steven Collins, *Selfless Persons*, Cambridge: Cambridge University Press, 1982, 57.

7 Ibid.

8 Surendranath Dasgupta, *History of Indian Philosophy*, vol. 2, 302.

9 David Gordon White, *The Alchemical Body: Siddha Traditions in Medieval India*, Chicago: University of Chicago Press, 1996, 27.

10 Ibid., 101.

11 The *Carakasaṃhitā*, for instance, is said by some scholars to be originally composed by Agniveśa, from before the seventh century B.C., and later enlarged upon by Caraka, although in fact Caraka is a name attributed to several figures and also to an entire school of mendicants who practiced medicine. See Priya Vrat Sharma, *History of Medicine in India, from Antiquity to 1000 A.D.*, New Delhi: Indian National Science Academy, 1992, 175–95. Also see Surendranath Dasgupta, *History of Indian Philosophy*, vol. 2; Dominik Wujastyk, *The Roots of Ayurveda*, 2nd ed., London: Penguin Classics, 2003. On connections between Āyurveda and philosophical traditions, see Viktoria Lyssenko, "The Human Body Composition in Statics and Dynamics: Āyurveda and the Philosophical Schools of Vaiśeṣika and Sāṃkhya," *Journal of Indian Philosophy* 32, 2004.

12 There are several partial translations of this text, including *Agniveśa's Caraka saṃhitā (Text with English Translation and Critial Exposition Based on Cakrapāṇi Datta's Āyurveda Dīpikā)*, trans. Ram Karan Sharma and Vaidya Bhagwan Dash, vol. 2, *Chowkhamba Sanskrit Studies*, Varanasi: Chowkhamba Press, 1976.

13 *Agniveśa's Caraka saṃhitā*, verse 4.1.151.

14 The *Suśruta-Saṃhitā* section on the human body can be found loosely translated in Dinkar Govind Thatte, *Śāryrasthānam Suśruta-Saṃhitā (Section on the Study of the Human body), Text with English Translation and Commentary, Kashi Ayurveda Series No. 16*, Varanasi: Chaukhambha Orientalia, 1994. Murthy notes that this text was translated into Arabic as early as the ninth century C.E. See his chapter on

Suśruta in Sharma, *History of Medicine in India*, 196–204. Also see Surendranath Dasgupta, *History of Indian Philosophy*, vol. 2.

15 Dominik Wujastyk, *Roots*, 193–194.

16 B. Rama Rao summarizes the debates over the identity of the medical writer named Vāgbhaṭa in his chapter on the figure in Sharma, *History of Medicine in India*, 205–221. Also see Surendranath Dasgupta, *History of Indian Philosophy*, vol. 2, 433–436; Claus Vogel, *Vāgbhaṭa's Aṣṭāṅgahṛdayasaṃhitā, the first five chapters of its Tibetan version, Abhanglungen fur die Kunde des Morgenlandes*, Wiesbaden: Deutsche Morgenlandische Gesellschaft, Komissionsverkag Franz Steiner GMBH, 1965 (the introduction of which has a lengthy discussion of the text's authorship); Dominik Wujastyk, *Roots*. Vāgbhaṭa is referred to in Tibetan medical literature by the names *pha khol, pha gol*, or simply *dpa' bo*.

17 Translations of other medical books in the Tibetan Tengyur include Bhagwan Dash, *Nāgārjuna's Yogasataka*, Library of Tibetan Works and Archives, 1976; R.E. Emmerick, "Ravigupta's Siddhasara," *Verzeichnis der orientalischen Handschriften in Deutschland* Supplemental Volume 23, 1980–1982, published in Sanskrit and Tibetan with an English translation. Also see the *Sman 'tsho ba'i mdo*, published in English translation with reconstructed Sanskrit in Bhagwan Dash and Doboom Tulku, *Positive Health in Tibetan Medicine*, Delhi: Sri Satguru Publications, 1991. For more on medical texts authored by Nāgārjuna and other Indians held in high regard by the Tibetan medical tradition, see Lobsang Rabgay, "The Origin and Growth of Medicine in Tibet," *Tibetan Medicine* 3, 1981. Also see Bhagwan Dash's essay on Tibetan medicine in Sharma, *History of Medicine in India*, 453–463. Twenty-two Indian medical texts are typically included in the Tibetan canon, although in this book I only refer to those that are of direct relevance to the study of embryology.

18 An auto-commentary, *Yan lag brgyad pa'i snying po shes bya ba'i sman dpyad kyi bshad pa*, and *Yan lag brgyad pa'i snying po'i rnam par 'grel pa tshig gi don zla zer*, by *Zla ba la dga' ba* or *zla ba mngon dga'* (Skt. *Candranandana* or possibly *Candrabhinandana*). These and other medical texts included in the Tibetan Tengyur have recently been published in book form in the four volume collection, *Gso ba rig pa'i rtsa 'grel bdam bsgrigs–bstan 'gyur nang gi gso ba rig pa'i skor gyi dpe tshogs*, Mi rigs dpe skrun khang gi rtsi 'khor, 1996. On the identity of the commentator Dawa Ngönga, see Manfred Taube, *Beitrage zur Geschichte der Medizinischen Literatur Tibets*, Sankt Augustin: VGH Wissenschaftsverlag, 1981, 28; Vogel, *Vāgbhaṭa*'s *Aṣṭāṅgahṛdayasaṃhitā*, 15–16.

19 Dawa Ngönga is also called Khaché Dawa Ngönga (kha che zla ba mngon dga') and sometimes Dawala Gawa (zla ba la dga' ba); corresponding in Sanskrit to Candranandana or possibly Candrābhinandana. According to Sanggyé Gyatso, Rinchen Zangpo taught the Indian texts to his student, Zhangzhungpa Sherab Ö. This student transmitted these teachings to one Gyatön Drapa Sherab, who wrote a commentary on the *Four Tantras* called *Gser gyi bang mdzod* and a history of medicine, neither of which are now extant. Gyatön Drapa Sherab passed the teachings on to Yuthok Gyagar Dorje, who passed them to Yuthok Jidpo, who passed them to Garpo. These and other figures are described at Sangs rgyas rgya mtsho, *Gso rig sman gyi khog 'bugs*, Dharamsala: Tibetan Medical and Astro Institute, 1994, 177–178. On Rinchen Zangpo's students, also see Roberto Vitali, "On some disciples of Rinchen Zangpo and Lochung Legpai Sherab, and their successors, who brought teachings popular in Ngari Korsum to Central Tibet," in *Tibet and Her Neighbours: A History*, ed. Alex McKay, London: Edition Hansjorg Mayer, 2003.

20 Sangs rgyas rgya mtsho, *Khog 'bugs*, 229.

21 For more on Āyurvedic views of conception and gestation, see Martha Ann Selby, "Narratives of Conception, Gestation, and Labour in Sanskrit Āyurvedic Texts," *Asian Medicine: Tradition and Modernity* 1, no. 2, 2005.

22 For example, see works by Rahul Peter Das, Surendranath Dasgupta, Louis De La Vallée Poussin, J.R. Haldar, Robert Kritzer, McDermott, Jyotir Mitra and O. Wijesekara.
23 These differences are summarized in J.R. Haldar, *Medical Science in Pali Literature*, Calcutta: Indian Museum, 1977, 29. Also see Jeffrey Hopkins and Lati Rinpoche, *Death, Intermediate State and Rebirth in Tibetan Buddhism*, Ithaca: Snow Lion Publications, 1979, 62.
24 O. Wijesekara, "Vedic Gandharva and Pali Gandhabba," *University of Ceylon Review* 1, 1945, 89–90.
25 Ibid., 92.
26 James P. McDermott, "Karma and Rebirth in Early Buddhism," in *Karma and Rebirth in Classical Indian Traditions*, ed. Wendy Doniger, Delhi: Motilal Banarsidass, 1983, 169–171. On related debates in early Indian Buddhist literature, also see Mathieu Boisvert, "Conception and Intrauterine Life in the Pali Canon," *Studies in Religion* 29, no. 3, 2000; David J. Kalupahana, *Causality: The Central Philosophy of Buddhism*, Honolulu: The University Press of Hawaii, 1975, 115–121; Wayman, "The Intermediate-State Dispute in Buddhism," 227–237. An interesting discussion of medieval Indian Buddhist notions of karma's role in rebirth can be found in Bruce Matthews, "Post-Classical Developments in the Concepts of Karma and Rebirth in Theravada Buddhism," in *Karma & Rebirth: Post-Classical Developments*, ed. Ronald W. Neufeldt, *SUNY Series in Religious Studies*, Albany: State University of New York Press, 1986.
27 Louis De La Vallée Poussin, *Abhidharmakośabhāṣyam*, trans. Leo M. Pruden, 4 vols., vol. 2, Berkeley: Asian Humanities Press, 1988, 380–381. Also see Khedrup Norsang Gyatso, *Ornament of Stainless Light*, ed. Thupten Jinpa, trans. Gavin Kilty, *The Library of Tibetan Classics*, Boston: Wisdom Publications and the Institute of Tibetan Classics, 2004, 164–165.
28 Bryan J. Cuevas, *The Hidden History of The Tibetan Book of the Dead*, Oxford: Oxford University Press, 2003, 39–44; Robert Kritzer, "Antarābhava in the Vibhāsā," *Nōtom Damu Joshi Daigaku Kirisutokyō Bunka Kenkyū Kiyō (Maranata)* 3, no. 5, 1993; Robert Kritzer, "Rūpa and the Antarābhava," *Journal of Indian Philosophy* 29, 2000; Robert Kritzer, "Semen, Blood, and the Intermediate Existence," *Journal of Indian and Buddhist Studies* 46, no. 2, 1998.
29 Louis De La Vallée Poussin, *Abhidharmakośabhāṣyam*, 395. For a detailed discussion of Vasubhandu's sources and earlier, conflicting Buddhist descriptions of conception, see Robert Kritzer, "The Four Ways of Entering the Womb (*garbhāvakrānti*)," *Bukkyi Bunka* 10, 2000; Robert Kritzer, "Rūpa," 248–258.
30 Louis De La Vallée Poussin, *Abhidharmakośabhāṣyam*, 397–398.
31 Robert Kritzer, "Four Ways," 10.
32 Louis De La Vallée Poussin, *Abhidharmakośabhāṣyam*, 400. For notes on Sūtric sources for this citation, see De La Vallée Poussin, *Abhidharmakośabhāṣyam*, 511, ff. 147. For a survey of debates in early Indian Buddhist literature on the mechanics of conception and early embryonic growth, also see Mathieu Boisvert, "Conception and Intrauterine Life."
33 Robert Kritzer identifies at least four Chinese translations: (1) in the Ratnakūṭa section of the sūtra-piṭaka is the *Pao-t'ai'ching* (T. 317), translated by Dharmarakṣa in the Western Chin dynasty; (2) also in the Ratnakūṭa section is the *Ju t'ai tsang hui* (T. 310 sūtra no. 14, 326b-336c); (3) a version identical to the *Ju t'ai tsang hui* but translated by I Ching and located in the Mūlasarvāstivādavinaya (T. 1451); and (4) the *Fu-wei-a-nan-shuo-jen-ch'u-t'ai-hui* (T. 310 sūtra no. 13: 322a-326b), translated by Bodhiruci in the Tang dynasty. See Robert Kritzer, "Garbhāvakrāntisūtra: A Comparison of the Contents of Two Versions," *Maranatha: Bulletin of the Christian*

Culture Research Institute (Kyoto) 6, 1998; G.P. Malalasekera, "Āyuśman-Nanda-Garbhāvakrānti-Nirdeśa-(Nāma-Mahayana-)Sūtra," in *Encyclopaedia of Buddhism*, Government of Ceylon, 1961, 480–481. A version of the sūtra has been translated into German in Huebotter, *Die Sutra Uber Empfangnis und Embryologie*, Tokyo: Deutsche Gesellschaft fur Natur- U. Volkerkunde Ostasiens, 1932.

34 Robert Kritzer, "Garbhāvakrāntisūtra"; Marcelle Lalou, "La Version Tibetain Du Ratnakūṭa," *Journal Asiatique* Octobre-Decembre, 1927; Mark Tatz, *Buddhism and Healing: Demiéville's Article "Byō" from Hōbōgirin*, Lanham: University Press of America, 1985, 92.

35 Marcelle Lalou, "La Version Tibetain Du Ratnakūṭa," 241–243.

36 This passage is not found in the Degé edition of the *Entering the Womb* sūtra but rather in the considerably longer *Abiding in the Womb*; "Tshe dang ldan pa dga' po la mngal na gnas pa bstan pa," in *The Sde-dge Black Bka'-'gyur: a reprint of a print from the Sde dge blocks originally edited by Si-tu Chos-kyi-'byung-gnas*, ed. Si tu pan chen chos kyi 'byung gnas, 211a (423). This text will be referred to henceforth as "Mngal na gnas pa (Degé edition)." Also see "Gcung mo'u dga' bo zhes bya ba theg pa chen po'i mdo," in *The Tog Palace manuscript of the Tibetan Kanjur*, Leh: Smanrtsis Shesrig Dpemzod, 1975–1980, 395b-396a (790–91). This text will be referred to from this point as "Mngal na gnas pa (Tog Palace)."

37 "Mngal na gnas pa (Degé edition)," 211b–212a (424–425); "Mngal na gnas pa (Tog Palace)," 396b-397a (792–793). Also see "'Phags pa tshe dang ldan pa dga' po la mngal du 'jug pa bstan pa zhes bya ba theg pa chen po'i mdo," in *The Sde-dge Black Bka'-'gyur: a reprint of a print from the Sde dge blocks originally edited by Si-tu Chos-kyi-'byung-gnas*, ed. Si tu pan chen chos kyi 'byung gnas, Chengdu, 237b (476). This latter text will be referred to from this point as "Mngal du 'jug pa (Degé edition)."

38 "Mngal na gnas pa (Degé edition)," 212a (425); "Mngal na gnas pa (Tog Palace)," 397b (794). A similar statement is made at "Mngal du 'jug pa (Degé edition)," 237b–38a (476–477).

39 Vesna Wallace, *The Inner Kālacakratantra: a Buddhist Tantric View of the Individual*, New York: Oxford University Press, 2001, 11.

40 Ibid., 57.

41 Ibid., 61.

42 Ibid., 22, 68, 87.

43 Ibid., 65.

44 Ibid., 183.

45 Sabine Wilms, "The Transmission of Medical Knowledge on 'Nurturing the Fetus' in Early China," *Asian Medicine: Tradition and Modernity* 1, no. 2, 2005, 276.

46 Ibid., 280–283.

47 Chen Ming, "Zhuan Nu Wei Nan Turning Female to Male: An Indian Influence on Chinese Gynaecology?" *Asian Medicine: Tradition and Modernity* 1, no. 2, 2005, 317–319.

48 Ibid., 323. On Buddhist texts in China that addressed gestation and pregnancy, also see Prabodh Chandra Bagchi, "A Fragment of the Kāśyapa-Saṃhitā in Chinese," *Indian Culture* 9, 1942.

49 Sabine Wilms, "Transmission," 311.

50 Anne Kinney, *Representations of Childhood and Youth in Early China*, Stanford: Stanford University Press, 2003, 349–350. Fascinating details on early Chinese textual traditions of embryology can also be found in Charlotte Furth, *A Flourishing Yin: Gender in China's Medical History, 960–1665*, Berkeley: University of California Press, 1999, 101–116.

51 Anne Kinney, *Childhood and Youth in Early China*, 359.

52 Charlotte Furth, *Flourishing Yin*, 101. Also see Charlotte Furth, "From Birth to Birth: the Growing Body in Chinese Medicine," in *Chinese Views of Childhood*, ed. Anne Behnke Kinney, Honolulu: University of Hawai'i Press, 1995.
53 Kenneth Zysk, *Asceticism and Healing in Ancient India*, New York: Oxford University Press, 1991. On the issue of whether medicine was practiced by monks in early Indian Buddhist monasteries, see Wetara Mahinda, "Medical Practices of Buddhist Monks: a Historical Analysis of Attitudes and Problems," in *Recent Researches in Buddhist Studies: Essays in Honour of Professor Y. Karunadasa*, ed. Kuala Lumpur Dhammajoti, Asanga Tilakaratne, and Kapila Abhayawansa, Columbo: Y. Karunadasa Felicitation Committee, 1997.

3 INTERACTIONS BETWEEN MEDICINE AND RELIGION IN TIBET

1 Skal bzang 'phrin las, *Bod kyi gso ba rig pa'i byung 'phel gyi lo rgyus gsal bar ston pa baidurya sngon po'i zhun thigs*, Krung go'i bod kyi shes rig dpe skrun khang, 1997, 32–39.
2 Sangs rgyas rgya mtsho, *Khog 'bugs*, 149.
3 Byams pa 'phrin las, *Bod kyi gso ba rig pa'i 'byung tshul dang 'phel rgyas skor gyi ngo sprod rags bdus*, Lhasa: Mentsikhang, 1986, 2; Byams pa 'phrin las, *Krung go'i bod kyi gso ba rig pa*, krung go'i bod kyi shes rig dpe skrun khang, 1996. Also see Sangs rgyas rgya mtsho, *Khog 'bugs*, 213.
4 Pasang Yonten, Tsepak Rigzin, and Phillippa Russell, "A History of the Tibetan Medical System," *Tibetan Medicine* 12, 1989, 34. Also see Sangs rgyas rgya mtsho, *Khog 'bugs*, 213.
5 Pasang Yönten points to Sa skya je btzun bsod nams rgyal mtsan, *Rgyal rabs gsal ba'i me long*, Peking edition, 1981, 61. See also Sangs rgyas rgya mtsho, *Khog 'bugs*, 149–150.
6 Ibid., 150.
7 Pasang Yonten, Tsepak Rigzin, and Phillippa Russell, "History," 33–36. On the possible relationships between Greek medicine and Tibetan medicine, see Christopher I. Beckwith, "The Introduction of Greek Medicine into Tibet in the 7th and 8th Century," *Journal of the American Oriental Society* 99, 1979; Marianne Winder, "Tibetan Medicine Compared with Ancient and Mediaeval Western Medicine," *Bulletin of Tibetology (Gangtok, Sikkim)* 1, 1981.
8 On Eurasian collaboration in early Tibetan medical history, see Frances Garrett, "Critical Methods in Tibetan Medical Histories," *Journal of Asian Studies* 66, no. 2, 2007.
9 For a detailed description of his contributions to the medical tradition, see Sangs rgyas rgya mtsho, *Khog 'bugs*, 163–169.
10 Ibid., 169.
11 The question of whether there are, in fact, two individuals named Yuthok Yönten Gönpo is debated by some Tibetan scholars. Samten Karmay notes that because the biography of the twelfth-century Yuthok Yönten Gönpo written by his student, Sumtön Yeshé Zung, does not mention an eighth century Yuthok, the existence of such a figure must be questioned. Karmay notes that Sodokpa Lodrö Gyeltsen (1552–1624) likewise does not accept the existence of two Yuthoks. See Samten G. Karmay, "Vairocana and the rgyud-bzhi," *Tibetan Medicine*, 1989, 21 and 29, ff 14. On this question, also see Rechung Rinpoche Jampal Kunzang, *Tibetan Medicine, Illustrated in Original Texts, Indian Medical Science Series No. 112*, Delhi: Sri Satguru Publications, 2001, vii. There is a sixteenth-century biographical sketch of Yuthok Yönten Gönpo in the *Mkhas pa'i dga' ston* mentioned in Barbara Gerke,

"The Authorship of the Tibetan Medical Treatise 'Cha lag bco brgyad' (Twelfth Century AD) and a Description of its Historical Background," *Traditional South Asian Medicine* 6, 2001, 34. Both Yuthoks are discussed at Sangs rgyas rgya mtsho, *Khog 'bugs*, 206–284.

12 Marcelle Lalou, "Les texts Bouddhiques au temps du Roi Khri-sron-lde-bcan," *Journal Asiatique* 261, 1953.

13 Sangs rgyas rgya mtsho, *Khog 'bugs*, 169. The names of nearly sixty medical texts are listed in Sangs rgyas rgya mtsho, *Khog 'bugs*, 156–160 and 171–174.The medical congress is also described in the eighth-century Yuthok's biography, translated by Rechung Rinpoche, beginning at Kunzang, *Tibetan Medicine*, 202. I do not know what location is meant by Drugu (*gru gu*).

14 Sangs rgyas rgya mtsho, *Khog 'bugs*, 175–176. The ten systems he lists that influ enced the make-up of Tibetan medicine are Kha che, Oyn, Dbus, Bal bo, Ta zig, Dol bo, Hor, Mi nyag, Li and Khrom. See Frances Garrett, "Critical Methods."

15 Frances Garrett, "Buddhism and the Historicizing of Medicine in Thirteenth Century Tibet," *Asian Medicine: Tradition and Modernity* 2, no. 2, 2007.

16 Rechung Rinpoche Jampal Kunzang, 19. Sangs rgyas rgya mtsho, *Khog 'bugs*, 178–79. For comments on Darma Gönpo in particular, see Sangs rgyas rgya mtsho, *Khog 'bugs*, 179. The four great Ngari doctors were Nyangdé Senggé Dra, Taktri Yeshé, Jungné, Ongmen Ayé, and Mangmo Mangtsün. One of these, Mangmo Mangtsün was especially renowned in this group, and his most prominent student was Chejé Tipa, who in turn taught Chejé Zhangtön Zhikpo. The latter composed a history of medicine that has only recently been found to be extant. Chejé Zhangtön Zhikpo's student was Darma Gönpo.

17 Sangs rgyas rgya mtsho, *Khog 'bugs*, 180–182.

18 The contributions to medical literature made by many figures active during this period are recorded at Ibid., 290–296, in addition to sections of Sanggyé Gyatso's text mentioned above. Many figures known primarily for their contributions to the religious canon are also mentioned here as authors of medical texts.

19 Rje btsun grags pa rgyal mtshan, *Gso dpyad rgyal po'i dkor mdzod*, Kan su'u mi rigs dpe skrun khang, 1993. This work is discussed in the contemporary medical history, Skal bzang 'phrin las, *Bod kyi gso ba rig pa'i byung 'phel gyi lo rgyus*, 314–317.

20 For discussion of editions of the *Four Tantras*, see Natalia D. Bolsokhoyeva, *Introduction to the Studies of Tibetan Medical Sources*, Kathmandu: Mandala Book Point, 1993, 25–26; Barbara Gerke and Natalia Bolsokhoeva, "Namthar of Zurkha Lodo Gyalpo (1509–1579)," *AyurVijnana* 6, 1999; Fernand Meyer, "Introduction: The Medical Paintings of Tibet," in *Tibetan Medical Paintings: Illustrations to the "Blue Beryl" treatise of Sangye Gyamtso (1653–1705)*, ed. Gyurme Dorje and Fernand Meyer, New York: Harry N. Abrams, Inc. Publishers, 1992, 6.

21 Sanggyé Gyatso's account of the twelfth-century Yuthok's life begins at Sangs rgyas rgya mtsho, *Khog 'bugs*, 225. For a list of texts authored by the twelfth-century Yuthok, see Sangs rgyas rgya mtsho, *Khog 'bugs*, 275–284. Manfred Taube's chapter on the *Eighteen Additional Practices* claims that it was of major importance from the twelfth-sixteenth centuries, until Sanggyé Gyatso's critique of it removed it from circulation. See Barbara Gerke, "Authorship," 27; Manfred Taube, *Medizinischen Literatur Tibets*, 39–50. A discussion of Sumtön Yeshé Zung begins at Sangs rgyas rgya mtsho, *Khog 'bugs*, 284. Sanggyé Gyatso quotes extensively from a biography of the twelfth-century Yuthok written by Sumtön Yeshé Zung, a text that exists as part of the *Eighteen Additional Practices* collection. Sanggyé Gyatso lists several other early biographies of Yuthok by figures named Yuthok Kharag Lharjé and Kongbo Degyel, neither of which are known to exist today. Sangs rgyas rgya mtsho, *Khog 'bugs*, 290.

22 Rechung Rinpoche Jampal Kunzang, *Tibetan Medicine*, 10. Sanggyé Gyatso dis-

cusses the controversy over the location of Tanaduk at Sangs rgyas rgya mtsho, *Khog 'bugs*, 55 onwards.

23 G.yu thog yon tan mgon po, *Bdud rtsi snying po yan lag brgyad pa gsang ba man ngag gi rgyud ces bya ba bzhugs so*, Bod ljongs mi dmangs dpe skrun khang, 2000, 4. In English, *The Quintessence Tantras of Tibetan Medicine*, trans. Barry Clark, Ithaca: Snow Lion Publishers, 1995, 26.

24 Olaf Czaja, "Zurkharwa Lodro Gyalpo (1509–1579) on the Controversy of the Indian Origin of the rGyud bzhi," *The Tibet Journal* 30 and 31, no. 4 and 1, 2005–2006; Frances Garrett, "Buddhism and the Historicizing of Medicine"; Janet Gyatso, "The Authority of Empiricism and the Empiricism of Authority: Medicine and Buddhism in Tibet on the Eve of Modernity," *Comparative Studies of South Asia, Africa and the Middle East* 24, no. 2, 2004.

25 This is the *Rnam thar bka' rgya cen*, also known as *Sku lnga lhun grub ma* and *Rnam thar med thabs med pa*. This is the first of three sub-documents within the twelfth text of the *Eighteen Additional Practices*, a collection typically attributed uncritically to Yuthok Yönten Gönpo. See Frances Garrett, "Buddhism and the Historicizing of Medicine"; Samten Karmay, "Vairocana and the rgyud-bzhi," 28, ff. 5.

26 Samten Karmay, "Vairocana and the rgyud-bzhi," 21. From *Rgyud bzhi'i bka' bsgrub nges don snying po*, vol. 2 (tha), 213–241, in *Collected writings of Sog-bzlog-pa Blo-gros-rgyal-mtshan. Reproduced from a unique but incomplete manuscript from the library of Bdud-'joms Rin-po-che*, New Delhi: Sanje Dorji, 1975, vol. 9, 235. Sanggyé Gyatso locates an early identification of Drapa Ngönshé as the discoverer of the *Four Tantras* in the fourteenth-century biography of Padmasambhava, the *Pad ma bka' thang*. Sangs rgyas rgya mtsho, *Khog 'bugs*, 202.

27 On historical problems with this scenario, see Marianne Winder, "Introduction," in *Tibetan Medicine, Illustrated in Original Texts*, ed. Rechung Rinpoche Jampal Kunzang, *Indian Medical Science Series No. 112*, Delhi: Sri Satguru Publications, 2001. On this lineage, see Byams pa 'phrin las, *Gang ljongs gso rig bstan pa'i nyin byed rim byon gyi rnam thar phyogs bsgrigs (Medical biographies of Tibet in chronological order)*, Dharamsala: Tibetan Medical and Astrological institute, no date, 98–99. Könchok Kyab is discussed at Sangs rgyas rgya mtsho, *Khog 'bugs*, 182 and 206. Könchok Kyab is likely the author of one of the texts from the *Eighteen Additional Practices*, the *Rtsod bzlog gegs sel*, a record of debates on the meaning of the root and branch and other theoretical aspects of medical theory; see Skal bzang 'phrin las, *Bod kyi gso ba rig pa'i byung 'phel gyi lo rgyus*, 319. This text is the sixth text in the *Eighteen Additional Practices*. See Frances Garrett, "Buddhism and the Historicizing of Medicine"; Barbara Gerke, "Authorship."

28 Manfred Taube, *Medizinischen Literatur Tibets*, 26–27. Vairocana's involvement in the medical tradition is discussed extensively in Sangs rgyas rgya mtsho, *Khog 'bugs*, 163–169.

29 According to Jampa Trinley, this student is Sumtön Yeshé Zung, who, ironically, is the author of a text mentioned above that maintains the *Four Tantras'* divine origins. Samten Karmay points to references to this text cited in works by Sodokpa Lodrö Gyeltsen and Sanggyé Gyatso. Karmay says this text is no longer extant, however Jampa Trinlé claims to have seen the text recently in Lhasa; he says that Sumton Yeshé Zung claims that Yuthok wrote the *Four Tantras* on page 2–4 of a text called *Lo rgyus dge ba'i lcags kyu*. Byams pa 'phrin las, *Krung go'i bod kyi gso ba rig pa*, 30.

30 Samten Karmay, "Vairocana and the rgyud-bzhi," 22–23.

31 Manfred Taube, *Medizinischen Literatur Tibets*, 33.

32 Cited by Ibid., 32. This topic is also discussed at Sangs rgyas rgya mtsho, *Khog 'bugs*, 275.

33 Bla ma skyabs, *Bod kyi mkhas pa rim byon gyi gso rig gsung 'bum dkar chag mu tig*

phreng ba, Kan su'u mi rigs dpe skrun khang, 1997; Taube, *Medizinischen Literatur Tibets*, 33.

34 José Ignacio Cabezón, "Authorship and Literary Production in Classical Buddhist Tibet," in *Changing Minds: Contributions to the Study of Buddhism and Tibet in Honor of Jeffrey Hopkins*, ed. Guy Newland, Ithaca: Snow Lion Publications, 2001, 236.

35 Sangs rgyas rgya mtsho, *Khog 'bugs*, 292 onwards.

36 Manfred Taube, *Medizinischen Literatur Tibets*, 37.

37 On the authorship of these texts, which are from the *Eighteen Additional Practices* collection, see Barbara Gerke, "Authorship." Sanggyé Gyatso discusses the texts' authorship at *Khog 'bugs*, 277–278. For a brief overview of these texts' contents, see Frances Garrett, "Buddhism and the Historicizing of Medicine."

38 This figure is discussed at Sangs rgyas rgya mtsho, *Khog 'bugs*, 285–289. Sumtön Yeshé Zung's explanation of causes of conception is divided into four subsections, a taxonomy that is not inherent to the *Four Tantras* itself (the causes of conception, defects that result in inability to conceive, how conception occurs in the womb, and a teaching on the generation of causes from effects), although I cannot say whether this organization may have been added by later editors. See Dzanya na dha ri (Sum ston ye shes gzung), *Bshad rgyud 'grel pa 'bum nag gsal sgron*, Pe cing: Mi rigs dpe skrun khang, 1998, 8–23.

39 My discussion of Longchenpa's work relies upon David Germano's extensive research. Germano reports that recently discovered early Nyingma texts suggest that much of Longchenpa's writings in fact largely duplicate earlier Nyingma works, suggesting a much earlier provenance for this embryological presentation. I have not had the opportunity to examine these earlier sources.

40 Sangs rgyas rgya mtsho, *Khog 'bugs*, 306–312.

41 Manfred Taube, *Medizinischen Literatur Tibets*, 53.

42 Barbara Gerke, "On the History of the Two Tibetan Medical Schools: Janglug and Zurlug," *AyurVijnana* 6, 1999, 20.

43 For more on this tradition, see Sangs rgyas rgya mtsho, *Khog 'bugs*, 329 onwards. Nyamnyi Dorjé is also called Abo Chöjé. See his biography in Bkra shis tshe ring, *Bod kyi gso ba rig pa'i ched rtsom gces btus*, Bod ljongs mi dmangs dpe skrun khang, 1994. Scores of additional texts produced at this time are listed at Sangs rgyas rgya mtsho, *Khog 'bugs*, 332–334.

44 Barbara Gerke and Natalia Bolksokhoyeva noted that recent editions of the text have been reorganized for modern medical students after the structure of the *Four Tantras*; the original chapter structure of the text, which does not follow the model of the *Four Tantras*, is recorded in Manfred Taube, 63. See Barbara Gerke and Natalia Bolsokhoyeva, "Namthar," 35.

45 Pasang Yonten, Tsepak Rigzin, and Phillipa Russell, "History," 43. Sanggyé Gyatso's history does not seem to mention this fact; see *Khog 'bugs*, 349–350. Pasang Yönten does not mention his source.

46 Pasang Yonten, Tsepak Rigzin, and Phillipa Russell, "History," 44; Sangs rgyas rgya mtsho, *Khog 'bugs*, 349; Also see Barbara Gerke and Natalia Bolsokhoyeva, "Namthar," 29–30.

47 Barbara Gerke and Natalia Bolsokhoyeva, "Namthar," 31, citing Pasang Yonten.

48 Todd Fenner, "The Origin of the rGyud bzhi: A Tibetan Medical Tantra," in *Tibetan Literature: Studies in Genre*, ed. José Ignacio Cabezón and Robert R. Jackson, Ithaca: Snow Lion Publications, 1996, 460.

49 For comments on this issue see José Ignacio Cabezón and Roger R. Jackson, "Editors' Introduction."

50 Personal communication with Yangga, Lhasa 2002; Dorje Dramdul, Sarnath, 2001; Jampa, Darjeeling, 2000.

51 For a summary, see Frances Garrett, "Buddhism and the Historicizing of Medicine."
52 Texts from this collection relevant to medicine are published in *Rin gter sman yig gces btus*. The entire collection is *Rin chen gter mdzod* of miscellaneous authorship, compiled and edited by Jamgon Kongtrul Lodrö Thayay, 111 volumes, Paro: Ngodrup and Sherab Drimey, 1976.
53 These are now published together as *Shel gong shel 'phreng*, *Pe cin: Mi rigs dpe skrun khang*, 1986. See also an article about this text, Dashang Luo, "History of Tibetan Medicine and *Crystal Pearl Materia Medica*," *Tibet Studies* 2, no. 1, 1990.
54 Frances Garrett, "Buddhism and the Historicizing of Medicine."
55 Fernand Meyer, "Medical Paintings of Tibet," 11. Some of these early sources for medical iconography are also mentioned in Natalia Bolsokhoyeva, *Introduction to the Studies of Tibetan Medical Sources*, 31–32. For an analysis of medical iconography in Tibet, including comments on its relationship to Chinese medical iconography, see Fernand Meyer, "Medical Paintings of Tibet," 7–12. For lists of texts with titles such as which lists texts with titles such as *Ro bgra 'phrul gyi me long, Ro bgra thu gu dgu sbyor*, and *Byang khog grems kyi mdo*, see Sangs rgyas rgya mtsho, *Khog 'bugs*, 154–155.

4 THE FETAL BODY, GENDER AND THE NORMAL

1 For a discussion of the study of anatomy in ancient Greek medicine and philosophy, see Ludwig Edelstein, *Ancient Medicine; Selected Papers of Ludwig Edelstein*, Baltimore: Johns Hopkins Press, 1967.
2 From Liz Wilson, *Charming Cadavers: Horrific Figurations of the Feminine in Indian Buddhist Hagiographic Literature*, Chicago: University of Chicago Press, 1996, 51. On the early Indian ascetic's knowledge of the human body, see also Kenneth Zysk, *Asceticism and Healing*, 34–37.
3 From Liz Wilson, *Charming Cadavers*, 56.
4 Joseph J. Loizzo and Leslie J. Blackhall, "Traditional Alternatives as Complementary Sciences: The Case of Indo-Tibetan Medicine," *The Journal of Alternative and Complementary Medicine* 4, no. 3, 1998, 313. On the term *doṣa* and the problem of using the translation "humors," see Hartmut Scharfe, "The Doctrine of the Three Humors in Traditional Indian Medicine and the Alleged Antiquity of Tamil Siddha Medicine," *Journal of the American Oriental Society* 119, no. 4, 1999. On this issue and also the tradition of speaking about the "balance" of the *doṣa*, also see Dominik Wujastyk, *Roots*, xli–xliv.
5 Chinese influences on Tibetan medicine appear to occur primarily in areas other than that of physiology, although it is likely that there are connections with the Chinese methods of classifying internal organs into solid and hollow organs. Moxibustion techniques are claimed to originate with Chinese medical traditions. The maturity of the Tibetan system of pulse analysis, a means of diagnosis not present in Āyurveda until the twelfth century, also suggests links with Chinese medicine. See Tom Dummer, *Tibetan Medicine and Other Holistic Health Care Systems*, New Delhi: Paljor Publications, 1998, Robert Svoboda and Arnie Lade, *Chinese Medicine and Āyurveda*, Delhi: Motilal Banarsidass, 1999.
6 Although I have not extensively researched this issue, I have not seen this type of presentation in Āyurvedic texts. A clear explanation of this presentation can be found in Namkhai Norbu, *On Birth and Life: A Treatise on Tibetan Medicine*, trans. Enrico Dell'Angelo, Tipographia Commerciale Venezia, 1983. This presentation is also found in the fifth chapter of the *Four Tantras' Explanatory Tantra*: Also see Thub bstan phun tshogs, *Gso bya lus kyi rnam bshad*, Pe cin: Mi rigs dpe skrun khang, 1999, 63.

7 The digestive physiology described here appears to be closely derived from Āyurvedic models of digestive physiology; see for instance, the graphic depiction of the process in Robert Svoboda and Arnie Lade, *Chinese Medicine and Āyurveda*, 56. Identification of subtle divergences between the two traditions would require further research beyond the scope of this project. On the variety of theories on humoral and digestive physiology among the three great Āyurvedic writers, see Surendranath Dasgupta, *History of Indian Philosophy*, 325–339. The metabolic process of Tibetan medicine is described in detail at Thub bstan phun tshogs, *Gso bya lus kyi rnam bshad*, 68–69.With more research an interesting comparison might be made here with a Middle Persian view in which semen is seen as "the very essence of all bodily matter, drawn from all parts of the body"; see Bruce Lincoln, "Physiological Speculation and Social Patterning in a Pahlavi Text," *Journal of the American Oriental Society* 108, no. 1, 1988, 139. Bruce's article makes the further correspondence between sexual reproduction and the sacred and creative action of the sacrifice linking articulations of physiology to social relations. Also see Bruce Lincoln, "Embryological Speculation and Gender Politics in a Pahlavi Text," *History of Religions* 27, no. 4, 1988. On the issue of it taking six days to complete the digestive process resulting in the reproductive fluids, it is noteworthy that this span of time is cited also by the Cikitsāsthāna and so this may be part of the view of metabolism inherited from Indian texts; see Rahul Peter Das, *The Origin of the Life of a Human Being: Conception and the Female According to Ancient Indian Medical and Sexological Literature*, ed. Dominik Wujastyk and Kenneth Zysk, vol. 6, *Indian Medical Tradition*, Delhi: Motilal Banarsidass, 2003, 57. For a detailed examination of Indian medical views on the metabolic process, see Rahul Peter Das, *Origin*, 108–221.

8 *Bdud rtsi snying po yan lag brgyad pa gsang ba man ngag gi rgyud*, Delhi: Bod kyi lcags po ri'i dran rten slob gner khang, 1993, 16–17. This edition will, henceforth, be referred to as *Rgyud bzhi* (1993); page numbers indicate Tibetan numbers, not the Arabic numerals also used in that edition. For an English translation, see *Quintessence Tantras*, 47–48.

9 Thub bstan phun tshogs, *Gso bya lus kyi rnam bshad*, 66.

10 Ibid., 107.

11 Sachen Kunga Nyingpo, "Explication of the Treatise for Nyak," in *Taking the Result as the Path: Core Teachings of the Sakya Lamdre Tradition*, ed. Cyrus Stearns, Boston: Wisdom Publications and Institute of Tibetan Classics, 2006, 52 and 634 ff 47.

12 Zur mkhar pa blo gros rgyal po, *Rgyud bzhi'i 'grel pa mes po'i zhal lung*, 2 vols., Krung go'i pod kyi shes rig dpe skrun khang, 1989, 132–134. Also see Tshul khrim rgyal mtshan, "Sman thang las 'brel pa rtsa yi gnas lugs kyi dpe ris skor gsal bar bshad pa," in *Krung go'i mtho rim bod sman shib 'jug bgro gleng 'dzin grwa'i rtsom yig gces bsdus*, Bod rang skyong ljongs sman rtsis khang nas bsgrigs, late 1990s, 88.

13 Tshul khrim rgyal mtshan, "Rtsa yi gnas lugs," 89. For more on this debate, see Frances Garrett and Vincanne Adams, "The Three Channels in Tibetan Medicine, with a translation of Tsultrim Gyaltsen's "A clear explanation of the principal structure and location of the circulatory channels as illustrated in the medical paintings"," in *Traditional South Asian Medicine*, forthcoming; Janet Gyatso, "Authority of Empiricism."

14 This discussion about the winds is at Grags pa rgyal mtshan, "Rgyud kyi mngon par rtogs pa rin po che'i ljon shing," in *The Complete Works of Grags pa rgyal mtshan*, ed. bsod nams rgya mtsho, *Sa skya bka' 'bum (The Complete Works of the Great Masters of the Sa skya Sect of the Tibetan Buddhism), vol. 3*, Tokyo: The Toyo Bunko, 1968, 63a-65b. For a discussion of the winds in religious traditions, see also Thub bstan phun tshogs, *Gso bya lus kyi rnam bshad*, 113–118.

15 Grags pa rgyal mtshan, "Rgyud kyi mngon par rtogs pa rin po che'i ljon shing," 65a.
16 Thub bstan phun tshogs, *Gso bya lus kyi rnam bshad*, 123–126.
17 For an overview of the circulatory system in classical Āyurveda, followed by a discussion of the same in Tantric texts, see Surendranath Dasgupta, *History of Indian Philosophy*, vol. 2: 344–357. Also see Kenneth Zysk, "The Science of Respiration and the Doctrine of the Bodily Winds in Ancient India," *Journal of the American Oriental Society* 113, no. 2, 1993. A comparison of Āyurvedic and Tibetan medical theories of the circulatory system is beyond the scope of this book, and the following section focuses only on Tibetan literature.
18 Thub bstan phun tshogs, *Gso bya lus kyi rnam bshad*, 80.
19 *Explanatory Tantra* discussion of the circulatory channels begins on *Rgyud bzhi (1993)*, 22.
20 Tubten Püntsok summarizes the *Four Tantras* presentation at Thub bstan phun tshogs, *Gso bya lus kyi rnam bshad*, 83–85.
21 Tshul khrim rgyal mtshan, "Rtsa yi gnas lugs," 84. This article has been translated in Garrett and Adams, "Three Channels in Tibetan Medicine."
22 Cited by Thubten Püntsok on the basis of Lodrö Gyelpo's *Transmission of the Elders*, 165. Thub bstan phun tshogs, *Gso bya lus kyi rnam bshad*, 108–109.
23 *Rgyud bzhi (1993)*, 23.
24 Thub bstan phun tshogs, *Gso bya lus kyi rnam bshad*, 101.
25 Ibid., 102.
26 Ibid., 103.
27 Tsultrim Gyeltsen attributes the former position to the medical scholar Tashi Bum, a student of Situ Panchen, who wrote a commentary on the *Four Tantras* (I have not been able to locate this text). Tshul khrim rgyal mtshan, "Rtsa yi gnas lugs," 85. Lodrö Gyelpo (132) does not identify these scholars by name.
28 Grags pa rgyal mtshan, "Rgyud kyi mngon par rtogs pa rin po che'i ljon shing," 60.
29 Klong chen pa, *Mkha' 'gro snying thig*, 11 vols., vol. 2, *Snying thig ya bzhi*, New Delhi: Trulku Tsewang, Jamyang and L. Tashi, 1971, 433. Cited in David Germano, "Poetic thought." Germano's translation with some minor terminological modifica tions.
30 Janet Gyatso, "One plus one makes three: Buddhist gender, monasticism, and the law of the non-excluded middle," *History of Religions* 43, no. 2, 2003.
31 *Rgyud bzhi (1993)*, 17; for English translation in context, see *Quintessence Tantras*, 48.
32 *Rgyud bzhi (1993)*, 17; *Quintessence Tantras*, 48–49.
33 Bruce Lincoln, "Embryological Speculation," 356.
34 K. Kaladhar, "Niruktopaniṣad and Garbhopaniṣad: The Vedic Sources of Studies on Human Embryology." For a discussion of various classical Greek views on sex determination, see Helen King, *Hippocrates' Woman: Reading the Female Body in Ancient Greece*, London: Routledge, 1998, 8–9.
35 Lakshmi Kapani, "Upanisad of the Embryo," 178. Cited in Bernard Faure, *The Power of Denial: Buddhism, Purity, and Gender*, ed. Stephen Teiser, *Buddhisms: A Princeton University Press Series*, Princeton: Princeton University Press, 2003, 85.
36 See reference to this model in *The Jewel Ornament of Liberation by Sgam.po.pa*, trans. Herbert V. Guenther, *The Clear Light Series*, Berkeley: Shambala Publications, 1971, 73, ff 42 and 43.
37 Zur mkhar pa blo gros rgyal po, *Mes po'i zhal lung*, 117. The passage referred to is at "Mngal du 'jug pa (Degé edition)," 237b-238a (476–477). See a similar account in Louis De La Vallée Poussin, *Abhidharmakośabhāṣyam*, 395.
38 For example see Grags pa rgyal mtshan, "Rgyud kyi mngon par rtogs pa rin po che'i

ljon shing," 59a; *Jewel Ornament*, 64. Longchenpa's *Tshig don mdzod* embryology does not mention sex identification at all

39 C.K. Ramachandran, "'Foetal Medicine' in Ancient India," *Aryavaidyan* 10, no. 3, 1997.

40 Skyem pa tshe dbang, *Rgyud bzhi'i rnam bshad*, Zi ling: Mtsho sngon rigs dpe skrun khang, 2000, 113; Zur mkhar pa blo gros rgyal po, *Mes po'i zhal lung*, 126. By contrast, Anne Kinney cites the Chinese *Taichan shu* to say that external rites can influ ence the sex of the fetus as late as the third *month* of gestation. Anne Kinney, *Childhood and Youth in Early China*, 365.

41 Yeshi Dhonden, "Embryology in Tibetan Medicine," *Tibetan Medicine* 1, 1980, 45–46.

42 *Rgyud bzhi (1993)*, 18; *Quintessence Tantras*, 50.

43 *Rgyud bzhi (1993)*, 20; *Quintessence Tantras*, 52.

44 Bruce Lincoln, "Embryological Speculation," 362.

45 *Rgyud bzhi (1993)*, 17; *Quintessence Tantras*, 49.

46 Carl Suneson, "Remarks on Some Interrelated Terms in the Ancient Indian Embryology," *WZKS* 35, 1991, 116; *The Kālacakratantra: The Chapter on the Individual together with the Vimalaprabhā*, ed. Robert A.F. Thurman, trans. Vesna A. Wallace, *Treasury of the Buddhist Sciences Series*, New York: American Institute of Buddhist Studies, Columbia University, 2004, 12; David Germano, "Poetic thought," 478, citing Klong chen pa, *Zab mo yang thig*, 11 vols., vol. 11, *Snying thig ya bzhi*, New Delhi: Trulku Tsewang, Jamyang and L. Tashi, 1971, 110.

47 Bernard Faure, *The Power of Denial: Buddhism, Purity, and Gender*, 83.

48 Skyem pa tshe dbang, *Rgyud bzhi'i rnam bshad*, 128.

49 Helen King, *Hippocrates' Woman*, 10. For a detailed study of attitudes toward the "third sex" in Buddhist and medical texts, see Janet Gyatso, "One plus one."

50 Janet Gyatso, "One plus one," 93.

51 Robert Kritzer, "Childbirth and the Mother's Body in the *Abhidharmakośabhāṣya* and Related Texts," forthcoming. Kritzer's translation.

52 "Mngal na gnas pa (Tog Palace)," 408a-408b (815–816); "Mngal na gnas pa (Degé edition)," 219b-220a (440–441). A part of this passage is also cited in Robert Kritzer, "Childbirth and the Mother's Body in the *Abhidharmakośabhāṣya* and Related Texts."

53 Thub bstan phun tshogs, *Gso bya lus kyi rnam bshad*, 69.

54 Skyem pa tshe dbang, *Rgyud bzhi'i 'grel pa*, 126. This topic is also addressed in the *Secret Oral Tantra*'s seventy-fourth chapter on women's diseases (*mo nad*).

55 Thub bstan phun tshogs, *Gso bya lus kyi rnam bshad*, 69.

56 Skyem pa tshe dbang, *Rgyud bzhi'i 'grel pa*, 126.

57 Ibid., 127.

58 See these views summarized in Thub bstan phun tshogs, *Gso bya lus kyi rnam bshad*, 108–109. Also see discussions of these debates in Frances Garrett and Vincanne Adams, "Three Channels in Tibetan Medicine"; Janet Gyatso, "Authority of Empiricism."

59 *Rgyud bzhi (1993)*, 17; *Quintessence Tantras*, 48.

60 Skyem pa tshe dbang, *Rgyud bzhi'i 'grel pa*, 126–127.

61 Zur mkhar pa blo gros rgyal po, *Mes po'i zhal lung*, 109–110.

62 Ibid., 110.

63 Rahul Peter Das, *Origin*, 17–18 and elsewhere.

64 Skyem pa tshe dbang, *Rgyud bzhi'i 'grel pa*, 127.

65 *Rgyud bzhi (1993)*, 17; *Quintessence Tantras*, 49.

66 Zur mkhar pa blo gros rgyal po, *Mes po'i zhal lung*, 121.

67 *Rgyud bzhi (1993)*, 20; *Quintessence Tantras*, 52.

68 Martha Ann Selby, "Narratives of Conception."
69 Pha khol, "Yan lag brgyad pa'i snying po bsdus pa," 258.
70 Ibid., 260.

5 GESTATION AND THE RELIGIOUS PATH

1 David Gordon White, *Alchemical Body*, 196. See also R. A. Stein, "Grottes-Matrices et Lieux Saints de la Deesse en Asie Orientale," *Bulletin de l'Ecole Francaise d'Extreme-Orient*, 1988, 37–43.
2 Francois Bizot, "La grotte de la naissance: Recherches sur le Bouddhisme Khmer II," *Bulletin de l'Ecole Francaise d'Extreme-Orient* LXVII, 1980.
3 Helen Hardacre, "The Cave and the Womb World," *Japanese Journal of Religious Studies* 10, no. 2–3, 1983. Also see Paul L. Swanson, "Shugendo and the Yoshino-Kumano Pilgrimage: An Example of Mountain Pilgrimage," *Monumenta Nipponica* 36, no. 1, 1981.
4 Manfred Jahn, "Narratology: A Guide to the Theory of Narrative," in *Poems, Plays, and Prose: A Guide to the Theory of Literary Genres*, ed. Manfred Jahn, English Department, University of Cologne: http://www.uni-koeln.de/~ame02/pppn.htm, 2002, Section N4.3.
5 Paul Ricoeur, "Narrative Time," in *On Narrative*, ed. W. J. T. Mitchell, Chicago and London: University of Chicago Press, 1980, 167.
6 D. Ezzy, "Theorizing Narrative Identity: Symbolic Interactionism and Hermeneutics," *Sociological Quarterly* 39, no. 2, 1998.
7 Robert E. Buswell Jr. and Robert M. Gimello note that asserting a direct equivalence between the concepts is problematic. See the discussion of the use of the term "soteriology" in the study of the Buddhist concept of "the path" in the introduction to Robert E. Jr. Buswell and Robert M. Gimello, eds., *Paths to Liberation: The Marga and its Transformations in Buddhist Thought, Kuroda Institute Studies in East Asian Buddhism*, Honolulu: University of Hawaii Press, 1992.
8 Ibid., 7. Not all religious path texts are about practices: in some cases, path structure formulations serve rather to classify diverse doctrinal positions. Such texts on the path commonly present a hierarchical, and often polemical, systematization of Buddhist doctrines.
9 *Rgyud bzhi (1993)*, 16; *Quintessence Tantras*.
10 *Rgyud bzhi (1993)*, 17; *Quintessence Tantras*, 48.
11 Cited in Skyem pa tshe dbang, *Rgyud bzhi'i 'grel pa*, 122; Zur mkhar pa blo gros rgyal po, *Mes po'i zhal lung*, 118.
12 "Mngal du 'jug pa (Degé edition)," 238b (478).
13 Skyem pa tshe dbang, *Rgyud bzhi'i 'grel pa*, 122.
14 Doniger and Spinner's article has a cross-cultural overview of this topic: Wendy Doniger and Gregory Spinner, "Misconceptions: Parental Imprinting," in *Science in Culture*, ed. Peter Galison; Stephen Graubard; Everett Mendelsohn, New Jersey: Transaction Publishers, 2001. On similar Chinese views also see Anne Kinney, *Childhood and Youth in Early China*.
15 John W. Pettit, *Mipham's Beacon of Certainty: Illuminating the View of Dzogchen, the Great Perfection*, Boston: Wisdom Publications, 1999, 159–160.
16 Cited in Thomas Yarnall, "The Emptiness that is Form: Developing the Body of Buddhahood in Indo-Tibetan Buddhist Tantra," Ph.D., Columbia University, 2003, 578. Yarnall creates a critical edition, which is presented in his dissertation, based on a study of three editions of the *Sngag rim chen mo*.
17 Cited in Ibid., 584–585.
18 Alex Wayman, "The Five-Fold Ritual Symbolism of Passion," in *Studies of Esoteric*

Buddhism and Tantrism, Koyosan, Japan: Koyosan University, 1995, 137. A sixteenth-century esoteric Sakya work by Jamyang Khyentsé Wangchuk, explains that the transmigrating consciousness "enters the mouth or anus of the father, and together with his white constituent…, it exits through his vajra into the mother's lotus." Jamyang Khyentse Wangchuk (1524–1568), "Profound Summarizing Notes on the Path Presented as the Three Continua," in *Taking the Result as the Path: Core Teachings of the Sakya Lamdre Tradition*, ed. Cyrus Stearns, *The Library of Tibetan Classics*, Boston: Wisdom Publications and Institute of Tibetan Classics, 2006, 420.

19 Cited in Thomas Yarnall, "Emptiness," 584–585.

20 These terms describing the shape of the newly conceived embryo, mentioned in the last chapter, are Tibetan translations of the Indic terms found in the Pāli Canon, the *Mahābhārata*, and other early Indian sources. For a summary of inconsistencies in usage of these terms in early Indian sources, see Carl Suneson, "Remarks on Some Interrelated Terms in the Ancient Indian Embryology."

21 The five solid organs (*don*) are the heart (*snying*), liver (*mchin pa*), kidney (*mkhal ma*), spleen (*mcher pa*), and lungs (*glo ba*). The five hollow organs (*snod*) are the stomach (pho ba), small intestine (*rgyu ma*), large intestine (*long ga*), urinary bladder (*lgang pa*), gall bladder (*mkhris thum*), and reproductive organs (*bsam se'u*).

22 The term *dwangs ma* sometimes refers to the nutritive essences, the first of the bodily constituents (*lus zungs*) to develop from the woman's food and drink intake in the stomach. The term *dwangs ma* can also refer to the *result* of the metabolic process, namely the seventh constituent, also called *khu ba*, which is the case here.

23 Zur mkhar pa blo gros rgyal po, *Mes po'i zhal lung*, 124. *Snying* is frequently better translated simply as "essence," as it is commonly used to refer to the essence of something, rather than to an internal organ; but the fact that Lodrö Gyelpo feels compelled to explain the term here suggests that its primary meaning in this case could be reasonably understood as the "heart."

24 Klong chen pa, *Tshig don mdzod*, 199. Germano's translation; David Germano, "Poetic thought." I am indebted to Germano's skillful translation and encyclopedic notes for my understanding of this esoteric text.

25 Giacomella Orofino, *Sacred Tibetan Teachings on Death and Liberation*, Great Britain: Prism Press, 1990, 54. On this text also see Bryan J. Cuevas, *Hidden History*, 62–64.

26 Grags pa rgyal mtshan, "Rgyud kyi mngon par rtogs pa rin po che'i ljon shing," 59b. Lodrö Gyelpo also describes this scheme, linking the ten incarnations of Viṣṇu with the ten months in the womb, as originating with the *Kālacakra*. Zur mkhar pa blo gros rgyal po, *Mes po'i zhal lung*, 129. This account is found in several Indian Tantric sources and is repeated in various Tibetan texts; some are mentioned in Alex Wayman, *Yoga of the Guhyasamajatantra: The Arcane Lore of Forty Verses, A Buddhist Tantra Commentary*, Delhi: Motilal Banarsidass, 1977, 215. For a narrative account of Viṣṇu's lives in these forms, see Khedrup Norsang Gyatso, *Stainless Light*, 166–167.

27 Buddhas complete ten grounds (*bhūmi*) and so are said to stay inside the womb for ten months. Grags pa rgyal mtshan, "Rgyud kyi mngon par rtogs pa rin po che'i ljon shing," 59b–60a.

28 Alex Wayman, *Yoga of the Guhyasamajatantra: The Arcane Lore of Forty Verses, A Buddhist Tantra Commentary*, 97. Also see the chart of "intrauterine correspondences," linking mental states, incarnations of Viṣṇu, winds, and origins of winds based on several Tantric sources in Wayman's *Yoga of the Guhyasamajatantra: The Arcane Lore of Forty Verses, A Buddhist Tantra Commentary*, 216. See also Alex Wayman, "The Five-Fold Ritual Symbolism of Passion," 140.

29 *The Kālacakratantra: The Chapter on the Individual together with the Vimalaprabhā*; Vesna Wallace, *Inner Kālacakratantra*, 38.
30 Khedrup Norsang Gyatso, *Stainless Light*, 168–172.
31 The scholar Ngawang Jinpa speculates that this is probably, although it is not specified in the text, the *samaya* substances (*amritas*) of highest yoga tantra: urine, excrement, blood, semen and brains. Personal communication, Darjeeling, 2000.
32 Grags pa rgyal mtshan, "Rgyud kyi mngon par rtogs pa rin po che'i ljon shing," 62b.
33 Jamyang Khyentse Wangchuk, "Profound Summarizing Notes on the Path Presented as the Three Continua," 420.
34 Ibid., 397.
35 James H. Sanford, "Wind, Waters, Stupas, Mandalas: Fetal Buddhahood in Shingon," *Japanese Journal of Religious Studies* 24, no. 1–2, 1997, 15 and 19–20.
36 Ibid., 26–28.
37 Ibid., 21–22.
38 Ibid., 6.
39 Ibid., 24. For more on Japanese Shingon embryological metaphors, also see Hardacre, "The Cave and the Womb World."
40 *The Lalita Vistara: Memoirs of the Early Life of Sakya Sinha*, trans. R. L. Mitra, Delhi: Sri Satguru Publications, 1998, 96. As cited in Vanessa Sasson, "A Womb with a View: the Buddha's Final Fetal Experience," in *The Fetus: the Religious Life of Very Small Things*, ed. Vanessa Sasson and Jane Marie Law, forthcoming.
41 For a discussion of this story and sources, see Jonathan A. Silk, "The Fruits of Paradox: On the Religious Architecture of the Buddha's Life Story," *Journal of the American Academy of Religion* 71, no. 4, 2003, 868. Also see Minoru Hara, "A Note on the Buddha's Birth Story"; Sasson, "Womb with a View."
42 Zur mkhar pa blo gros rgyal po, *Mes po'i zhal lung*, 116–117.
43 This is recounted in Ibid., 117–118.
44 This early Indian Buddhist tradition is described in Ibid., 119–120. Also see Janet Gyatso, "One plus one," 101. There is a detailed analysis of this foursome in Robert Kritzer, "Four Ways."
45 Giacomella Orofino, *Sacred Tibetan Teachings*, 53.
46 Padmasambhava, *The Tibetan Book of the Dead*, trans. Robert A. F. Thurman, *Mystical Classics of the World*, New York: Bantam Books, 1994, 184.
47 Ibid., 185.
48 Ibid., 187.
49 The awareness of a carriage (*bzhon pa'i 'du shes*), a storied house (*khang bu brtsegs pa'i 'du shes*), a throne (*khri stan kyi 'du shes*), a spring (*chu mig gi 'du shes*), a pool (*rdzing gi 'du shes*), a lake (*chu bo'i 'du shes*), enjoyment (*kun dga' ra ba'i 'du shes*), and a pleasure garden (*skyed mos tshal gyi 'du shes*). "Mngal na gnas pa (Tog Palace)," 407a–407b (813–814); "Mngal du 'jug pa (Degé edition)," 243b (488); "Mngal na gnas pa (Degé edition)," 219a (439).
50 "Mngal du 'jug pa (Degé edition)," 244a. The *Abiding in the Womb* only lists three distorted conception here; "Mngal na gnas pa (Tog Palace)," 408a (815); "Mngal na gnas pa (Degé edition)," 219b (440).
51 Cited in Khedrup Norsang Gyatso, *Stainless Light*, 170.
52 Ibid., 171.
53 Skyem pa tshe dbang, *Rgyud bzhi'i 'grel pa*, 125; Thub bstan phun tshogs, *Zab mo nang gi don 'grel ba'i lus sems gsal ba'i me long*, Lha sa: Bod ljongs mi dmangs dpe skrun khang, 2003, 47.
54 Cited in Herbert V. Guenther, *Philosophy and Psychology in the Abhidharma*, Berkeley: Shambhala, 1974, 173–174.
55 "Mngal du 'jug pa (Degé edition)," 239b (480). A more expansive form of this

passage is found at "Mngal na gnas pa (Degé edition)," 213b (428). A Chinese version of the passage is cited at Robert Kritzer, "Life in the Womb: Conception and Gestation in Buddhist Scripture and the Classical Indian Medical Literature," unpublished manuscript.

56 From *Jewel Ornament*, 68–69.

57 Herbert V. Guenther notes that a similar account is found in the Great Perfection text, the *Rdzogs chen kun bzang bla ma*. Ibid., 73 ff. 45.

58 Ibid., 65–66.

59 Ibid., 66. On a similar attitude toward the womb in the Hindu epic, the *Mahābhārata*, see Harold G. Coward, "Purity in Hinduism: With Particular Reference to Pataìjali's *Yoga Sátras*," in *Hindu Ethics: Purity, Abortion, and Euthanasia*, ed. Harold G. Coward, Julius J. Lipner, and Katherine K. Young, *McGill Studies in the History of Religions*, Albany: State University of New York Press, 1989, 17.

60 Cited in Mathieu Boisvert, "Conception and Intrauterine Life," 309.

61 This text is translated in Ngorchen Konchog Lhundrup, *The Beautiful Ornament of the Three Visions: An exposition of the preliminary practices of the path which explains the instructions of the "Path Including its Result" in accordance with the Root Treatise of the Vajra Verses of Virupa*, trans. Lobsang Dagpa and Jay Goldberg, Ithaca: Snow Lion Publications, 1991, 40.

62 *The Kālacakratantra: The Chapter on the Individual together with the Vimalaprabhā*, 14.

63 Ibid., 15.

64 Gian Giuseppe Filippi, "The Secret of the Embryo According to the *Garbha Upaniṣad*," 301.

65 Bryan J. Cuevas, *Hidden History*, 67.

66 For a discussion of this transmission see Ibid., 49–57.

67 Tsong-ka-pa, *The Six Yogas of Naropa: Tsongkhapa's commentary entitled A Book of Three Inspirations: A Treatise on the Stages of Training in the Profound Path of Naro's Six Dharmas, commonly referred to as The Three Inspirations*, trans. Glen H. Mullin, Ithaca: Snow Lion Publications, 2005, 182–90; also see Mullin's Introduction, 35–39.

68 Padmasambhava, *Tibetan Book of the Dead*, 190.

69 Ibid., 193–94.

70 This is debated. For a survey by Jeffrey Hopkins of Tibetan views on the purpose of the four tantra classes see Tsong-ka-pa, *Tantra in Tibet: The Great Exposition of Secret Mantra – Volume 1*, trans. Jeffrey Hopkins, *The Wisdom of Tibet Series*, London: George Allen & Unwin, 1977, 201–209. Also see Tsong-ka-pa, *The Yoga of Tibet: The Great Exposition of Secret Mantra – 2 and 3*, trans. Jeffrey Hopkins, *The Wisdom of Tibet Series*, London: George Allen & Unwin, 1981. For a presentation of highest yoga tantra according to the Geluk system as articulated by the nineteenth-century Mongolian scholar Ngawang Belden, see Daniel Cozort, *Highest Yoga Tantra: An Introduction to the Esoteric Buddhism of Tibet*, Ithaca: Snow Lion Publications, 1986.

71 Blo bzang rgyal mtshan seng ge, *Dpal rdo rje 'jigs byed dpa' bo gcig pa'i rdzogs rim gyi rnam bzhag 'jam dpal dgyes pa'i mchod sprin*, Delhi: 1972, 3a. Translated in Jeffrey Hopkins and Lati Rinpoche, *Death, Intermediate State and Rebirth*, 31–32.

72 Jeffrey Hopkins and Lati Rinpoche, *Death, Intermediate State and Rebirth*, 32.

73 For charts detailing the stages of dissolution with the external and internal signs, and for a description of each stage, see Ibid., 17–18 and 32–46.

74 Ibid., 45. Also see Nga wang mkhas grub (1779–1838), *Skye shi bar do'i rnam bzhag*, The Collected Works, vol. 1, Leh: S.W. Tashigangpa, 1972, 464.6; Geshe

Kelsang Gyatso, *Essence of Vajrayana: The Highest Yoga Tantra Practice of Heruka Body Mandala*, Delhi: Motilal Banarsidass, 2000, 78–79.

75 Jeffrey Hopkins and Lati Rinpoche, *Death, Intermediate State and Rebirth*, 19 and 45–46. See 45–46 for exceptions to this general rule where certain people may remain in the state of clear light for less than or more than three days.

76 Ibid., 60.

77 Thomas Yarnall, "Emptiness," 326.

78 Cited in Ibid., 583.

79 Geshe Kelsang Gyatso, *Essence of Vajrayana*, 86.

80 Ibid., 88.

81 Gyatrul Rinpoche, *The Generation Stage in Buddhist Tantra*, trans. Sangye Khandro, Ithaca: Snow Lion Publications, 1996, 59.

82 Jeffrey Hopkins and Lati Rinpoche, *Death, Intermediate State and Rebirth*, 69–70. A discussion of the practices of taking the three bodies into the path is also at Geshe Kelsang Gyatso, *Essence of Vajrayana*, 77–88. Also see Yangchen Gawai Lodoe, *Paths and Grounds of Guhyasamaja According to Arya Nagarjuna (With Commentary by Geshe Losang Tsephel)*, ed. David Ross Komito and Andrew Fagan, trans. Tenzin Dorjee, Library of Tibetan Works and Archives, 1995; Thomas Yarnall, "Emptiness"; also see Tsong-ka-pa, *Six Yogas*, 35–39.

83 Yael Bentor, "Identifying the Unnamed Opponents of Tsong kha pa and Mkhas grub rje Concerning the Transformation of Ordinary Birth, Death and Intermediate State into the Three Bodies," forthcoming, ff19.

84 Ibid., ff. 22. For an English language description of how to purify the four modes of rebirth, see Gyatrul Rinpoche, *Generation Stage*, 57–63.

85 From Thomas Yarnall, "Emptiness," 586.

86 Cited by Longchenpa in Klong chen pa, "Theg mchog mdzod," in *Mdzod chen bdun*, Gangtok, Sikkim: Sherab Gyaltsen and Khyentse Labrang, 1983, 112.2. See David Germano, "Poetic thought," 476.

87 Gyatrul Rinpoche, *Generation Stage*, 50.

88 Vesna Wallace, *Inner Kālacakratantra*, 160–161.

89 Ibid., 166–167.

90 Alex Wayman cites also the *Āryasaṃdhinirmocana-sūtrasya vyākhyāna*; Alex Wayman, "The Five-Fold Ritual Symbolism of Passion," 136.

91 Khedrup Norsang Gyatso, *Stainless Light*, 165.

92 Gyatrul Rinpoche, *Generation Stage*, 69–70.

93 Ibid., 51.

94 Geshe Lharampa Ngawang Dhargyey, *A Commentary on the Kalacakra Commentary*, Dharamsala: Library of Tibetan Works and Archives, 1985, 102.

95 Grags pa rgyal mtshan, "Rgyud kyi mngon par rtogs pa rin po che'i ljon shing," 60.

96 Klong chen pa, *Mdzod chen bdun*, 6 vols., Gangtok, Sikkim: Sherab Gyaltsen and Khyentse Labrang, 1983, 279 (vol 2). David Germano's translation, cited in "Poetic thought," 473.

97 Cited in Klong chen pa, "Theg mchog mdzod," 112.2. David Germano's translation, in "Poetic thought," 467–468.

98 Klong chen pa, *Tshig don mdzod*, 196. David Germano's translation, in "Poetic thought," 188.

99 Klong chen pa, "Theg mchog mdzod," 111.6–7. See David Germano, "Poetic thought," 456. In still another model of this type of correlation, M. Broido reports that Sönam Tsemo (1142–1182) and Tashi Namgyel (1512–1587) both link four stages (*gnas pa bzhi*) of the development of the fetus (*gong bu*, *chu*, *gzugs*, and *gzugs las 'das pa*) to the four Buddha Bodies, the *sambhogakāya*, *dharmakāya*,

nirmāṇakāya and *svabhāvikakāya*, respectively. M. Broido, "bsad thabs: Some Tibetan Methods of Explaining the Tantras," paper presented at the Csomo de Koros Symposium, Velm-Vienna, Austria, 1981, 17 ff. 13.

100 Klong chen pa, "Theg mchog mdzod," 344.2. David Germano's translation, in "Poetic thought," 456.

101 The transition of the enlightened essence from its home at the heart outwards is described using the terminology of the "four lamps," discussed in detail in the *Treasury's* sixth chapter. The "far-ranging lasso water lamp" (*rgyang zhags chu yi sgron ma*), which refers to the light channels running from the heart to the eyes and also more generally to the entire network of light channels, is described at Klong chen pa, *Tshig don mdzod*, 263–265. Translated in David Germano, "Treasury of Precious Words (1994 manuscript)," 115–119.

102 *Rgyud bcu bdun*, 3 vols., New Delhi: Sanje Dorje, 1973, 291. Cited in Klong chen pa, *Tshig don mdzod*, 261. In translation (with some minor terminological changes) at David Germano, "Treasury of Precious Words (1994 manuscript)," 113–114.

103 Klong chen pa, *Bla ma yang thig*, 11 vols., vol. 1, *Snying thig ya bzhi*, New Delhi: Trulku Tsewang, Jamyang and L. Tashi, 1971, 239. Cited in David Germano, "Notes to the translation of Longchenpa's *Treasury of Words and Meanings*," 9/13/94 manuscript, 960.

104 Grags pa rgyal mtshan, "Rgyud kyi mngon par rtogs pa rin po che'i ljon shing," 59b.

105 Zur mkhar pa blo gros rgyal po, *Mes po'i zhal lung*, 138.

106 He writes, "Vasubandhu's Commentary on the 'Treasury of Knowledge' and the Sūtra of Teaching to Nanda on Entry to the Womb [switch the order of the names] for the first of the five stages, leaving the latter three as before; whereas Asanga's Actuality of the Levels reverses the first two [as was done in this explanation]. However, it is said that, except for there being different orders in the designation of the names, there is no contradiction in the meaning." From Jeffrey Hopkins and Lati Rinpoche, *Death, Intermediate State and Rebirth*, 62.

107 For more on the various uses of the Sanskrit terms, see Carl Suneson, "Remarks on Some Interrelated Terms in the Ancient Indian Embryology."

108 Kyempa Tsewang's summary of Tantric embryological narratives is at Skyem pa tshe dbang, *Rgyud bzhi'i 'grel pa*, 139–140.

109 Paul Ricoeur, "Narrative Time," 167.

6 GROWTH, CHANGE AND CONTINUITY

1 David Seyford Ruegg, *Buddha-nature, Mind and the Problem of Gradualism in a Comparative Perspective: On the Transmission and Reception of Buddhism in India and Tibet*, New Delhi: Heritage Publishers, 1992, 19.

2 See a summary of theories of causality in W. S. Karunaratne, *The Theory of Causality in Early Buddhism*, Nugegoda, Sri Lanka: Indumati Karunaratne, 1988, 1–17. For comments on the primacy of causality theories in Buddhism generally, see David J. Kalupahana, *Causality: The Central Philosophy of Buddhism*, W.S. Karunaratne, *The Theory of Causality in Early Buddhism.*

3 David J. Kalupahana, *Causality: The Central Philosophy of Buddhism*, 110.

4 D. Ezzy, "Theorizing Narrative Identity."

5 Paul Ricoeur, "Narrative Time," 167.

6 For a summary, see Lobsang Dargyay, "Tsong-Kha-Pa's Concept of Karma," in *Karma and Rebirth: Post Classical Developments*, ed. Ronald W. Neufeldt, *SUNY Series in Religious Studies*, Albany: State University of New York Press, 1986, 169. For a brief overview of how this issue is considered according to Tibetan philosophers see Lobsang Dargyay, "Tsong-Kha-Pa's Concept of Karma," 169–171. For

an interesting discussion of medieval Theravāda views on karma's relationship to rebirth, see Bruce Matthews, "Post-Classical Developments."

7 Luis Gomez, "Purifying Gold: The Metaphor of Effort and Intuition in Buddhist Thought and Practice," in *Sudden and Gradual: Approaches to Enlightenment in Chinese Thought*, ed. Peter Gregory, Honolulu: University Press of Hawaii, 1987, 131.

8 See summaries in Surendranath Dasgupta, *History of Indian Philosophy*; James McDermott, *Development in the Early Buddhist Concept of Kamma/Karma*, New Delhi: Munishiram Manoharlal Publishers Pvt. Ltd., 1984; James P. McDermott, "Karma and Rebirth."

9 The twelve links are explained clearly in Jeffrey Hopkins, *Meditation on Emptiness*, London: Wisdom Publications, 1983, 275–283. The doctrine of interdependent origination is also represented iconographically by the "wheel of life" (*srid pa'i 'khor lo*). See, for example, Geshe Sopa, "The Tibetan Wheel of Life: Iconography and Doxography," *The Journal of the International Association of Buddhist Studies* 7, no. 1, 1984. See also David M. Williams, "The Translation and Interpretation of the Twelve Terms in the Paticcasamuppada," *Numen* 21, 1974.

10 This explanation is treated more expansively in Jeffrey Hopkins, *Meditation on Emptiness*, 275–283.

11 Klong chen pa, *Tshig don mdzod*, 192–195.

12 Vesna Wallace, *Inner Kālacakratantra*, 197.

13 Ibid., 21.

14 From the *Rdo rje sems dpa' snying gi me long gi rgyud*, as cited in Klong chen pa, *Tshig don mdzod*, 191. Translation by David Germano, in "Poetic thought," 180.

15 James H. Sanford, "Wind, Waters," 9.

16 Ibid., 15.

17 Charlotte Furth, *Flourishing Yin*, 101. Also see Charlotte Furth, "From Birth to Birth."

18 For a discussion of Vedic traditions of rebirth demonstrating this correlation, see Herman W. Tull, *The Vedic Origins of Karma: Cosmos as Man in Ancient Indian Myth and Ritual*, ed. Wendy Doniger, *SUNY Series in Hindu Studies*, Albany: State University of New York Press, 1989. C. S. F. Burnett describes the effects of planets and the activities of the natural elements on monthly embryogenesis in texts of the European Middle Ages and Antiquity; C. S. F. Burnett, "The Planets and the Development of the Embryo," in *The Human Embryo, Aristotle and the Arabic and European Traditions*, ed. G. R. Dunstan, Exeter: University of Exeter Press, 1990. For comments on the links between embryology and cosmology in Middle Persian literature, see the final pages of Bruce Lincoln, "Embryological Speculation.

19 Akira Sadakata, *Buddhist Cosmology, Philosophy and Origins*, Tokyo: Kosei Publishing Company, 1997, 20, ff. 2.

20 Zur mkhar pa blo gros rgyal po, *Mes po'i zhal lung*, 107.

21 *Jewel Ornament*, 73 ff. 43. Also see James P. McDermott, "Karma and Rebirth," 169.

22 Skyem pa tshe dbang, *Rgyud bzhi'i 'grel pa*, 125. In the sūtra this is at "Mngal du 'jug pa (Degé edition)," 238b (478).

23 Skyem pa tshe dbang, *Rgyud bzhi'i 'grel pa*, 128.

24 Zur mkhar pa blo gros rgyal po, *Mes po'i zhal lung*, 105. He specifics three types of causes: tangible or identifiable causes, conditions unfavorable for causing conception, and special causes (*rgyu ngos bzung*, *rgyu'i 'gal rkyen*, and *rgyu'i khyad par*). Zur mkhar pa blo gros rgyal po, *Mes po'i zhal lung*, 103.

25 About the identity of these claimants, Sherab Gyeltsen, a Sakya scholar in Sarnath, does not know who the first position might be attributed to; he suggests that the second is a Hindu subsect called the 'U phrug pa, the third is the is Bye brag smra ba

(Vaibhasika), the fourth is Mdo sde ba (Sautrantika), and the fifth is a Hindu subsect called Drang chen pa. (Personal communication, Sarnath, 2000); Grags pa rgyal mtshan, "Rgyud kyi mngon par rtogs pa rin po che'i ljon shing," 59b.

26 Zur mkhar pa blo gros rgyal po, *Mes po'i zhal lung*, 116.

27 Ibid., 117.

28 Tsele Natsok Rangdrol, *The Mirror of Mindfulness: The Cycle of the Four Bardos*, trans. Erik Pema Kunsang, New Delhi: Rupa, 2002, 71–72.

29 *Jewel Ornament*, 63–64; Zur mkhar pa blo gros rgyal po, *Mes po'i zhal lung*, 106–107 and 116–117.

30 Tsele Natsok Rangdrol, *The Mirror of Mindfulness: The Cycle of the Four Bardos*, 71–72. Also see a similar account in Padmasambhava, *Tibetan Book of the Dead*, 188–189.

31 Zur mkhar pa blo gros rgyal po, *Mes po'i zhal lung*, 106–107 and 116–117.

32 Ibid., 119–120.

33 Ibid., 104.

34 Vāgbhaṭa's *Heart of Medicine* does describe other rituals to ensure the birth of a male child that involve propitiation of Hindu deities, to be performed prior to conception, but these were not replicated in the *Four Tantras*, not surprisingly given their Hindu orientation. See *Vāgbhaṭa's Aṣṭāṇga Hṛdayam Sūtrasthāna*, Varanasi: Krishnadas Academy, 1996, 365–366. More research would be required to discover where in the Tibetan Buddhist corpus there might be rituals for changing fetal sex that involve propitiation of deities; I would assume that there are such rituals, although I have not seen them.

35 He cites a medicinal formulation described in the *Four Tantras* from the *'Bum nag*, a *Four Tantras* commentary by the student of Yuthok Yönten Gönpo, Yeshé Zung. He also provides extensive commentary on the use of the sea buckthorn and grape from an unidentified commentary on the *Bdud rtsi bam po brgyad pa* by Vimalamitra. Skyem pa tshe dbang, *Rgyud bzhi'i 'grel pa*, 133–134. The Tibetan doctor, Jampa, living in Darjeeling in 2000, suggested that Kyempa Tsewang is explaining how one may use substitutes such as these for the originally intended ritual substances, namely, a woman's first menstrual blood and a man's first seminal emission (personal communication, 2000). Tantric ritual texts may provide more information.

36 See, for example, Sanggyé Gyatso's reference to his *White Beryl* astrological work for techniques for predicting fetal sex, Sangs rgyas rgya mtsho, *Gso ba rig pa'i bstan bcos sman bla'i dgongs rgyan rgyud bzhi'i gsal byed bai durya sngon po'i malli ka zhes bya ba bzhugs so*, 2 vols., Dharamsala: Tibetan Medical and Astro Institute, 1994, 66.

37 Lodrö Gyelpo also explains here why the *Entering the Womb* mentions four elements, and the *Four Tantras* and other Tibetan sources describe five. Zur mkhar pa blo gros rgyal po, *Mes po'i zhal lung*, 107–108.

38 Ibid., 122.

39 Citing the the *Mahāmūdra Quintessence Tantra* (*Phyag rgya chen po thig le'i rgyud*), Ibid., 120–121.

40 Neither I nor the Tibetan scholars I consulted could identify this text, referred to simply as the "Second Inquiry of the Root Tantra" (*Rtsa ba'i rgyud brtag pa gnyis pa*), beyond confirming that it is not the *Four Tantras*. Cited in Ibid., 121. Lodrö Gyelpo also cites here a similar presentation from Rangjung Dorjé.

41 Khedrup Norsang Gyatso, *Stainless Light*, 165–166.

42 Zur mkhar pa blo gros rgyal po, *Mes po'i zhal lung*, 120.

43 Klong chen pa, *Tshig don mdzod*, 200–208.

44 David Germano, "Poetic thought," 871–872.

45 Kenneth Zysk, "Science of Respiration," 201.

46 Giacomella Orofino, *Sacred Tibetan Teachings*, 54; *Rgyud bcu bdun*, vol. 3, 232. Also cited in Klong chen pa, *Tshig don mdzod*, 199. For translation and commentary on this passage, see David Germano, "Poetic thought," 192 and 474–476.
47 Grags pa rgyal mtshan, "Rgyud kyi mngon par rtogs pa rin po che'i ljon shing," 59.
48 David Seyford Ruegg, *Buddha-nature, Mind and the Problem of Gradualism*, 3.
49 David Germano, "Pure Lands and Creative Buddhas in Renaissance Tibet," in *Mysticism and Rhetoric in the Great Perfection (rDzogs chen)*, 3/22/02 manuscript, 1.
50 See, for example, Wendy Doniger O'Flaherty, ed., *Karma and Rebirth in Classical Indian Traditions*, Delhi: Motilal Barnarsidass, 1983; Ronald W. Neufeldt, ed., *Karma and Rebirth: Post Classical Developments*, *SUNY Series in Religious Studies*, Albany: State University of New York Press, 1986.
51 See, for example, Faure's claim to this effect at Bernard Faure, *The Power of Denial: Buddhism, Purity, and Gender*, 88, 334 and elsewhere.
52 D. Ezzy, "Theorizing Narrative Identity."

EPILOGUE: HISTORIOGRAPHY RECAPITULATES EMBRYOLOGY

1 Manfred Jahn, "Narratology," Section N4.3.
2 Hayden White, "The Value of Narrativity," 14. Also see Georg G. Iggers, *Historiography in the Twentieth Century, From Scientific Objectivity to the Postmodern Challenge*, Hanover: Wesleyan University Press, 1997; Frank Ankersmit and Hans Kellner, ed., *A New Philosophy of History*, Chicago: University of Chicago Press, 1995; Dominick LaCapra, *Rethinking Intellectual History: Texts, Contexts, Language*, Ithaca: Cornell University Press, 1983.
3 Zeff Bjerken, "The Mirrorwork of Tibetan Religious Historians: A Comparison of Buddhist and Bon Historiography," Ph.D. Dissertation, University of Michigan, 2001, 5. Inspired by Hayden White's analysis of historical writing, Bjerken's book identifies three distinct genres of historiography in Tibetan literature: annals, chronicles, and narratives. Describing annals and chronicles primarily for comparative purposes, Bjerken's discussion focuses mainly on historical narratives (*chos 'byung*).
4 Ibid., 85.
5 D. Ezzy, "Theorizing Narrative Identity."
6 According to Tucci, none of these medical students of Rinchen Zangpo are even mentioned in the *Blue Annals'* lists of his students; nor are they mentioned in the *Chos 'byung* of Pema Karpo. Giuseppe Tucci, *Rin-chen-bzang-po and the Renaissance of Buddhism in Tibet around the Millenium*, ed. Lokesh Chandra, trans. Nancy Kipp Smith, *õata-Piïaka Series, Indo-Asian Literatures, Volume 348*, New Delhi: Aditya Prakashan, 1988. See also *Pod kyi gso ba rig pa'i byung 'phel gyi lo rgyus gsal bar ston pa baidurya sngon po'i shun thigs*, 317–319.
7 Sangs rgyas rgya mtsho, *Khog 'bugs*, 226–229. While Losang Chödrag's biography of Yuthok provides a more dramatic rendition of his religious and medical experiences in India, Sanggyé Gyatso's description of the later Yuthok's stay there is limited to an accounting of the various texts he studied in each region he visited.
8 *The Blue Annals*, trans. George N. Roerich, Delhi: Motilal Banarsidass, 1976, 74.
9 *Quintessence Tantras*, 53–54.
10 Fernand Meyer, "Medical Paintings of Tibet," 8.
11 Zeff Bjerken, "Mirrorwork," 65.
12 Matthew T. Kapstein, *The Tibetan Assimilation of Buddhism: Conversion, Contestation, and Memory*, New York: Oxford University Press, 2000, 34.
13 Ibid., 44.
14 Ibid., 54.

APPENDIX

Transliteration of Tibetan proper nouns

This book follows the Tibetan and Himalayan Digital Library's Simplified Phonetic Transcription of Standard Tibetan scheme for phonetic representation of Tibetan proper nouns, and Extended Wylie for the transliteration of Tibetan words.

Phonetics	**Wylie transliteration**
Abo Chöjé	a bo chos rje
Akhu Rinpoche	a khu rin po che (shes rab rgya mtsho)
Barawa	'ba' ra ba
Biji	bi ji
Biji Gajé	bi byi dga' byed
Bilha Gadzé	bi lha dga' mdzes
Bodong Choklé Namgyel	bo dong phyogs las rnam rgyal
Butön Rinchen Drub	bu ston rin chen grub
Chakpori	lcags po ri
Cheje Tipa	cher rje ti pa
Cheje Zhangtön Zhikpo	che rje zhang ston zhig po
Chöbar	chos 'bar
ChÖrub	chos grub
Darma Gönpo	dar ma mgon po
Dawa Ngönga	zla ba mngon dga'
Denkar	ldan dkar
Dharamradza	dha rma ra dza
Deumar Tendzin Puntsok	de'u dmar bstan 'dzin phun tshogs
Drangti	brang ti
Drangti Jampel Zangpo	brang ti 'jam dpal bzang po
Drangti Penden Tsojé	brang ti dpal ldan 'tsho byed
Drakpa Gyeltsen	grags pa rgyal mtshan
Drapa Ngönshé	grwa pa mngon shes
Drogmi	'brog mi (lo tsa ba)

Dungi Torchak	dung gi thor cag
Gampopa	sgam po pa (bsod nams rin chen)
Galenö	ga le nos
Garpo	mgar po
Gendün Gyatso	dge 'dun rgya mtsho
Gyatön Drapa Sherab	rgya ston grags pa shes rab
Hantipata	han ti pa ta
Hashabala	ha sha ba la
Hasheng Mahakhyinda	ha sheng ma hra khyin da
Jangdak Namgyel Drakzang (byang pa rnam	byang dag rnam rgyal grags bzang rgyal grags pa bzang po)
Jungné	'byung gnas
Kadam	bka' gdams
Kagyü	bka' rgyud
Kangyur	bka' 'gyur
Khedrub Jé	mkhas grub rje (dge legs dpal bzang)
Khyölma Rutsi	khyol ma ru tsi
Khyungpo Nenjor	khyung po rnal 'byor
Kimsheng Kongcho	kim sheng kong co/khyim shang kong jo
Könchok Kyab	dkon mchog skyabs; rog ston dkon mchog skyabs; tsho byed dkon mchog skyabs
Kongbo Degyel	kong bo bde rgyal
Kyempa Tsewang	skyem pa tshe dbang
Lang Darma	glang dar ma
Lha Totori Nyentsen	lha mtho mtho ri gnyan brtsan
Lodrö Sengyön	blo gros seng yon
Longdöl Lama	klong rdol bla ma
Longchen Rabjampa	klong chen (rab 'byams) pa
Mangmo Mangtsün	mang mo mang btsun
Mangsong Mentsen	mang srong man btsan
Marpa	mar pa (lo tsa ba)
Mé Agtsom	mes ag tshom
Mikyö Dorjé	(rgyal ba karma pa) mi bskyod rdo rje
Mipam	mi pham (rgya mtsho)
Namri Songtsen	gnam ri srong btsan
Ngawang Lozang Gyatso	nga dbang blo bzang rgya mtsho
Ngog Legpé Sherab	ngog legs pa'i shes rab
Ngorchen Könchok Lhündrub	ngor chen dkon mchog lhun grub
Nyangdé Senggé Dra	myang 'das seng ge sgra
Nyingma	rnying ma
Ongmen Ayé	'ong sman 'a ye
Orgyen Lingpa	o rgyan gling pa
Pema Karpo	pad ma dkar po

Pasang Yönten	pa sangs
Rangjung Dorjé	rang byung rdo rje
Rikpé Yeshé	rig pa'i ye shes
Rinchen Zangpo	rin chen bzang po
Sachen Künga Nyingpo	sa chen kun dga' snying po
Sakya	sa skya
Sanggyé Gyatso	sangs rgyas rgya mtsho
Sarma	gsar ma
Sengdo Öchen	seng mdo 'od chen
Sodokpa Lodrö Gyeltsen	sog zlog pa blo gros rgyal mtshan
Sonam Tsemo	(sa skya pa) bsod nams rtse mo
Songtsen Gampo	srong btsan sgam po
Sumpa Khenpo Yeshé Penjor	sum pa mkhan po ye shes dpal 'byor
Sumtön Yeshé Zung	sum ston ye shes gzungs
Taktri Yeshé	stag bri ye shes/shag khri ye shes
Takthang Lotsawa Sherab Rinchen	stag sthang lo tsa ba shes rab rin chen
Tanaduk	lta na sdug
Tashi Namgyel	(sgam po pa) bkra shis rnam rgyal
Tenpé Gönpo	bstan pa'i mgon po
Tendzin Püntsok	bstan 'dzin phun tshogs
Tengyur	btsan 'gyur
Tönmi Sambhota	thon mi sambhota
Tongsum Gangba	stong gsum gang ba
Tri Detsuktsen	khri lde gtsug btsan
Tri Songdetsen	khri srong lde btsan
Tsampashila	tsam pa shi la
Tselé Natsok Rangdröl	rtse le sna tshogs rang grol
Tsong Khapa	tsong kha pa (blo bzang grags pa)
Tsultrim Gyeltsen	tshul khrim rgyal mtshan
Tsurpu	mtsur pu
Tubten Püntsok	thub bstan phun tshogs
Üpa Dardrak	dbus pa dar grags
Yangchen Gawé Lodrö	dbyangs can dga' ba'i blos gros
Yeshé Ö	ye shes 'od
Yilekyé	yid las skyes
Yuthok Drejé Besa	g.yu thog 'dre rje bad sra
Yuthok Gyagar Dorje	g.yu thog rgya gar rdo rje
Yuthok Jidpo	g.yu thog brjid po
Yuthok Kharag Lharjé	g.yu thog kha rag lha rje
Yuthok Yönten Gönpo	g.yu thog yon tan mgon po
Zhang Zijibar	('khrungs pa) zhang gzi brjid 'bar
Zhangzhungpa Sherab Ö	zhang zhung pa shes rab 'od
Zurkhar Lodrö Gyelpo	Zur mkhar blo gros rgyal po
Zurkhar Nyamnyi Dorjé	zur mkhar mnyam nyid rdo rje

BIBLIOGRAPHY

Chief Tibetan sources referred to in English

When multiple editions are noted, the edition to which page numbers in this book refer is listed first, followed by alternate editions consulted

Blue Beryl by Sanggyé Gyatso
Sang rgyas rgya mtsho, *Gso ba rig pa'i bstan bcos sman bla'i dgongs rgyan rgyud bzhi'i gsal byed bai durya sngon po'i malli ka zhes bya ba bzhugs so*, 2 vols., Dharamsala: Tibetan Medical and Astro Institute, 1994.

Four Tantras
Bdud rtsi snying po yan lag brgyad pa gsang ba man ngag gi rgyud, Delhi: Bod kyi lcags po ri'i dran rten slob gner khang, 1993. Page numbers in Tibetan script are referred to from this edition (these do not correspond to the editor's Arabic numerals); the Tibetan script page numbers for this edition are identical to page numbers in G.yu thog yon tan mgon po, *Bdud rtsi snying po yan lag brgyad pa gsang ba man ngag gi rgyud ces bya ba bzhugs so*, Bod ljongs mi dmangs dpe skrun khang, 2000.

Four Tantras Commentary by Kyempa Tsewang
Mkhas dbang skyem pa tshe dbang mchog gis mdzad pa'i rgyud bzhi'i 'grel pa bzhugs so, vol. 1, New Delhi: Bod gshung sman rtsis khang, no date.

Eighteen Additional Practices
G.yu thog gsar ma yon tan mgon po, *G.yu thog cha lag bco brgyad bzhugs so*, 2 vols., Kan su'u mi rigs dpe skrun khang, 1999.

Entering the Womb/Abiding in the Womb sūtras
Tibetan page numbers are referred to first, with the editor's Arabic numerals following in parentheses.
"'Phags pa tshe dang ldan pa dga' bo la mngal du 'jug pa bstan pa zhes bya pa theg pa chen po'i mdo," in *The Sde-dge Black Bka'-'gyur: a reprint of a print from the Sde dge blocks originally edited by Si-tu Chos-kyi-'byung-gnas,*

Chengdu, no date, vol. 41, 237–248 (Tibetan page numbers), 475–498 (TBRC Arabic numeral page numbers), TBRC vol. 926. Referred to in short as "Mngal du 'jug pa (Degé edition)."

"'Phags pa dga' bo la mngal na gnas pa bstan ba zhes bya ba theg pa chen po'i mdo," in *The Sde-dge Black Bka'-'gyur: a reprint of a print from the Sde dge blocks originally edited by Si-tu Chos-kyi-'byung-gnas*, Chengdu, no date, vol. 41, 412–474 (TBRC page numbers), TBRC vol. 926. Referred to in short as "Mngal na gnas pa (Degé edition)."

"Dga' bo mngal du 'jug pa bstan pa zhes bya ba theg pa chen po'i mdo," in *The Tog Palace manuscript of the Tibetan Kanjur*, Leh: Smanrtsis Shesrig Dpemzod, vol. 37, 369–435 (Tibetan page numbers), 737–775 (editor's page numbers), 1975–1980. Referred to in short as "Mngal du 'jug pa (Tog Palace)."

"Gcung mo'u dga' bo zhes bya ba theg pa chen po'i mdo", in *The Tog Palace manuscript of the Tibetan Kanjur*, Leh: Smanrtsis Shesrig Dpemzod, vol. 37, 308–435 (Tibetan page numbers), 775–869 (editor's page numbers), 1975–1980. This is the *Mngal na gnas pa*; it is referred to in short as "Mngal na gnas pa (Tog Palace)."

"'Phags pa dga' bo la mngal na gnas pa bstan pa bzhes bya ba theg ba chen po'i mdo," in *The Nyingma Edition of the sDe-dge bKa'-'gyur and bsTan-'gyur*, Oakland: Dharma Press, vol. 16, text 57: 411–473, 1981.

"'Phags pa tshe dang ldan ldan pa dga' bo la mngal du 'jug pa bstan pa zhes bya ba theg pa chen po'i mdo," in *The Nyingma Edition of the sDe-dge bKa'-'gyur and bsTan-'gyur*, Oakland: Dharma Press, vol. 16, text 58, 1981.

"'Phags pa tshe dang ldan ldan pa dga' bo la mngal du 'jug pa bstan pa zhes bya ba theg pa chen po'i mdo," *Peking edition of the Tibetan Tripiṭaka*, ed. D.T. Suzuki, Tokyo-Kyoto: Suzuki Research Foundation, vol. 23, no. 760.

Feast for the Learned
Gtsug lag 'phreng ba, *Chos 'byung mkhas pa'i dga' ston*, New Delhi International Academy of Indian Culture, 1959–62.

Great Jeweled Wishing Tree by Drakpa Gyeltsen
Grags pa rgyal mtshan, "Rgyud kyi mngon par rtogs pa rin po che'i ljon shing" in *The Complete Works of Grags pa rgyal mtshan*, ed. Bsod nams rgya mtsho, 1, 1–139, Tokyo: The Toyo Bunko, 1968.

Heart Essence of Yuthok
Mkha' spyod dgyes pa'i rdo rje, ed., *G.yu thog snying thig skor (g.yu thog snin thig gi yig cha: the collected basic texts and ritual works of the medical teachings orally passed from g.yu-thog yon-tan-mgon-po)*, Leh: D. L. Tashigang, 1981.

Heart of Medicine by Vāgbhaṭa
Pha khol, "Yan lag brgyad pa'i snying po bsdus pa," in Rdo rje rgyal po, ed.,

Bstan 'gyur nang gi gso ba rig pa'i skor gyi dpe tshogs: gso rig pa'i rtsa 'grel bdam bsgrigs, Mi rigs dpe skrun khang, 1: 112–756, 1989.

Interior Analysis of Medicine by Sanggyé Gyatso
Sangs rgyas rgya mtsho, *Gso rig sman gyi khog 'bugs*, Dharamsala: Tibetan Medical and Astro Institute, 1994.

Jewel Ornament of Liberation by Gampopa
Dam chos yid bzhin nor bu thar pa rin po che'i rgyan, Sde dge: Sde dge par khang chen mo, 1998.

Profound Inner Meaning by Rangjung Dorjé
Rang byung rdo rje, *Zab mo nang don zhes bya ba'i bzhung gzhugs*, Sikkim: Rumtek Karma chos sgar, 1970.
Thub bstan phun tshogs, *Zab mo nang gi don 'grel ba'i lus sems gsal ba'i me long*, Lha sa: Bod ljongs mi dmangs dpe skrun khang, 2003. This commentary also reproduces the root text.

Transmission of the Elders by Zurkhar Lodrö Gyelpo
Zur mkhar pa blo gros rgyal po, *Rgyud bzhi'i 'grel pa mes po'i zhal lung*, 2 vols.: Krung go'i pod kyi shes rig dpe skrun khang, 1989.

Treasury of Precious Words and Meanings by Longchen Rabjampa
Klong chen pa, *Tshig don mdzod*, Gangtok, Sikkim: Sherab Gyeltsen and Khyentse Labrang, 1983. Page numbers refer to Arabic numerals inserted by the editors in order to correspond to the partial translation of this work in Germano, David, "Poetic thought, the intelligent universe, and the mystery of self: the tantric synthesis of rdzogs chen in fourteenth-century Tibet," Ph.D. Dissertation, University of Wisconsin, 1992.

Tibetan sources arranged alphabetically

"'Phags pa dga' bo la mngal na gnas pa bstan pa bzhes bya ba theg ba chen po'i mdo," in *The Nyingma Edition of the sDe-dge bKa'-'gyur and bsTan-'gyur*, Oakland, Dharma Press, vol. 16, text 57: 411–473, 1981.

"'Phags pa tshe dang ldan ldan pa dga' bo la mngal du 'jug pa bstan pa zhes bya ba theg pa chen po'i mdo," in *The Nyingma Edition of the sDe-dge bKa'-'gyur and bsTan-'gyur*, Oakland, Dharma Press, vol. 16, text 58, 1981.

Sman dpyad zla ba'i rgyal po, Dharamsala, Tibetan Medical and Astro Institute, 1994.

Gso ba rig pa'i rtsa 'grel bdam bsgrigs – bstan 'gyur nang gi gso ba rig pa'i skor gyi dpe tshogs, Mi rigs dpe skrun khang gi rtsi 'khor, 1996.

Śrī Kālacakratantrarāja: Collated with the Tibetan Version, ed. S. Bishwanath, *Bibliotheca Indica: A Collection of Oriental Works*, Calcutta: The Asiatic Society, 1985.

Kālacakra-tantra and Other Texts, 2 vols., ed. R. Vira and L. Chandra, *Śatapiṭaka Series*, vols. 69–70, New Delhi: International Academy of Indian Culture.

The Tibetan Tripiṭaka: Peking Edition, ed. D.T. Suzuki, Tokyo-Kyoto: Tibetan Tripiṭaka Research Institute, 1955–1961.

Bdud rtsi snying po yan lag brgyad pa gsang ba man ngag gi rgyud, Delhi: Bod kyi lcags po ri'i dran rten slob gner khang, 1993.

Bkra shis tshe ring, *Bod kyi gso ba rig pa'i ched rtsom gces btus*, Bod ljongs mi dmangs dpe skrun khang, 1994.

Bla ma skyabs, *Bod kyi mkhas pa rim byon gyi gso rig gsung 'bum dkar chag mu tig phreng ba*, Kan su'u mi rigs dpe skrun khang, 1997.

Blo bzang rgyal mtshan seng ge, *Dpal rdo rje 'jigs byed dpa' bo gcig pa'i rdzogs rim gyi rnam bzhag 'jam dpal dgyes pa'i mchod sprin*, Delhi, 1972.

Byams pa 'phrin las, *Bod kyi gso ba rig pa'i 'byung tshul dang 'phel rgyas skor gyi ngo sprod rags bdus*, Lhasa: Mentsikhang, 1986.

——, *Krung go'i bod kyi gso ba rig pa*, Krung go'i bod kyi shes rig dpe skrun khang, 1996.

——, *Gang ljongs gso rig bstan pa'i nyin byed rim byon gyi rnam thar phyogs bsgrigs (Medical biographies of Tibet in chronological order)*, Dharamsala: Tibetan Medical and Astrological Institute, no date.

Byang pa rnam rgyal grags pa bzang po, *Bshad rgyud kyi 'grel chen bdud rtsi'i chu rgyun*, Pod kyi gso rig dpe rnying phyogs bsgrigs, no. 2, Si khron mi rigs dpe skrun khang, 2001.

De'u dmar bstan 'dzin phun tshogs, "Gso ba rig pa'i chos 'byung rnam thar rgya mtsho'i rba rlabs drang srong dgyes pa'i 'dzum phreng," in *Gso rig gces btus rin chen phreng ba bzhugs so*, Zi ling: Mtsho sngon mi rigs dpe skrun khang, 1993.

——, "Gso ba rig pa'i thob yig byin rlabs myu gu," in *Gso rig gces btus rin chen phreng ba bzhugs so*, Zi ling: Mtsho sngon mi rigs dpe skrun khang, 1993.

Doniger, Wendy and Gregory Spinner, "Misconceptions: Parental Imprinting," in *Science in Culture*, ed. Peter Galison, Stephen Graubard, Everett Mendelsohn, New Jersey: Transaction Publishers, 2001.

Dza ya pandita blo bzang 'phrin las, *Chos kyi thob yig gsal ba'i me long*, New Delhi, International Academy of Indian Culture, 1981.

Dzanya na dha ri (sum ston ye shes gzung), *Bshad rgyud 'grel pa 'bum nag gsal sgron*, Pe cing: Mi rigs dpe skrun khang, 1998.

'Gos lo gzhon nu dpal, *Deb ther sngon po*, Si khron mi rigs dpe skrun khang, 1985.

Gtsug lag 'phreng ba, *Chos 'byung mkhas pa'i dga' ston*, New Delhi International Academy of Indian Culture, 1959–1962.

G.yu thog gsar ma yon tan mgon po, *G.yu thog cha lag bco brgyad bzhugs so*, 2 vols., Kan su'u mi rigs dpe skrun khang, 1999.

Grags pa rgyal mtshan, "Rgyud kyi mngon par rtogs pa rin po che'i ljon shing," in *The Complete Works of Grags pa rgyal mtshan*, ed. Bsod nams rgya mtsho, 1, 1–139, Tokyo: The Toyo Bunko, 1968.

Gso ba rig pa'i rtsa 'grel bdam bsgrigs – bstan 'gyur nang gi gso ba rig pa'i skor gyi dpe tshogs, Mi rigs dpe skrun khang gi rtsi 'khor, 1996.

Klong chen pa, "Theg mchog mdzod," in *Mdzod chen bdun*, Gangtok, Sikkim: Sherab Gyeltsen and Khyentse Labrang, 1983.

——, "Bla ma yang thig," in *Snying thig ya bzhi*, 11 vols., vol. 1, New Delhi: Trulku Tsewang, Jamyang and L. Tashi, 1971.

——, "Mkha' 'gro snying thig," in *Snying thig ya bzhi*, 11 vols., vol. 2, New Delhi: Trulku Tsewang, Jamyang and L. Tashi, 1971.

——, "Tshig don mdzod," in *Mdzod chen bdun*, Gangtok, Sikkim: Sherab Gyaltsen and Khyentse Labrang, 1983.

——, "Zab mo yang thig," in *Snying thig ya bzhi*, 11 vols., vol. 11, New Delhi: Trulku Tsewang, Jamyang and L. Tashi, 1971.

Mkha' spyod dgyes pa'i rdo rje, ed. *G.yu thog snying thig skor (g.yu thog snin thig gi yig cha: the collected basic texts and ritual works of the medical teachings orally passed from g.yu-thog yon-tan-mgon-po)*, arranged and largely restructured by Khams smyon dharma senge, Leh: D. L. Tashigang, 1981.

Padma dkar po, "Rgyud bzhi'i 'grel pa gzhan la phan dter bzhigs so," in *Collected Works of Kun mkhyen padma dkar po*, vol. 1, Darjeeling: Kargyud Sungrab Nyamso Khang, 1973.

Pha khol, "Yan lag brgyad pa'i snying po bsdus pa," in ed., Rdo rje rgyal po, *Bstan 'gyur nang gi gso ba rig pa'i skor gyi dpe tshogs: gso rig pa'i rtsa 'grel bdam bsgrigs*, Mi rigs dpe skrun khang, vol. 1, 112–756, 1989.

Rang byung rdo rje, *Zab mo nang don zhes bya ba'i bzhung gzhugs*, Sikkim: Rumtek Karma chos sgar, 1970.

Rje btsun grags pa rgyal mtshan, *Gso dpyad rgyal po'i dkor mdzod*, Kan su'u mi rigs dpe skrun khang, 1993.

Sang rgyas rgya mtsho, *Gso ba rig pa'i bstan bcos sman bla'i dgongs rgyan rgyud bzhi'i gsal byed bai durya sngon po'i malli ka zhes bya ba bzhugs so*, 2 vols., Dharamsala, Tibetan Medical and Astro Institute, 1994.

——, *Gso rig sman gyi khog 'bugs*, Dharamsala: Tibetan Medical and Astro Institute, 1994.

Skal bzang 'phrin las, *Bod kyi gso ba rig pa'i byung 'phel gyi lo rgyus gsal bar ston pa baidurya sngon po'i zhun thigs*, Krung go'i bod kyi shes rig dpe skrun khang, 1997.

Sgam po pa, *Dam chos yid bzhin nor bu thar pa rin po che'i rgyan*, Sde dge: sde dge par khang chen mo, 1998.

Skyem pa tshe dbang, *Mkhas dbang skyem pa tshe dbang mchog gis mdzad pa'i rgyud bzhi'i 'grel pa bshugs so*, 3 vols., New Delhi, Bod gshung sman rtsis khang, no date.

Sman dpyad zla ba'i rgyal po, transl. Bai ro tsa na, Dharamsala, Tibetan Medical and Astro Institute, 1994.

Thub bstan phun tshogs, *Gso bya lus kyi rnam bshad*, Pe cin: Mi rigs dpe skrun khang, 1999.

Tshul khrim rgyal mtshan, "Sman thang las 'brel pa rtsa yi gnas lugs kyi dpe ris skor gsal bar bshad pa," in *Krung go'i mtho rim bod sman shib 'jug bgro gleng 'dzin grwa'i rtsom yig gces bsdus*, 83–91, Bod rang skyong ljongs sman rtsis khang nas bsgrigs, late 1990s.

Zla ba mngon par dga' ba, "Sman dpyad yan lag brgyad pa'i snying po'i rnam par 'grel pa'i tshig gi don gyi zla zer zhes bya ba 'zhugs so," in ed., 'Gan 'khur pa, *Gso ba rig pa'i rtsa 'grel bdam bsgrigs*, Mi rigs dpe skrun khang, vol. 3, 1992.

Zur mkhar pa blo gros rgyal po, *Rgyud bzhi'i 'grel pa mes po'i zhal lung*, 2 vols., Krung go'i pod kyi shes rig dpe skrun khang, 1989.

——, *Sman pa rnams kyis mi shes su mi rung ba'i shes bya spyi'i khog dbubs*, Si khron mi rigs dpe skrun khang, 2001.

Secondary sources

Agniveśa's Caraka saṃhitā (Text with English Translation and Critial Exposition Based on Cakrapāṇi Datta's Áyurveda Dīpikā), transl. Ram Karan Sharma and Vaidya

Bhagwan Dash, vol. 2, *Chowkhamba Sanskrit Studies*, Varanasi: Chowkhamba Press, 1976.

The Blue Annals, transl. George N. Roerich, Delhi: Motilal Banarsidass, 1976.

Caraka saṃhitā, transl. A. Chandra Kaviratna and P. Sharma, 2nd ed., vol. 2, *Indian Medical Science Series No. 42*, Delhi: Sri Satguru Publications, 1996.

The Kālacakratantra: The Chapter on the Individual together with the Vimalaprabhā, transl. Vesna A. Wallace, ed. Robert A.F. Thurman, *Treasury of the Buddhist Sciences Series*, New York: American Institute of Buddhist Studies, Columbia University, 2004.

The Lalita Vistara: Memoirs of the Early Life of Sakya Sinha, transl. R. L. Mitra, Delhi: Sri Satguru Publications, 1998.

The Quintessence Tantras of Tibetan Medicine, transl. Barry Clark, Ithaca: Snow Lion Publishers, 1995.

Vāgbhaṭa's Aṣṭāṅga Hṛdayam Sūtrasthāna, Varanasi: Krishnadas Academy, 1996.

Vāgbhaṭa's Aṣṭāṅga Hṛdayam (Text, English translation, Notes, Appendix and Indices), transl. K.R. Srikantha Murthy, vol. 1, *Krishnadas Ayurveda Series*, Varanasi: Krishnadas Academy, 1991.

Adams, Vincanne, "The sacred in the scientific: Ambiguous practices of science in Tibetan medicine," *Cultural Anthropology* 16, no. 4, 2001, 542–575.

Almond, Philip C., *The British Discovery of Buddhism*, Cambridge: Cambridge University Press, 1988.

Anderson, Pamela Sue, *A Feminist Philosophy of Religion: The Rationality and Myths of Religious Beliefs*, Oxford: Blackwell Publishers, 1998.

Bagchi, Prabodh Chandra, "A Fragment of the Kāśyapa-Saṃhitā in Chinese," *Indian Culture* 9, 1942, 53–64.

Bates, Don, ed., *Knowledge and the Scholarly Medical Traditions*, Cambridge: Cambridge University Press, 1995.

Beckwith, Christopher I., "The Introduction of Greek Medicine into Tibet in the 7th and 8th Century," *Journal of the American Oriental Society* 99, 1979, 97–313.

Bentor, Yael, "Identifying the Unnamed Opponents of Tsong kha pa and Mkhas grub rje Concerning the Transformation of Ordinary Birth, Death and Intermediate State into the Three Bodies," forthcoming.

Bizot, Francois, "La grotte de la naissance: Recherches sur le Bouddhisme Khmer II," *Bulletin de l'Ecole Francaise d'Extreme-Orient* LXVII, 1980, 221–269.

Bjerken, Zeff, "The Mirrorwork of Tibetan Religious Historians: A Comparison of Buddhist and Bon Historiography," Ph.D. Dissertation, University of Michigan, 2001.

Boisvert, Mathieu, "Conception and Intrauterine Life in the Pali Canon," *Studies in Religion* 29, no. 3, 2000, 301–311.

Bolsokhoyeva, Natalia D., *Introduction to the Studies of Tibetan Medical Sources*, Kathmandu: Mandala Book Point, 1993.

Broido, M., "bsad thabs: Some Tibetan Methods of Explaining the Tantras," paper presented at the Csomo de Koros Symposium, Velm-Vienna, Austria 1981.

Brooke, John Hedley, *Science and Religion: Some Historical Perspectives*, Cambridge: Cambridge University Press, 1991.

Bruner, Jerome, *Actual Minds, Possible Worlds*, Cambridge: Harvard University Press, 1986.

Burnett, C. S. F., "The Planets and the Development of the Embryo," in *The Human Embryo, Aristotle and the Arabic and European Traditions*, ed. G. R. Dunstan, Exeter: University of Exeter Press, 1990.

Burrell, D., and S. Hauerwas, "From System to Story: An Alternative Pattern for Rationality in Ethics," in *Why Narrative? Readings in Narrative Theology*, ed. S. Hauerwas and L. G. Jones, 159–190, Grand Rapids, MI: Eerdmans, 1977.

Buswell, Robert E. Jr., and Robert M. Gimello, eds., *Paths to Liberation: The Marga and its Transformations in Buddhist Thought*, *Kuroda Institute Studies in East Asian Buddhism*, Honolulu: University of Hawaii Press, 1992.

Cabezón, José Ignacio, "Authorship and Literary Production in Classical Buddhist Tibet," in *Changing Minds: Contributions to the Study of Buddhism and Tibet in Honor of Jeffrey Hopkins*, ed. Guy Newland, Ithaca: Snow Lion Publications, 2001.

——, "Buddhism and Science: On the Nature of the Dialogue," in *Buddhism and Science: Breaking New Ground*, ed. B. Alan Wallace, 35–70, New York: Columbia University Press, 2003.

Cabezón, José Ignacio, and Roger R. Jackson, "Editors' Introduction," in *Tibetan Literature: Studies in Genre*, ed. José Ignacio Cabezón and Roger R. Jackson, Ithaca: Snow Lion Publishers, 1996.

Caillat, C., "Sur les doctrines medicales dans le Tandulaveyāliya," *Indologica Taurenesia* 2, 1975, 45–55.

Collins, Steven, *Selfless Persons*, Cambridge: Cambridge University Press, 1982.

Coward, Harold G., "Purity in Hinduism: With Particular Reference to Pataijali's *Yoga Sátras*," in *Hindu Ethics: Purity, Abortion, and Euthanasia*, ed. Harold G. Coward, Julius J. Lipner and Katherine K. Young, 9–41, Albany: State University of New York Press, 1989.

Cozort, Daniel, *Highest Yoga Tantra: An Introduction to the Esoteric Buddhism of Tibet*, Ithaca: Snow Lion Publications, 1986.

Cuevas, Bryan J., *The Hidden History of The Tibetan Book of the Dead*, Oxford: Oxford University Press, 2003.

Czaja, Olaf, "Zurkharwa Lodro Gyalpo (1509–1579) on the Controversy of the Indian Origin of the rGyud bzhi," *The Tibet Journal* 30 and 31, no. 4 and 1, 2005–2006, 131–153.

Dargyay, Lobsang, "Tsong-Kha-Pa's Concept of Karma," in *Karma and Rebirth: Post Classical Developments*, ed. Ronald W. Neufeldt, Albany: State University of New York Press, 1986.

Das, Rahul Peter, *The Origin of the Life of a Human Being: Conception and the Female According to Ancient Indian Medical and Sexological Literature*, Delhi: Motilal Banarsidass, 2003.

Dasgupta, Surendranath, *A History of Indian Philosophy*, 5 vols., New Delhi: Motilal Banarsidass, 1975.

Dash, Bhagwan, *Embryology and Maternity in Ayurveda*, New Delhi: Delhi Diary, 1975.

——, *Nāgārjuna's Yogasataka*, Library of Tibetan Works and Archives, 1976.

Dash, Bhagwan, and Doboom Tulku, *Positive Health in Tibetan Medicine*, Delhi: Sri Satguru Publications, 1991.

Davidson, Ronald M., *Indian Esoteric Buddhism: A Social History of the Tantric Movement*, New York: Columbia University Press, 2002.

De La Vallée Poussin, Louis, *Abhidharmakośabhāṣyam*, transl. Leo M. Pruden, 4 vols., vol. 2, Berkeley: Asian Humanities Press, 1988.

Dhonden, Yeshi, "Embryology in Tibetan Medicine," *Tibetan Medicine* 1, 1980, 43–48.

Dix, R., "Organic Theories of Art: The Importance of Embryology," *Notes and Queries*, 1985.

Dorje, Gyurme, and Fernand Meyer, eds., *Tibetan Medical Paintings: Illustrations to the*

"Blue Beryl" Treatise of Sangye Gyamtso (1653–1705), 2 vols., New York: Harry N. Abrams, Inc. Publishers, 1992.

Dummer, Tom, *Tibetan Medicine and Other Holistic Health Care Systems*, New Delhi: Paljor Publications, 1998.

Edelstein, Ludwig, *Ancient Medicine; Selected Papers of Ludwig Edelstein*, Baltimore: Johns Hopkins Press, 1967.

Ezzy, D., "Theorizing Narrative Identity: Symbolic Interactionism and Hermeneutics," *Sociological Quarterly* 39, no. 2, 1998, 239–253.

Faure, Bernard, *The Power of Denial: Buddhism, Purity, and Gender*, Princeton: Princeton University Press, 2003.

Fenner, Todd, "The Origin of the rGyud bzhi: A Tibetan Medical Tantra," in *Tibetan Literature: Studies in Genre*, ed. José Ignacio Cabezón and Robert R. Jackson, 458–470, Ithaca: Snow Lion Publications, 1996.

Figlio, Karl, "The Historiography of Scientific Medicine: An Invitation to the Human Sciences," *Comparative Studies in Society and History* 19, no. 3, 1977, 262–286.

——, "The Metaphor of Organization: An Historiographical Perspective on the Bio-Medical Sciences of the Early Nineteenth Century," *History of Science* 14, 1976, 17–53.

Filippi, Gian Giuseppe, "The Secret of the Embryo According to the *Garbha Upaniṣad*," *Annali di Ca' Foscari* 31, 1992, 271–307.

Ford, Norman, *When Did I Begin? Conception of the Human Individual in History, Philosophy and Science*, Cambridge: Cambridge University Press, 1988.

Furth, Charlotte, *A Flourishing Yin: Gender in China's Medical History, 960–1665*, Berkeley: University of California Press, 1999.

——, "From Birth to Birth: the Growing Body in Chinese Medicine," in *Chinese Views of Childhood*, ed. Anne Behnke Kinney, 157–192, Honolulu: University of Hawai'i Press, 1995.

Garrett, Frances, "Buddhism and the Historicizing of Medicine in Thirteenth Century Tibet," *Asian Medicine: Tradition and Modernity* 2, no. 2, 2007.

——, "Critical Methods in Tibetan Medical Histories," *Journal of Asian Studies* 66, no. 2, 2007.

Garrett, Frances, and Vincanne Adams, "The Three Channels in Tibetan Medicine, with a translation of Tsultrim Gyaltsen's "A clear explanation of the principal structure and location of the circulatory channels as illustrated in the medical paintings"," *Traditional South Asian Medicine*, forthcoming.

Gerke, Barbara, "The Authorship of the Tibetan Medical Treatise 'Cha lag bco brgyad' (Twelfth Century AD) and a Description of its Historical Background," *Traditional South Asian Medicine* 6, 2001, 27–50.

——, "On the History of the Two Tibetan Medical Schools: Janglug and Zurlug," *AyurVijnana* 6, 1999.

Gerke, Barbara, and Natalia Bolsokhoyeva, "Namthar of Zurkha Lodo Gyalpo (1509–1579)," *AyurVijnana* 6, 1999, 26–38.

Germano, David, "Notes to the translation of Longchenpa's *Treasury of Words and Meanings*," 9/13/94 manuscript.

——, "Poetic thought, the intelligent universe, and the mystery of self: the tantric synthesis of Rdzogs Chen in fourteenth-century Tibet," Ph.D. Dissertation, University of Wisconsin, 1992.

——, "Pure Lands and Creative Buddhas in Renaissance Tibet," in *Mysticism and Rhetoric in the Great Perfection (rDzogs chen)*, 3/22/02 manuscript.

——, translator, "Longchenpa's The Treasury of Precious Words and Meanings," 9/13/94 manuscript.

Gomez, Luis, "Purifying Gold: The Metaphor of Effort and Intuition in Buddhist Thought and Practice," in *Sudden and Gradual: Approaches to Enlightenment in Chinese Thought*, ed. Peter Gregory, Honolulu: University Press of Hawaii, 1987.

Grant, Edward, *Science and Religion, 400 B.C. to A.D. 1550: From Aristotle to Copernicus*, Baltimore: Johns Hopkins University Press, 2004.

Guenther, Herbert V., *Philosophy and Psychology in the Abhidharma*, Berkeley: Shambhala, 1974.

Gyatrul Rinpoche, *The Generation Stage in Buddhist Tantra*, transl. Sangye Khandro, Ithaca: Snow Lion Publications, 1996.

Gyatso, Geshe Kelsang, *Essence of Vajrayana: The Highest Yoga Tantra Practice of Heruka Body Mandala*, Delhi: Motilal Banarsidass, 2000.

Gyatso, Janet, "The Authority of Empiricism and the Empiricism of Authority: Medicine and Buddhism in Tibet on the Eve of Modernity," *Comparative Studies of South Asia, Africa and the Middle East* 24, no. 2, 2004, 83–96.

——, "One plus one makes three: Buddhist gender, monasticism, and the law of the non-excluded middle," *History of Religions* 43, no. 2, 2003, 89–115.

Halbfass, Wilhelm, *India and Europe, An Essay in Understanding*, Albany: State University of New York Press, 1988.

Haldar, J. R., *Medical Science in Pali Literature*, Calcutta: Indian Museum, 1977.

Hamda, Sarita, and Jyotirmitra, "Agnipurana ka garbhakranti sarir," *Journal of Research in Indian Medicine* 13, no. 3, 1978, 67–76.

Hara, Minoru, "A Note on the Buddha's Birth Story," in *Indianisme et bouddisme: melanges offerts a Mgr Etienne Lamotte*, 143–157, Louvain-la-Neuve: Universite catholique de Louvain, Institut orientaliste, 1980.

Hardacre, Helen, "The Cave and the Womb World," *Japanese Journal of Religious Studies* 10, no. 2–3, 1983.

Herbert V. Guenther (transl.), *The Jewel Ornament of Liberation by Sgam.po.pa*, Berkeley: Shambala Publications, 1971.

Hopkins, Jeffrey, *Meditation on Emptiness*, London: Wisdom Publications, 1983.

Hopkins, Jeffrey, and Lati Rinpoche, *Death, Intermediate State and Rebirth in Tibetan Buddhism*, Ithaca: Snow Lion Publications, 1979.

Huebotter (transl.), *Die Sutra Uber Empfangnis und Embryologie*, Tokyo: Deutsche Gesellschaft fur Natur- U. Volkerkunde Ostasiens, 1932.

Hunter, "Narrative, Literature and the Clinical Exercise of Practical Reason," *Journal of Medicine and Philosophy* 21, 1996.

Iggers, Georg G., *Historiography in the Twentieth Century, From Scientific Objectivity to the Postmodern Challenge*, Hanover: Wesleyan University Press, 1997.

Jahn, Manfred, "Narratology: A Guide to the Theory of Narrative," in *Poems, Plays, and Prose: A Guide to the Theory of Literary Genres*, ed. Manfred Jahn, English Department, University of Cologne: http://www.uni-koeln.de/~ame02/pppn.htm, 2002.

Jamyang Khyentse Wangchuk, "Profound Summarizing Notes on the Path Presented as the Three Continua," in *Taking the Result as the Path: Core Teachings of the Sakya Lamdre Tradition*, ed. Cyrus Stearns, 395–477, Boston: Wisdom Publications and Institute of Tibetan Classics, 2006.

Kaladhar, K., "Niruktopaniṣad and Garbhopaniṣad: The Vedic Sources of Studies on

Human Embryology," *Bulletin of the Indian Institute of History of Medicine: Hyderabad* 24, no. 1, 1994, 1–4.
Kalupahana, David J., *Causality: The Central Philosophy of Buddhism*, Honolulu: The University Press of Hawaii, 1975.
Kapani, Lakshmi, "Upanisad of the Embryo and Notes on the Garbha-Upanisad," in *Fragments for a History of the Human Body*, ed. Michael Feher, 177–196, Urzone, Inc., 1989.
Kapstein, Matthew T., *The Tibetan Assimilation of Buddhism: Conversion, Contestation, and Memory*, New York: Oxford University Press, 2000.
Karmay, Samten G., "Vairocana and the rgyud-bzhi," *Tibetan Medicine*, 1989.
Karunaratne, W. S., *The Theory of Causality in Early Buddhism*, Nugegoda, Sri Lanka: Indumati Karunaratne, 1988.
Kellner, Frank, and Hans Ankersmit, eds., *A New Philosophy of History*, Chicago: University of Chicago Press, 1995.
Khedrup Norsang Gyatso, *Ornament of Stainless Light*, transl. Gavin Kilty, ed. Thupten Jinpa, *The Library of Tibetan Classics*, Boston: Wisdom Publications and the Institute of Tibetan Classics, 2004.
King, Helen, *Hippocrates' Woman: Reading the Female Body in Ancient Greece*, London: Routledge, 1998.
Kinney, Anne, *Representations of Childhood and Youth in Early China*, Stanford: Stanford University Press, 2003.
Kritzer, Robert, "Antarābhava in the Vibhāsā," *Nōtom Damu Joshi Daigaku Kirisutokyō Bunka Kenkyū Kiyō (Maranata)* 3, no. 5, 1993, 69–91.
——, "Childbirth and the Mother's Body in the *Abhidharmakośabhāṣya* and Related Texts," forthcoming.
——, "The Four Ways of Entering the Womb (*garbhāvakrānti*)," *Bukkyi Bunka* 10, 2000, 1–41.
——, "Garbhāvakrāntisūtra: A Comparison of the Contents of Two Versions," *Maranatha: Bulletin of the Christian Culture Research Institute (Kyoto)* 6, 1998, 4–13.
——, "Life in the Womb: Conception and Gestation in Buddhist Scripture and the Classical Indian Medical Literature," unpublished manuscript.
——, "Rūpa and the Antarābhava," *Journal of Indian Philosophy* 29, 2000, 235–272.
——, "Semen, Blood, and the Intermediate Existence," *Journal of Indian and Buddhist Studies* 46, no. 2, 1998, 1025–1031.
Kunzang, Rechung Rinpoche Jampal, *Tibetan Medicine, Illustrated in Original Texts, Indian Medical Science Series No. 112*, Delhi: Sri Satguru Publications, 2001.
Kurke, Leslie, *Coins, Bodies, Games, and Gold: The Politics of Meaning in Archaic Greece*, Princeton: Princeton University Press, 1999.
Kutumbiah, P, *Ancient Indian Medicine*, Calcutta: Orient Longmans Ltd., 1962.
LaCapra, Dominick, *Rethinking Intellectual History: Texts, Contexts, Language*, Ithaca: Cornell University Press, 1983.
Lalou, Marcelle, "La Version Tibetain Du Ratnakūṭa," *Journal Asiatique* Octobre–Decembre, 1927, 233–59.
——, "Les texts Bouddhiques au temps du Roi Khri-sron-lde-bcan," *Journal Asiatique* 261, 1953, 317–18.
Larson, Gerald, "The Concept of Body in Āyurveda and the Hindu Philosophical Systems," in *Self as Body in Asian Theory and Practice*, ed. Roger Ames, Thomas P. Kasulis, Wimal Dissanayake, Albany: State University of New York Press, 1993.

Leslie, Charles, and Allen Young, eds., *Paths to Asian Medical Knowledge*, Berkeley: University of California Press, 1992.

Lhundrup, Ngorchen Konchog, *The Beautiful Ornament of the Three Visions: An exposition of the preliminary practices of the path which explains the instructions of the "Path Including its Result" in accordance with the Root Treatise of the Vajra Verses of Virupa*, transl. Lobsang Dagpa and Jay Goldberg, Ithaca: Snow Lion Publications, 1991.

Lincoln, Bruce, "Embryological Speculation and Gender Politics in a Pahlavi Text." *History of Religions* 27, no. 4, 1988, 355–365.

——, "Physiological Speculation and Social Patterning in a Pahlavi Text," *Journal of the American Oriental Society* 108, no. 1, 1988, 135–140.

Loizzo, Joseph J., and Leslie J. Blackhall, "Traditional Alternatives as Complementary Sciences: The Case of Indo-Tibetan Medicine," *The Journal of Alternative and Complementary Medicine* 4, no. 3, 1998, 311–319.

Luo, Dashang, "History of Tibetan Medicine and *Crystal Pearl Materia Medica*," *Tibet Studies* 2, no. 1, 1990, 145–153.

Lyssenko, Viktoria, "The Human Body Composition in Statics and Dynamics: Āyurveda and the Philosophical Schools of Vaiśeṣika and Sāṃkhya," *Journal of Indian Philosophy* 32, 2004, 31–56.

MacIntyre, A., *After Virtue: A Study in Moral Theory*, Notre Dame: University of Notre Dame Press, 1981.

Mahinda, Wetara, "Medical Practices of Buddhist Monks: a Historical Analysis of Attitudes and Problems," in *Recent Researches in Buddhist Studies: Essays in Honour of Professor Y. Karunadasa*, ed. Kuala Lumpur: Dhammajoti, Asanga Tilakaratne and Kapila Abhayawansa, Columbo: Y. Karunadasa Felicitation Committee, 1997.

Malalasekera, G. P., "Āyuśman-Nanda-Garbhāvakrānti-Nirdeśa-(Nāma-Mahayana) Sūtra," in *Encyclopaedia of Buddhism*, Government of Ceylon, 1961.

Martin, Wallace, *Recent Theories of Narrative*, Ithaca: Cornell University Press, 1986.

Masuzawa, Tomoko, *The Invention of World Religions: Or, How European Universalism Was Preserved in the Language of Pluralism*, Chicago: University of Chicago Press, 2005.

Matthews, Bruce, "Post-Classical Developments in the Concepts of Karma and Rebirth in Theravada Buddhism," in *Karma & Rebirth: Post-Classical Developments*, ed. Ronald W. Neufeldt, 123–43, Albany: State University of New York Press, 1986.

McDermott, James, *Development in the Early Buddhist Concept of Kamma/Karma*, New Delhi: Munishiram Manoharlal Publishers Pvt. Ltd., 1984.

McDermott, James P., "Karma and Rebirth in Early Buddhism," in *Karma and Rebirth in Classical Indian Traditions*, ed. Wendy Doniger, 165–192, Delhi: Motilal Banarsidass, 1983.

Meyer, Fernand, "Introduction: The Medical Paintings of Tibet," in *Tibetan Medical Paintings: Illustrations to the "Blue Beryl" treatise of Sangye Gyamtso (1653–1705)*, ed. Gyurme Dorje and Fernand Meyer, 2–13, New York: Harry N. Abrams, Inc. Publishers, 1992.

Ming, Chen, "Zhuan Nu Wei Nan Turning Female to Male: An Indian Influence on Chinese Gynaecology?" *Asian Medicine: Tradition and Modernity* 1, no. 2, 2005, 315–334.

Mitra, Jyotir. *A Critical Appraisal of Ayurvedic Material in Buddhist Literature*. Varanasi: The Jyotiralok Prakashan, 1985.

Moore, James R., *The Post-Darwinian Controversies: A Study of the Protestant Struggle to Come to Terms with Darwin in Great Britain and America, 1870–1900*, Cambridge: Cambridge University Press, 1979.

Neufeldt, Ronald W., ed., *Karma and Rebirth: Post Classical Developments*, Albany: State University of New York Press, 1986.

Ngawang Dhargyey, Geshe Lharampa, *A Commentary on the Kalacakra Commentary*, Dharamsala: Library of Tibetan Works and Archives, 1985.

Norbu, Namkhai, *On Birth and Life: A Treatise on Tibetan Medicine*, transl. Enrico Del-l'Angelo: Tipographia Commerciale Venezia, 1983.

Nussbaum, M. C., *Love's Knowledge: Essays on Philosophy and Literature*, New York: Oxford University Press, 1990.

O'Flaherty, Wendy Doniger, ed., *Karma and Rebirth in Classical Indian Traditions*, Delhi: Motilal Barnarsidass, 1983.

Olson, Richard G., *Science and Religion, 1450–1900: From Copernicus to Darwin*, Baltimore: Johns Hopkins University Press, 2004.

Orofino, Giacomella, *Sacred Tibetan Teachings on Death and Liberation*, Great Britain: Prism Press, 1990.

Padmasambhava, *The Tibetan Book of the Dead*, transl. Robert A. F. Thurman, *Mystical Classics of the World*, New York: Bantam Books, 1994.

Pettit, John W., *Mipham's Beacon of Certainty: Illuminating the View of Dzogchen, the Great Perfection*, Boston: Wisdom Publications, 1999.

Pinto-Correia, Clara, *The Ovary of Eve: Egg and Sperm and Preformation*, Chicago: University of Chicago Press, 1997.

Polkinghorne, Donald, *Narrative Knowing and the Human Sciences*, Albany: State University of New York Press, 1988.

Punday, Daniel, "A Corporeal Narratology?" *Style* 34, no. 2, 2000.

Rabgay, Lobsang, "The Origin and Growth of Medicine in Tibet," *Tibetan Medicine* 3, 1981, 3–21.

Ramachandran, C. K., "'Foetal Medicine' in Ancient India," *Aryavaidyan* 10, no. 3, 1997, 140–143.

Ricoeur, Paul, "Narrative Time," in *On Narrative*, ed. W. J. T. Mitchell, 165–186, Chicago and London: University of Chicago Press, 1980.

Rolland, P., "Un fragment medical vedique; Le premier khaṇḍa du Vārāhapariśiṣṭa bhūtotpatti," *Munchener Studien zur Sprachwissenschaft* 30, 1972, 129–130.

Ruegg, David Seyford, *Buddha-nature, Mind and the Problem of Gradualism in a Comparative Perspective: On the Transmission and Reception of Buddhism in India and Tibet*, New Delhi: Heritage Publishers, 1992.

Russell, Colin A., "The Conflict of Science and Religion," in *Science and Religion: A Historical Introduction*, ed. Gary Ferngren, 3–12, Baltimore: Johns Hopkins University Press, 2002.

Sachen Kunga Nyingpo, "Explication of the Treatise for Nyak," in *Taking the Result as the Path: Core Teachings of the Sakya Lamdre Tradition*, ed. Cyrus Stearns, 23–127, Boston: Wisdom Publications and Institute of Tibetan Classics, 2006.

Sadakata, Akira, *Buddhist Cosmology, Philosophy and Origins*, Tokyo: Kosei Publishing Company, 1997.

Sanford, James H., "Wind, Waters, Stupas, Mandalas: Fetal Buddhahood in Shingon," *Japanese Journal of Religious Studies* 24, no. 1–2, 1997, 1–38.

Sasson, Vanessa, "A Womb with a View: the Buddha's Final Fetal Experience," in *The*

Fetus: the Religious Life of Very Small Things, ed. Vanessa Sasson and Jane Marie Law, forthcoming.

Scharfe, Hartmut, "The Doctrine of the Three Humors in Traditional Indian Medicine and the Alleged Antiquity of Tamil Siddha Medicine," *Journal of the American Oriental Society* 119, no. 4, 1999, 609–629.

Selby, Martha Ann, "Narratives of Conception, Gestation, and Labour in Sanskrit Āyurvedic Texts," *Asian Medicine: Tradition and Modernity* 1, no. 2, 2005, 254–276.

Sharma, Priya Vrat, *History of Medicine in India, from Antiquity to 1000 A.D.*, New Delhi: Indian National Science Academy, 1992.

Silk, Jonathan A., "The Fruits of Paradox: On the Religious Architecture of the Buddha's Life Story," *Journal of the American Academy of Religion* 71, no. 4, 2003, 863–881.

Sopa, Geshe, "The Tibetan Wheel of Life: Iconography and Doxography," *The Journal of the International Association of Buddhist Studies* 7, no. 1, 1984.

Sorabji, Richard, "Foreword," in *The Human Embryo: Aristotle and the Arabic and European Traditions*, ed. G. R. Dunstan, Exeter: University of Exeter Press, 1990.

Stein, R. A., "Grottes-Matrices et Lieux Saints de la Deesse en Asie Orientale," *Bulletin de l'Ecole Francaise d'Extreme-Orient*, 1988.

Suneson, Carl, "Remarks on Some Interrelated Terms in the Ancient Indian Embryology," *Wiener Zeitschrift für die Kunde Südasiens* 35, 1991, 109–191.

Svoboda, Robert, and Arnie Lade, *Chinese Medicine and Āyurveda*, Delhi: Motilal Banarsidass, 1999.

Swanson, Paul L., "Shugendo and the Yoshino-Kumano Pilgrimage: An Example of Mountain Pilgrimage," *Monumenta Nipponica* 36, no. 1, 1981, 515–584.

Tatz, Mark, *Buddhism and Healing: Demiéville's Article "Byō" from Hōbōgirin*, Lanham: University Press of America, 1985.

Taube, Manfred, *Beitrage zur Geschichte der Medizinischen Literatur Tibets*, Sankt Augustin: VGH Wissenschaftsverlag, 1981.

Thatte, Dinkar Govind, *Śāryrasthānam Suśruta-Saṃhitā (Section on the Study of the Human body), Text with English Translation and Commentary, Kashi Ayurveda Series No. 16*, Varanasi: Chaukhambha Orientalia, 1994.

Tselé Natsok Rangdröl, *The Mirror of Mindfulness: The Cycle of the Four Bardos*, transl. Erik Pema Kunsang, New Delhi: Rupa, 2002.

Tsong-ka-pa, *The Six Yogas of Naropa: Tsongkhapa's commentary entitled A Book of Three Inspirations: A Treatise on the Stages of Training in the Profound Path of Naro's Six Dharmas, commonly referred to as The Three Inspirations*, transl. Glen H. Mullin, Ithaca: Snow Lion Publications, 2005.

——, *Tantra in Tibet: The Great Exposition of Secret Mantra – Volume 1*, transl. Jeffrey Hopkins, *The Wisdom of Tibet Series*, London: George Allen & Unwin, 1977.

——, *The Yoga of Tibet: The Great Exposition of Secret Mantra – 2 and 3*, transl. Jeffrey Hopkins, *The Wisdom of Tibet Series*, London: George Allen & Unwin, 1981.

Tucci, Giuseppe, *Rin-chen-bzang-po and the Renaissance of Buddhism in Tibet around the Millenium*, transl. Nancy Kipp Smith, ed. Lokesh Chandra, *Sata-Pitaka Series, Indo-Asian Literatures, Volume 348*, New Delhi: Aditya Prakashan, 1988.

Tull, Herman W., *The Vedic Origins of Karma: Cosmos as Man in Ancient Indian Myth and Ritual*, ed. Wendy Doniger, *SUNY Series in Hindu Studies*, Albany: State University of New York Press, 1989.

van der Eijk, Philip, "Introduction," in *Magic and Rationality in Ancient Near Eastern and Graeco-Roman Medicine*, ed. H. F. J. Horstmanshoff and M. Stol, 1–10, Leiden: Brill, 2004.

Vitali, Roberto, "On some disciples of Rinchen Zangpo and Lochung Legpai Sherab, and their successors, who brought teachings popular in Ngari Korsum to Central Tibet," in *Tibet and Her Neighbours: A History*, ed. Alex McKay, 71–83, London: Edition Hansjorg Mayer, 2003.

Vogel, Claus, *Vāgbhaṭa's Aṣṭāṅgahṛdayasaṃhitā, the first five chapters of its Tibetan version, Abhanglungen fur die Kunde des Morgenlandes*, Wiesbaden: Deutsche Morgenlandische Gesellschaft, Komissionsverkag Franz Steiner GMBH, 1965.

Wallace, B. Alan, "Introduction: Buddhism and Science – Breaking Down Barriers," in *Buddhism and Science: Breaking New Ground*, ed. B. Alan Wallace, 1–30, New York: Columbia University Press, 2003.

Wallace, Vesna, *The Inner Kālacakratantra: a Buddhist Tantric View of the Individual*, New York: Oxford University Press, 2001.

Wayman, Alex, "The Five-Fold Ritual Symbolism of Passion," in *Studies of Esoteric Buddhism and Tantrism*, 117–144, Koyosan, Japan: Koyosan University, 1995.

——, "The Intermediate-State Dispute in Buddhism," in *Buddhist Studies in Honour of I. B. Horner*, Dordrecht: D. Reidel, 1974.

——, *Yoga of the Guhyasamajatantra: The Arcane Lore of Forty Verses, A Buddhist Tantra Commentary*, Delhi: Motilal Banarsidass, 1977.

White, David Gordon, *The Alchemical Body: Siddha Traditions in Medieval India*, Chicago: University of Chicago Press, 1996.

White, Hayden, "The Value of Narrativity in the Representation of Reality," in *On Narrative*, ed. W. J. T. Mitchell, 1–25, Chicago: University of Chicago Press, 1980.

Wijesekara, O., "Vedic Gandharva and Pali Gandhabba," *University of Ceylon Review* 1, 1945.

Williams, David M., "The Translation and Interpretation of the Twelve Terms in the Paticcasamuppada," *Numen* 21, 1974.

Wilms, Sabine, "The Transmission of Medical Knowledge on 'Nurturing the Fetus' in Early China," *Asian Medicine: Tradition and Modernity* 1, no. 2, 2005, 276–314.

Wilson, David B., "The Historiography of Science and Religion," in *Science and Religion: A Historical Introduction*, ed. Gary Ferngren, 13–29, Baltimore: Johns Hopkins University Press, 2002.

Wilson, Liz, *Charming Cadavers: Horrific Figurations of the Feminine in Indian Buddhist Hagiographic Literature*, Chicago: University of Chicago Press, 1996.

Winder, Marianne, "Introduction," in *Tibetan Medicine, Illustrated in Original Texts*, ed. Rechung Rinpoche Jampal Kunzang, Delhi: Sri Satguru Publications, 2001.

——, "Tibetan Medicine Compared with Ancient and Mediaeval Western Medicine." *Bulletin of Tibetology (Gangtok, Sikkim)* 1, 1981, 5–22.

Wujastyk, Dominik, *The Roots of Ayurveda*, 2nd ed., London: Penguin Classics, 2003.

Yangchen Gawai Lodoe, *Paths and Grounds of Guhyasamaja According to Arya Nagarjuna (With Commentary by Geshe Losang Tsephel)*, transl. Tenzin Dorjee, ed. David Ross Komito and Andrew Fagan, Library of Tibetan Works and Archives, 1995.

Yarnall, Thomas, "The Emptiness that is Form: Developing the Body of Buddhahood in Indo-Tibetan Buddhist Tantra," Ph.D., Columbia University, 2003.

Yonten, Pasang, Tsepak Rigzin, and Phillippa Russell, "A History of the Tibetan Medical System," *Tibetan Medicine* 12, 1989, 32–51.

Zammito, John, *The Genesis of Kant's Critique of Judgement*, Chicago: Chicago University Press, 1992.

Ziegler, Joseph, *Medicine and Religion c. 1300, The Case of Arnau de Vilanova*, Oxford: Clarendon Press, 1998.

Zysk, Kenneth, *Asceticism and Healing in Ancient India*, New York: Oxford University Press, 1991.

——, "The Science of Respiration and the Doctrine of the Bodily Winds in Ancient India," *Journal of the American Oriental Society* 113, no. 2, 1993, 198–213.

INDEX

Figures are indicated by bold page numbers, tables by italics.